PROJECTING A
CAMERA

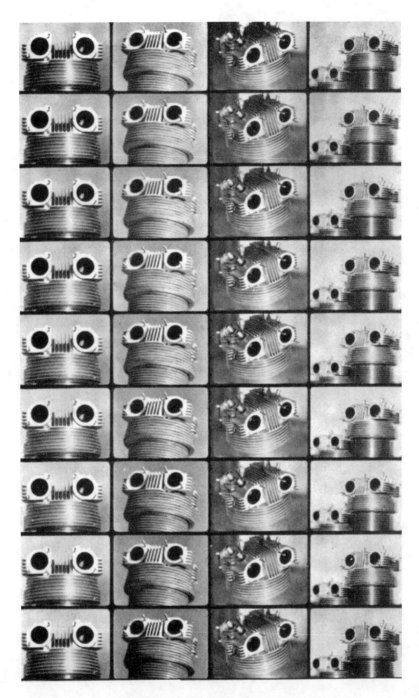

CAMERA APPROACH

PROJECTING A CAMERA

Language-Games in Film Theory

EDWARD BRANIGAN

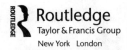

Routledge
Taylor & Francis Group
New York   London

Published in 2006 by
Routledge
Taylor & Francis Group
270 Madison Avenue
New York, NY 10016

Published in Great Britain by
Routledge
Taylor & Francis Group
2 Park Square
Milton Park, Abingdon
Oxon OX14 4RN

© 2006 by Taylor & Francis Group, LLC
Routledge is an imprint of Taylor & Francis Group

Printed in the United States of America on acid-free paper
10 9 8 7 6 5 4 3 2 1

International Standard Book Number-10: 0-415-94253-5 (Hardcover) 0-415-94254-3 (Softcover)
International Standard Book Number-13: 978-0-415-94253-9 (Hardcover) 978-0-415-94254-6 (Softcover)

Library of Congress Cataloging-in-Publication Data

Catalog record is available from the Library of Congress

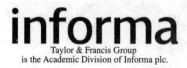

Taylor & Francis Group
is the Academic Division of Informa plc.

Visit the Taylor & Francis Web site at
http://www.taylorandfrancis.com

and the Routledge Web site at
http://www.routledge-ny.com

For Melinda, with radial love.

Contents

Contents

Cover and Frontispiece Illustrations

COVER ILLUSTRATION (TOP):

A vagabond Charlie Chaplin is amazed to discover that he is embedded in a new life. *The Idle Class* (Chaplin, 1921). The spectator is amazed by the games of frames. See chapter 4.

COVER ILLUSTRATION (BOTTOM):

A camera follows two characters but runs into bushes and halts. *Chinese Roulette* (Rainer Werner Fassbinder, 1976). See chapter 2.

FRONTISPIECE:

Although Rudolf Arnheim in his 1933 book, *Film*, does not explicitly state the purpose of the illustration entitled "Camera Approach," the following passage may be suggestive:

> [The film artist] shows the world not only as it appears objectively but also subjectively. He creates new realities, in which things are duplicated [multiplied], turns their movements and actions backwards, distorts them, retards or accelerates them. He calls into existence magical kingdoms where the force of gravity disappears, and mysterious powers move inanimate objects, and make whole things that are broken. He brings into being mystical bridges between events and objects that have never had any connection in reality. He intervenes in the structure of nature to make quivering, disintegrate [sic] ghosts of concrete bodies and spaces. He arrests the progress of the world and of things, and changes them to stone. He breathes life into stone [into a machine? into a camera?] and bids it move. Of chaotic and illimitable space he creates pictures beautiful in form and of profound significance, as subjective and rich in technical possibilities as painting. (134; see also 135; cf. *Film as Art* [1957], 133; the illustration does not appear in the German edition, *Film als Kunst* [1932], 153–55)

Figures

Preface

"A theory of cinema is not 'about' cinema, but about the concepts
that cinema gives rise to and which are themselves related to
other concepts corresponding to other practices, the practice of
concepts in general having no privilege over others, any more
than one object has over others. It is at the level of the interference of many practices that things happen, beings, images,
concepts, all the kinds of events. . . . Cinema's concepts are not
given in cinema."[1]

— Gilles Deleuze

"Wittgenstein's principal contrast with the metaphysical is what
he calls the ordinary or the everyday. . . . Where Wittgenstein
describes his effort in philosophy as one of 'returning words from
their metaphysical to their everyday use,' I habitually speak of
the task of accepting finitude. The attempt to satisfy the demand
for the absolute makes what we say inherently private (as though
we withheld the sense of our words even, or especially, from
ourselves), a condition in which the good city we would inhabit cannot be constructed, since it exists only in our intelligible
encounters with each other. . . . Wittgenstein's disappointment
with knowledge is not that it fails to be better than it is (for example, immune to skeptical doubt), but rather that it fails to
make us better than we are, or provide us with peace."[2]

— Stanley Cavell

Film theory needs to be rethought. It must seek a new relationship
to its own language. I will pursue this goal by examining the many
tangled, abstract languages that have been crafted by film theorists. What are the purposes of such languages? Are they meant to

become gradually more perfect at describing cinema? What work do they do for us? What sort of knowledge do we expect? In this book I will analyze the complicated sets of meanings devised for the word "camera." My analysis aims to expose the diverse ways of talking through which theorists have made their claims, chosen their metaphors, and staked their conceptions of film. The analysis will also reveal the basic approaches through which theories generate their languages. We will discover that the various conceptual networks proposed by theorists have materialized not from metaphysical principles but from competing figures of mind arising from differing ways of life.

This book will survey the numerous ways we talk about a "camera," including such stand-ins for a camera as a shot, image, frame, motion, motion picture, motivation, point of view, and narration. The idea is that the lines of an image (solid, broken, hypothetical) taken together bespeak the presence of an apparent "guide" that makes prominent certain streams of thought in a spectator. The reasons for a spectator's thought, however, are less photographic and less visual, indeed less causal, than might be supposed. Through a wide-ranging engagement with the work of Ludwig Wittgenstein and classical and contemporary theorists of film, I will argue that the patterns we find important in film have been projected through our linguistic behavior (our language-games) as well as through a multitude of embodied, schematic descriptions. The result is a folk theory of film and implicit folk psychology that guide our decisions about how to look at an image, imagine its completion, form prototypes, make revisions, and recall meanings. As Gilles Deleuze notes above, "Cinema's concepts are not given in cinema." This book aims to examine the conditions under which a spectator fashions numerous designs that later will be credited to a fictitious camera — a hypothetical camera that drives how we think, discuss, and marvel about the films we see.

Wittgenstein believes that it is fruitless to search for a metaphysical framework — an ultimate foundation or absolute definition — for a thing. Accordingly, I believe that such questions as, "what is cinema?," "what is cinema's specificity? (i.e., what are the elements that make cinema be cinema?),” and “what is a camera? (or, what is an image?),” are mistaken for they seem to call for a final, metaphysical answer. Wittgenstein argues that the task of a philosopher is to rearrange what already lies open to view, to remind oneself of some facts of the everyday, of how we speak to one another about what is ordinary and contingent in our lives. What are the *continuities* we project that allow us to speak of an ‘everyday’? The task is to create “a synopsis of *many* trivialities.”[3] Wittgenstein’s later writings demonstrate an approach to doing philosophy that does not involve acts of ‘building’ or construction from first principles.[4] For Wittgenstein, language is used — and objects appear within a dense nexus — relative to the concrete problems and circumstances of a particular world. I believe that the language of film theory, too, is public, open to view, and directed at particular problems framed by specific social purposes and values. For this reason, a given film theory may be found to be composed of several incompatible language-games (e.g., “suture” in chapter 4) or latent metaphorical projections (e.g., an “invisible observer” and cinematic “excess” in chapter 4). In short, as Stanley Cavell observes, Wittgenstein’s project is one of “returning words from their metaphysical to their everyday use,” because a search for “the absolute makes what we say inherently private.”

One of the methods I will employ in analyzing the everyday aspects of theoretical language comes from the work of George Lakoff and Mark Johnson. They assert that the abstract entities that supposedly ground our knowledge are in fact metaphorical projections derived from common bodily experience and from our interactions with surroundings. These projections of language reach into a person’s world to form groups of significant things.

> From Thales to Heraclitus, Plato to Aristotle, Descartes to Kant, Russell to Quine, it is the core metaphors at the heart of each philosopher’s thought that define its metaphysics. Each of those source-to-target mappings project the ontology of a given source domain to form the ontology of the relevant target domain. For example, ... when Descartes

appropriated the Understanding Is Seeing metaphor, he thereby accepted an ontology of the mental realm that required mental counterparts to visible objects, people who see, natural light sources, and so forth. His metaphysics of mind is populated with metaphorical counterparts to these entities, and he reasons about them using patterns of inference imported from the domain of vision to the domain of mind and thought.[5]

As we shall see (!), it is often claimed that our understanding of film springs from a seeing on the screen, or perhaps a seeing *through* the screen, due to the essentially visible, photographic, pictorial, and/or visual nature ascribed to film. In this Cartesian-inspired metaphor, light is the "source" of knowledge and the camera is the facilitating and vigilant "eye" (cf. the frontispiece). We will find, however, that there are many other ways to project an entity that can be designated as a "camera" (see, e.g., figure 3.2).

I have so far been discussing "language" on the one hand and "film" on the other. It is but a short step to the unruly problem of "film as language." How does our "talk" about film connect to film? Are verbal descriptions, metaphors, and interpretations of film only talk — talk that is removed from film itself? Many theorists think so. Their reaction, I believe, stems from an impoverished notion of language. Although it is generally accepted in the humanities nowadays that language is not simply a neutral and transparent instrument, the human mind is still viewed as being somehow separate from both language and film when a spectator is watching and comprehending. The mind is regarded as merely an instrument that operates with sense-data and simple names, and then digests information from a place above or beyond (or below). Alternatively, some theorists are convinced that the mind simply becomes pictorial and silent, though it may continue to listen, when confronted with film. In sum, for all of these theorists who are wary of language, a world of sensation (stimuli on/from the screen) is decisively *separated* from an intelligible world (a meaning or vision or value) rather than, for example, imagining a simple 'fold or crease' in the fabric of life where sensation and interpretation are part of a whole, which is not to say that they must be linear or 'unified.'[6] Where will the camera be found in such a metaphysical dualism: with sensation or with reason? (Compare the top cover illustration that offers a spectacle for our senses with the one at the bottom that hints at imperfect reasoning, a 'camera plan' gone awry.) The sensation/intelligence split raises a further question: Are there two kinds of language, a public one to 'converse' with the external world by reacting to stimuli and a second one for 'thinking' in private, for 'experiencing' the visual qualities of a film? Perhaps it would make sense to speak of a 'language' of sense-impressions.[7]

I hope in this book to suggest ways in which there is only a single language — one that is public — a language that has intricate links to our sense perceptions, thoughts, outlooks, intentions, bodies, emotions, and actions, and hence to the films we watch.[8] As Lakoff and Johnson emphasize, for a second-generation cognitive science the mind is fully "embodied." What is important, I believe, is to reject the idea that a thing is composed of a phenomenal surface (the source of stimuli) that conceals a deeper nature (meaning, essence, inner being). One should forgo appraisals of semiotic presence and absence, set aside facets of the imaginary, and avoid drawing up taxonomies of hybridity. Instead, a theorist should be assessing how and when an object is being framed by our cognitive, inferential, and emotive dispositions, which themselves arise from situations. This makes an object relative to various *descriptions of events* or rationalizations under which it is, or may be, seen, rather than the object being denoted by a simple name or sign that contains an inner sense. A spectator is not simply "placed" or "positioned" by a film, but *speaks* in response.

Evidence of the embodiment of mind may also be found in the many invisible, metaphorical projections that we live by. These projections are readily available to select and arrange what we see when watching a film, allowing us to draw inferences, make evaluations, and find the properties of things we need. Importantly, projections concern the future: what remarkable tales we may weave when our clothes are the threads of metaphor, and dressed to travel.

The idea of an embodied mind identical with a person's actions within settings raises the issue of causality. How do we use the word "causation"? Some writers continue to build theories of film around a single kind of causation — photographicity. Clearly, we will need to investigate the concept of cause-effect: what justifies or makes appropriate the "hyphen" in this word? My approach will be premised on thinking about causation as a public "language-game" (another hyphen. . .) derived from a person's intuitive and immediate awareness of a prototypical situation(s). This, I believe, makes the basic meaning of causation nonconscious, embodied, and radial (see figure 4.1).[9] In chapter 5 I will begin with relatively simple cases of causation involving motion on the screen and movement in a world before probing more complex cases involving the motivation of a fiction and the animation of a camera (cf. the frontispiece). Also relevant to the use of the word "causation" is the context that makes a given cause become prominent (become causal). Chapter 4 will analyze the word "context" in terms of fifteen major types of "frames" and "framing." It will be seen that causality and framing are tied to a multiplicity of human practices, thus supporting Deleuze's claim that it is because of "the interference of many practices that things happen, beings, images, concepts, all the kinds of events." Again, we will find that "Cinema's concepts are not given in cinema," but in ordinary and everyday practices that are distinctively human.

Those readers who would like a more detailed preview of each of the following chapters should skip to the last section of chapter 1. Here I will briefly mention some general themes to be found in this book along with my previous two books:

1. Character subjectivity
2. Point of view
3. Narration
4. Narrative
5. Fiction
6. Camera
7. Language
8. Film theory

All three of my books deal with all eight topics though the main emphasis in *Point of View in the Cinema* is on 1–3; *Narrative Comprehension and Film*, 3–5; and this book, 5–8. Each book maps a different decade of scholarly work: the 1970s, 1980s, and 1990s.

And, for what it's worth, here are the writers whose ideas and spirits have had a salutary influence on the content of the present book: Barbara Anderson; Joseph Anderson; Dudley Andrew; Rudolf Arnheim; Roland Barthes; André Bazin; David Black; David Bordwell; O.K. Bouwsma; Warren Buckland; Noël Burch; Noël Carroll; Daniel Dennett; Sergei Eisenstein; Thomas Elsaesser; Nelson Goodman; Torben Grodal; Stephen Heath; Paul Hernadi; Mark Johnson; John Kurten; George Lakoff; Peter Larsen; Christian Metz; Hugo Münsterberg; Steven Pinker; Carl Plantinga; Richard Rorty; Murray Smith; Melinda Szaloky; Kristin Thompson; George Wilson; Ludwig Wittgenstein; and Charles Wolfe.

Acknowledgments

Whether a book gets written is a matter of weather. The prevailing wind has been favorable for me due to the warmhearted contributions of many persons. Of first importance has been the support of my parents, Evelyn and Henry Odell, as steady and wise downwind as up. To them I owe most everything. I am also grateful to my parents-in-law, Dr. Terézia Tóth and Dr. Pál Szalóky, as well as to Klára Tóth.

I have taught about 6,000 students in more than 20 years and I have appreciated every one of them. Chapters 1 and 2 appeared first as brief class handouts. Those who have taught me include David Bordwell who has been a mentor, friend, generous scholar, incisive analyst, and model for me for over 30 years and who inspired, among many other of my writings, chapter 3 below; the inestimable Charles Wolfe from whom I learn daily and have for 20 years; John Kurten with his unerring eye for a film's aesthetic bristlings and for smart technical help; Stephen Heath there at the beginning; Mary Sirridge who decades ago in a philosophy class raised questions about the mysterious word "context" (to which I respond in the context of the word "frame" in chapter 4 below); Murray Smith who years ago suggested that I expand my ideas on narrative causality found in *Narrative Comprehension and Film* (for which see chapter 5 below); Richard Allen for a number of discussions about Wittgenstein; and Warren Buckland and Melinda Szaloky for detailed commentary on the manuscript. Early teachers in the art of writing fiction and nonfiction were my mother Evelyn, my uncle and aunt, Rice Odell and Audrey Erickson, and the stalwart Nick Blatchford of the *Washington Daily News*. Mien and mind have been shaped by two special fathers, Henry and Robert. Others who have contributed to this book have been left out, but not intentionally.

I have received sterling support from the Dean of Humanities and Fine Arts in the College of Letters and Science, David Marshall; from the Chair of the Department of Film Studies, Janet Walker;

and from the Academic Senate of the University of California, Santa Barbara.

I am fortunate to have the best critical studies colleagues one could imagine: Allison Anders, Peter Bloom, Kwame Braun, Anna Brusutti, JungBong Choi, Donna Cunningham, Dana Driskel, Anna Everett, Cynthia Felando, Willis Flachsenhar, Victor Fuentes, Naomi Greene, Dick Hebdige, Nancy Kawalek, Harry Lawton, Paul Lazarus, Suzanne Jill Levine, Lisa Parks, Constance Penley, Paul Portuges, Laurence Rickels, Bhaskar Sarkar, Alexander Sesonske, and Cristina Venegas. And little would be accomplished in the film studies department without the invaluable assistance of the staff presided over with unmatched professional skill by Kathryn Carnahan: Patrick Chose, Flora Furlong, Benjamin Kim, Joe Palladino, Sue Verhasselt, and Christy Zolla.

There is also a wider circle of scholars to thank: Porter Abbott, Rick Altman, Dudley Andrew, Tino Balio, Janet Bergstrom, Ben Brewster, Susan Derwin, Mary Ann Doane, Nataša Ďurovičová, James Elkins, Thomas Elsaesser, Arild Fetveit, Douglas Gomery, Ronald Gottesman, Jostein Gripsrud, Torben Grodal, Paul Hernadi, Christopher Husted, Anikó Imre, Lea Jacobs, Henry Jenkins, Kathryn Kalinak, Vance Kepley, Marsha Kinder, Tone Kolbjørnsen, András Bálint Kovács, Allan Langdale, Peter Larsen, Martin Lefebvre, Peter Lehman, Arnt Maasø, Stephen Mamber, Alison McMahan, Russell Merritt, Carl Plantinga, Michael Renov, David Rodowick, Philip Rosen, Jonathan Rosenbaum, Jeffrey Saver, Vivian Sobchack, Ove Solum, Bjørn Sørenssen, Guillaume Soulez, Janet Staiger, Garrett Stewart, László Tarnay, Kristin Thompson, Maureen Turim, Diane Waldman, and Kay Young.

I have again been exceptionally well-served by the editorial and production staff at Routledge. Bill Germano, a man of insight and wit who handles the English language like the buttons on his shirt, has fortunately been at hand for 15 years on a variety of projects. I also appreciate the skills of his editorial assistant, Frederick Veith, project editor Marsha Hecht, copyeditor Kristin Jones, compositor Mark Manofsky, and cover designer Elise Weinger. Chapters 3, 4, and 5 have specific histories given at the beginning of the endnotes.

My brother and sisters invariably understand: Will, Carol, Alison, and Suzie. Lorel and Laura are greatly missed. I write always with my beloved and admired sons in mind, Alex, Evan, Liam, and Nicholas, each a unique and permanent inspiration for me. I am grateful to Roberta Kimmel, the caring mother of Alex, Evan, and Liam.

The book is dedicated lovingly to my wife, Melinda Szaloky, a meticulous theorist, a loving mother for Nicholas, and she who enlivens me, of whom Edgar Allan Poe might have said:

So with the world thy gentle ways,

Thy grace, thy more than beauty,

Shall be an endless theme of praise

And love—a simple duty.

Oak Park, California
An agreeable day
May 2005

Terminological Note

SINGLE AND DOUBLE QUOTATION MARKS:

It is important that I explain how I will employ single and double quotation marks in this book. If I am in the midst of discussing *and quoting* an author's ideas (using double quote marks), then I will use single quote marks to show that something is *not* a quote from that author but is either my use of the author's term in a new (special) sense or my use of a general concept in a new (special) sense or my new term. This greatly reduces the number of endnotes that would otherwise be needed to distinguish every quote from an author from every highlighting of a word or concept attributable to me *when* quotes from an author and my special terms appear together in the text. If, however, the context is perfectly clear (i.e., I am *not* discussing another author and quoting his or her concepts), then I only use double quote marks for indicating words with special meanings.

Chapter 1: **The Life of a Camera**

"I think of [my] book [*Ways of Worldmaking*] as belonging in that mainstream of modern philosophy that began when Kant exchanged the structure of the world for the structure of the mind, continued when C. I. Lewis exchanged the structure of the mind for the structure of concepts, and that now proceeds to exchange the structure of concepts for the structure of the several symbol systems of the sciences, philosophy, the arts, perception, and everyday discourse. The movement is from unique truth and a world fixed and found to a diversity of right and even conflicting versions or worlds in the making."[1]

— Nelson Goodman

"When the film close-up strips the veil of our imperceptiveness and insensitivity from the hidden little things and shows us the face of objects, it still shows us man, for what makes objects expressive are the human expressions projected on to them. The objects only reflect our own selves. . . . "[2]

— Béla Balázs

"The concept of a 'cinematographic grammar' is very much out of favor today; one has the impression, indeed, that such a thing cannot exist. But that is only because it has not been looked for in the right place. Students have always implicitly referred them-selves to the *normative grammar of particular languages . . .*, but the linguistic and grammatical phenomenon is much vaster than any single language and is concerned with the *great and fundamental figures of the transmission of all information*. Only a general linguistics and a general semiotics . . . can provide the

1

study of cinematographic language with the appropriate methodological 'models.'"[3]

— Christian Metz

"[I]t is language which speaks, not the author; to write is, through
a prerequisite impersonality (not at all to be confused with the . . .
objectivity of the realist novelist), to reach that point where only
language acts, 'performs,' and not 'me.' . . . We know now that a
text is not a line of words releasing a single 'theological' meaning
(the 'message' of the Author-God) but a multi-dimensional space
in which a variety of writings, none of them original, blend and
clash. The text is a tissue of quotations drawn from the innumerable centres of culture."[4]

— Roland Barthes

"Gott im Himmel, it has spoken!"

— John Kruesi, assistant to Thomas Edison, on first hearing
Edison's voice coming from the "Talking-Machine"

"*Essence* is expressed by grammar. . . . Grammar tells what kind
of object anything is."[5]

— Ludwig Wittgenstein

THE DEATH OF THE AUTHOR

Roland Barthes famously announced the passing away of the literary author. What was lost was the sense of an identifiable Agent,
an origin (an original) — the One who had infused sense into a
work, creating meanings and unity. Critics used to have "the important task of discovering the Author (or its hypostases: society,
history, psyché, liberty) *beneath* the work: when the Author has
been found, the text is 'explained'. . . . "[6] Barthes refers to this
task of peering into the depths of a text's meaning to search for
the Author as an effort of "decipherment." The aim was to trace

2

back along the causal chain from the surface of a text to its hidden point-source.

For Barthes, the Author's death heralded "the birth of the reader," which meant an empowerment of a common language and way of thinking, a recognition that writing was actually a meshwork of "quotations" from a community rather than the private and unique utterance of an Author.[7] The newly born reader, however, was not conceived as a private individual:

> "[A] text's unity lies not in its origin but in its destination. Yet this destination cannot any longer be personal: the reader is without history, biography, psychology; he is simply that *someone* who holds together in a single field all the traces by which the written text is constituted."[8]

It is important that for Barthes the reader has simply evolved into a "someone" — that is, someone who is *impersonal*. In fact, the same thing has happened to the author: the state of being-an-Author for Barthes did not dissolve into nothing but instead found a new place within a life of letters in the form of an "impersonality,"[9] a kind of "Talking-Machine." As we shall see, however, a general form of impersonality is not a 'universal' form (every one) but instead is relative to 'a set of readings' produced through the discourse of a particular community, that is, relative to the dimensions of a specialized use of language.

Film, too, may be thought to have an Author, or its hypostasis behind the image: the Camera. This is true even if the Camera is said to be merely a thing that objectifies the world. The reason is that, for Barthes, "objectivity" is just a pretext or ruse that conceals the Author (or its hypostases: society, history, psyché, liberty).[10] For Barthes, the Author's death was also the death of "objectivity." The Author, and now presumably the Camera, have been replaced by a simple impersonality. But what is "impersonality"? Barthes seems to interpret the impersonal as a form of *indefiniteness*, so that rather than one Author, there will be many authors, not all of whom can be identified. A text, whether composed of words or pictures, would be thought of as a vast imbrication of quotations,

3

allusions, beliefs, and values arising from a community or communities. A particular "image," then, would actually be a composite or summation of many possible images, stereotypes, and verbal descriptions.[11]

An indefinite mode of speaking may be illustrated by the utterance, "it rains." I believe that the indefinite subject of this utterance (the "it" of raining) may also be applied to an *image* of rain. What is being said through *it* (the image) is that "it rains." The relationship of "rains" to "it" is the same as "it rains" to a camera-it that precipitates the meaning "rain." There is a subtle distinction to be made here. Even though a film may show rain, one should resist saying that the film depicts literally that "it *is* raining" or that "it *was* raining." This is because the "is" or "was" progressive tenses are appropriate only when one is thinking fictionally (e.g., "the character looks out the window and sees that it *is* raining") or else when one is tracing back along the causal chain from an image on the screen to its hidden point-source (e.g., "it *was* raining when the camera filmed the scene in the script"). The progressive tenses apply when the artifact is assumed to be transparent (i.e., when one thinks about what is happening "inside" the fiction) or the artifact is taken to be opaque (i.e., when one thinks about its manufacture as an object with an outside and an inside). By contrast, the "is" and "was" progressive tenses are not appropriate, I believe, when one is thinking about a novel or film as a product from which a thing ("rain") is being identified ("I understand there is rain" or "I see it is rain"). An indefinite mode of address emerges when we confront the sheer "flatness" of a text and discover that no privileged focus (beneath or above) authorizes our descriptions: the only focus for our language is hypothetical or potential, a product of our ability to speak — or, more exactly, a product of how we and others *have typically spoken* about a thing. Or else, how we have made a thing recognizable by recalling how we have spoken about "similar" things.[12]

For Barthes, a 'fact' in a text is not attributable to an author's unique vision, which supposedly bubbles upward through force of will and is often filtered through a character. Barthes is more concerned with the way that a 'fact' comes into being when put under descriptions in the act of interpretation. A 'text,' then, is not so much 'out there' as it is a mental process intimately connected with creating and assessing resemblances, metaphors, and projections deemed appropriate within or against the norms of a community. The purpose in searching for 'resemblances' (i.e., in searching for how a fact is simplified and sorted into one or many categories) is not to discover which individual or author is making a given interpretation, or to measure the truth of an interpretation, but rather to juxtapose an interpretation with the conditions that make it possible. Writing is an experiment in reading; to write is to be the first reader. Filming is an experiment in seeing; to film is to be the first spectator. Writing and filming are alike in that each depends on a common set of mental operations by which *knowledge* is being represented, retrieved, manipulated, and revised. Thus, a text's 'impersonality,' finally, has to do with the *commonness* and *intelligibility* of the knowledge being expressed. What is expressed is not due to an Author or Camera, but is the result of a person speaking about his or her knowledge and feelings on an *occasion* of reading or seeing.

Let me put the idea of 'commonness' and 'intelligibility' in a different light. In order to make sense, one must use a grammar; that is, one must communicate by following or bending the rules of a linguistic grammar. For Wittgenstein, however, there are still 'larger grammars' at work when we speak. These larger grammars select and shape local linguistic rules into special sets of rules that create patterned ways of speaking and thinking. Each of these special grammars possesses a rich 'vocabulary.' In turn, the vocabulary (usually composed of ordinary words employed in a special way) corresponds to a manner of acting in the world — to making the world seem. For Wittgenstein, each grammar is a kind of map created to help solve a set of closely related problems. In fact, for Wittgenstein we make a world by accumulating a large number of these sets of problems and their associated grammars. That is, we fashion a significant world out of problems and grammars into which our various desires and acts may be fitted and made significant. Wittgenstein proposes that these many grammars should be understood as a series of "language-games" where each game requires one to learn specific rules in order to be able to make a significant "move" (i.e., to play, or act in, the "game"). Playing a game is a practice, though we may also practice playing a game.

What counts in making a particular "move," according to John Ellis, is the "relation to other possible moves in that game rather than to the mental states of the speakers or to ideas or independent 'facts' that exist outside the structure of the game."[13] A language-game specifies the moves that can be made by us as well as by the objects in the game. A language-game specifies what can be meaningfully said about an object (and its range of movements) and hence determines what kind of object something is — its nature or essence.[14] To inquire about essence is to ask what a particular grammar allows one to *do* with an object or to see the object do. A language-game thus functions as a kind of *frame* for an object by creating a standard of rationality believed to be appropriate to the object. In chapters 4 and 5 we will look more closely at the notions of "frame" and "radial meaning," which result from a certain multiplicity of frames. (Radial meaning is a type of ambiguity that arises when the same word appears in different language-games, including the word "frame" itself.[15]) We will also examine how particular language-games are played out in film theory: for example, games concerning fictiveness, mobility, causation, subjectivity, and what will count as "concrete reality." Indeed, we will need to revise substantially some traditional ideas about the nature of "film theory" as individual film theories are seen to be an imbrication of games.

In the chapters to follow, I will seek to build on Barthes's argument that the personal Author has been replaced by impersonality. I will seek to demonstrate that this "impersonal," or 'indefinite,' mode of speaking in a text should be understood in terms of moves in one or more "language-games" that we are being invited to play. (See figure 1.1.) Indeed, the personal Author and the (gregarious) Narrator were themselves created through a language-game. The traditional way of describing the qualities of texts was often based on the notion that a text was a *conversation* with an Author or at least a condensed sort of message from the Author, even though this message was incomplete and contained exculpatory ambiguities.

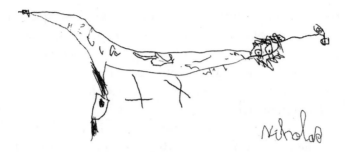

FIGURE 1.1   A Reader-Author
A reader-author makes a move (as conceived by five-year-old Nicholas Branigan).

Just as Barthes's notion of "the birth of the reader" means a new freedom for reading, where responses and criticisms are no longer limited to the rules of a conversation or to the rules of reading a kind of 'telegram,' so one may imagine that the death of the Author means that an author no longer needs to impersonate a narrator, a character, or a 'nobody' (i.e., appear in the guise of a disembodied "objectivity"), in order to be able to speak. After death, the author becomes simply another reader, occupying the same ground as any reader, including readers not yet born. Being an impersonal voice permits an author to work close up to a reader — in a place where language-games are being lived.

A CAMERA AS IMPERSONAL SUBJECT

This book is about a camera in its impersonal mode. A camera is most evident during its movements and long-held shots, so we will examine these events closely (in chapters 2 and 5). The impersonal mode, however, seems ever-present even when the *screen* is blank or black, and so we will need to examine theories about the general nature of the film *medium* (chapters 3 and 4). To complicate matters further, an "impersonal utterance" must still be an utterance *about* something and in this book the "something" will be taken to be an element of *narrative* discourse. Thus, we will need to consider a variety of general issues bearing on storytelling techniques in relation to camera movement and the long take (chapters 2 and 4).

Narrative discourse, however, cannot be analyzed apart from a particular choice of a theory of narrative. Thus, we will be led to consider various narrative theories and the relationship each establishes with a "camera" (chapters 2 and 3). Ultimately, we will be led to weigh various theories of film, each of which seeks to identify a unique place for a camera to occupy in the medium of film with the result that — by virtue of a particular film theory and narrative theory — a person will be able to talk confidently, and even boldly, about a camera as being *the* camera (chapter 3).

One may also say that because a camera occupies a "point" in space and "points" at things, it has a "point of view." But, of course, questions soon arise about the nature of the "space" in which a camera exists and about the nature of the pointing that produces a "point of view." One will need to ask, for example, how literal the "pointing" must be for a camera to *have* a point of view, which amounts to asking how literal a "camera" must be for it to have a point of view (chapter 2). For example, it is often said that an image appears onscreen for some (particular) reason and therefore must have a "point," must represent an attitude or viewpoint. Another issue is whether a sound track should be included in the description of a visual point of view. For instance, after we hear a sound we may be shown the source of the sound through a camera movement or in the next shot, and this sound may point to several meanings relevant to the image. How is the sound to be part of the point of view? There are still other issues involved in weighing the nature of the act of "pointing" at things. These sorts of issues suggest that an analysis of "point of view" (more exactly, the point of being in a field of view) will go far beyond specifying the location of a physical camera and the direction in which a lens is pointed. We will discover that problems concerning the nature of "point of view" lead back to narrative theories and their intersection with film theories. Also, we will discover that it does not simplify matters to say that a camera merely "frames" an object. As we shall see, the meaning of "frame" is anything but self-evident and, like a film theory, is caught in a tangle of philosophical issues and language-games (chapter 4).

A given film theory seeks to define the sensual, formal, cognitive, emotional, and aesthetic qualities of a camera. A theory will also attempt to discover the important narrative effects of a moving camera on a spectator/auditor so as to propose a vocabulary and method for conducting a critical analysis (chapter 2). We will find that a camera is (usually) enmeshed in character, place, atmosphere, action, reaction, events, connections among events, causality, enigmas, rhetoric, theme, narrative, and narration, though not necessarily all of these to the same degree in a particular film (chapter 3). We will also find that one of the functions of a moving camera is (often) to give volume and density to a locale through the *kinetic depth effect*, which is a perceptual cue about space that arises exclusively from the movement of a camera. Another function of a moving camera is (often) to create a sense of the continuous *presence of the present*, an omnipresence of time through a long-held shot. By allowing plot time to develop without interruption, the spectator is able to witness the full causal interaction of persons and objects. Nevertheless, on occasion a moving camera will function not to accumulate space or time for us (by building up details, acts, motives, changes, plot events, views, etc.) but instead will function to radically disconnect, subtract, interrogate, or even stop the constructive activities of a spectator. In brief, we will need to investigate both the standard and extraordinary effects of a moving camera if we wish to understand the range of a camera's impersonal address.

In examining the movements of a camera, we will begin to wonder exactly what a camera "is." What is the entity that we imagine to be in movement behind the motion that we see on the screen? Do we, for example, try to imagine the actual, unique camera used to make a shot? Or do we, instead, merely imagine a generalized camera and a procedure for making shots during production (for example, a dolly accompanied by tracks and chalk marks on the floor, and an indoor set)? Or, perhaps, we imagine an idealized camera made up of a set of physical laws and mechanical principles — a lightproof box with an aperture, shutter, lens, and light-sensitive emulsion. Or, perhaps, we think of more abstract ways of "looking" and "moving" connected to a filmmaker, narrator,

9

character, or, indeed, *connected to our own desires* (where, for example, the camera becomes a kind of "eye" or even "inner eye"). And there are still other ways to think about what it is that moves on the screen and creates a reaction in a spectator. Eventually we must inquire what the "thing," the entity, really is that we are naming with the word "camera." I will argue that this question depends upon what we intend to do with the word "camera." What language-game(s) will we play?

Finally, *why* does a camera move (or fail to move)? Does a camera ever *lie* to us? Does it conceal as well as reveal? If so, how and when? For instance, doesn't the camera lie to us in the sequence from Alfred Hitchcock's *Psycho* (1960) in which Norman carries his mother down from the upstairs bedroom to the basement? Recall that the camera has chosen *not* to move into the bedroom for the conversation between Norman and his mother but instead moves to frame the empty hallway and stairs, ironically, from an "ideal overhead view." In this case, however, the chosen view is the perfect view for concealing a crucial fact about "Mother" and, especially, for concealing the fact that something is being concealed. (Mother says to Norman: "Norman, what do you think you're doing? Don't you touch me! Don't! Norman! Put me down, put me down! I can walk with my own [two feet].") Note also that the camera has moved to frame the action on the stairs *in advance of* Norman carrying his mother out of the bedroom; that is, the camera "knows" what will happen and what must be concealed. In light of these questions, and the multiple functions of a camera, perhaps it might be better to ask *how many* types of cameras may exist in a film, rather than to imagine just one, or *the* one. Perhaps the question should be *when* is there one type of camera rather than another in a film (chapter 5), that is, at what point within a stream of conscious thought about a film is a person characterizing one sort of camera rather than another for that film.

Questions about what a camera *is* will lead us toward other problems, such as what an "image" is and where it is. Is an image *in* the film emulsion? Is it projected through the air? On the screen? In the mind? In memory? If so, in *whose* mind or memory? Ours?

The filmmaker's? A narrator's? A character's? An invisible observer's? For that matter, where is the *motion* that we perceive on the screen? Recall that literally only *still* frames — 24 per second, each flashed 3 times — are projected onto the screen. Each individual frame on a strip of film is moving through the projector only while the shutter of the projector is blacking out the screen (which is about 40 percent of the time). In fact, literally nothing is moving on the screen in front of us — not images, characters, objects, or a camera; if it were otherwise, there would be only a moving vertical blur on the screen as the film strip raced past the projector lamp.

Thus, we will need to examine how a series of unmoving frames flashed onto the screen can create an impression of motion and what implications there may be for a theory of film viewing (chapter 5). Furthermore, even a sequence of still *shots* will sometimes create for us a sense of motion, for example, the famous three-shot sequence in Sergei Eisenstein's *Potemkin* (1925) in which a stone lion "awakens." This fact illustrates that the nature of a camera and our perception of motion are closely related to what at first would seem a quite different mode of film production — animation. In an animated film, static *ink drawings* routinely create a sensation of motion for the spectator while bringing a "camera" into existence that, moreover, may sometimes be seen to act independently of the action in the drawings and be seen to move *through* a scene. An animated camera that follows the action and moves around a scene is quite distinct from the immobile one that once photographed the ink drawings from a fixed position on an animation stand.

I have stressed above the importance of narrative and film theories when we think about the nature of a camera. I have also maintained that a camera represents an impersonal kind of address related to the form of grammar we adopt when we make a move within a specific language-game. In this book I hope to show that it is essential to investigate *how we move* within one or more theories and grammars: how we create *through our talk* an unseen camera-entity that may itself seemingly begin to move within our words like the objects that (seem to) move on the screen. A camera may throw a series of still images of its own movement onto the screen, which we will then perceive as motion inside and through images on the screen. A spectator will explain this motion on the screen with reasons drawn from theories and grammars. These reasons, in turn, will direct our attention, shape our seeing, and specify significance. I believe, therefore, that it will be beneficial to analyze in close detail how we speak about a camera and its movements — how we think, discuss, and marvel about a camera we see in action. I believe that we will thereby gain insight into broader and deeper issues about the institution of cinema, because film itself is often felt to be something "in motion," a "motion picture" creating meaning and emotion, a moving experience par excellence.

HOW SHOULD ANALYSIS PROCEED? VERTICAL DISSECTION VERSUS HORIZONTAL INTERSECTION

> "Suppose you said: 'one thing must rest on another — the cushion on the chair, the chair on the earth . . . but in the end something must rest on itself.' You can say this, but it produces puzzlement because it is not a normal statement. One would rather say 'it rests on nothing'; but this gives a feeling of insecurity, whereas the other gives a sense of security. 'If the earth rests on nothing, you might as well have no foundation to your house.' — This is the source of the idea of 'a priori.'"[16]

> — Ludwig Wittgenstein

If we are to analyze and understand what a camera means to us when we confidently declare that we have seen a certain "something" on the screen (moving or not), how should our analysis proceed — with what principles? P. F. Strawson argues that there are two basic approaches to analysis: "reduction" and "connection."[17] Reduction is a method of "dismantling" a thing whereby something is broken into simpler pieces, ultimately, into pieces that are the simplest possible. The idea is to discover the fundamental, irreducible constituents of a thing — what makes up that thing, makes it be that thing and no other. The simple pieces will show how the various parts of the thing interact with one another to make it work. The pieces will also allow one to judge which parts are necessary for that thing, which parts are optional, and which parts are sufficiently similar to parts found in other things that they may be exchanged, or nearly exchanged, for example, when we say, "this shot (or scene) is just like a shot (or scene) I saw in another film." In general, the method of "reduction" searches for the necessary and sufficient conditions for the existence of a thing, for an a priority. In the case of analyzing a "concept," the reduction method searches for the necessary and sufficient conditions for the proper application or use of the concept. The reduction method also correlates to our perception of a thing. According to Charles Stevenson, when we are thinking of a thing's individual pieces, we exhibit a "dissective" attention, and when we are thinking of the thing as a perfect whole — when all of its parts are intact — we exhibit a "synoptic" attention that yields a "net impression."[18]

There is a second kind of analysis that Strawson refers to as "connection." What is important here is that a thing is understood in terms of its connections, links, and relations to a large group of other things. Rather than dissecting or breaking down a thing on the basis of arbitrary criteria, one focuses on how a thing is being juxtaposed with a variety of situations and contexts. Whereas the reduction approach is like an autopsy, finding "connections" is like doing geography: One is projecting, mapping, and charting.[19] The difference is between a search for there to be a being and a search for a being to be *there*.

It is important to note that "metaphorical language" will have a different status in these two kinds of analysis. In the reductive approach, a metaphor is seen as merely a convenient way of speaking and/or as a "surface decoration." A metaphor becomes a veil that must be pierced in order to glimpse what lies below. A metaphor must be penetrated in order to confront, for example, the "content" of a statement, the "truth," the "foundation," the "literal" nature of a thing or its "substance." By contrast, in a connectionist approach, a metaphor acts as an important "road" or "association" that links two *areas*, bringing together two complexes (two domains of use), and thus is neither simple nor expendable. In the connectionist approach a metaphor states or shows a way forward for thinking. It may be an important aid in tracing and disentangling multiple uses of a word or in highlighting interlocking practices.

Strawson generally favors the "connection" approach to analysis. He argues as follows:

> But now let us consider a quite different model of philosophical analysis. This new model [connection] I am going to declare more realistic and more fertile than the one just discussed [reduction]. . . . Let us abandon the notion of perfect simplicity in concepts; let us abandon even the notion that analysis must always be in the direction of greater simplicity. Let us imagine, instead, the model of an elaborate network, a system, of connected items, concepts, such that the function of each item, each concept, could, from the philosophical point of view, be properly understood only by grasping its connections with the others, its place in the system — perhaps better still, the picture of a set of interlocking systems of such a kind. If this becomes our model, then there will be no reason to be worried if, in the process of tracing connections from one point to another of the network, we find ourselves returning to, or passing through, our starting-point. We might find, for example, that we could not fully elucidate the concept of knowledge without reference to the concept of sense perception; and that we could not explain all the features of the concept of sense perception without reference to the concept of knowledge. But this might be an unworrying and unsurprising fact. So the general charge of circularity would lose its sting, for we might have moved in a wide, revealing, and illuminating circle.[20]

Strawson's example of how a 'connectionist' approach might work is particularly apt, considering that one of the major claims in this book will be that our notion of a 'camera' cannot be based on "sense perception" alone "without reference to the concept of knowledge." I will argue that our *perception* of, for example, the photographicity of an image, the motion of objects on the screen, and the motion of a moving camera onscreen cannot alone define what we mean by the concept of a 'camera' or how we use the concept of a 'camera' to explain our reactions to a motion picture. "Sense perception" is not enough. Instead, our talk about a camera is firmly linked with our implicit *knowledge* of everyday practices, aesthetic discourses, film theories, and narrative theories. Our talk about film and the work of the 'camera' is not simply a rephrasing of "sense perception" (e.g., 'the camera pans left') but is already a modeling and projection of how a film and its 'camera' fit into our lives and system of values.

Here is an example of talking about a camera, not in terms of sense perception alone but as being connected to our "knowledge" of the world: to the problems we face in making a world significant. Gilberto Perez, speaking broadly, contrasts a number of these cameras:

> The dramatic camera knows exactly what to show us, knows the extent of what matters. The epic camera of Mizoguchi, the devil's camera Hitchcock employs, not only knows what to show us but makes palpable to us its stance of knowledge. The explorer's camera Flaherty employs has scouted the territory for us, has discovered what to show us. Renoir's camera is another kind of explorer, one who hasn't gone ahead of us into the territory and can't presume to know exactly what to show us. Antonioni's camera is like Renoir's in this respect, an inquiring rather than a knowing camera, though Renoir's camera takes the point of view of a friend rather than a stranger.[21]

A reduction method might dismiss Perez's claims as merely extravagant statements about the (concealed) creative intentions of the five auteurs. A connection method, however, would take seriously the metaphorical descriptions of the cameras. It would weigh how such descriptions might project beyond sense perception toward other areas of experience summoned through memory and felt similarities. For connectionism, the proper name of an author is employed not to identify a person and his or her traits, but to build a large, loose collection of meanings to anchor a spectator's responses (i.e., not Mizoguchi, but "Mizoguchi").

In this book I will primarily be concerned with Strawson's second kind of analysis, based on "connection," not "reduction." I will refer to "connection" as a method that works "horizontally," searching for appropriate links and knots (ribbons, kinks, clumps) among systems. This movement of analysis will be across and through a network, from item to item, rather than either downward toward ever-smaller pieces of a thing (*sub*sets) or upward toward an ideal overview that gives a synoptic panorama. Later we will examine the far-reaching consequences of adopting a connectionist method that searches laterally for how things intersect rather than adopting a reductive method that dissects and dismantles a thing while looking for a hidden essence. The choice of a connectionist method will have important consequences for reconceiving theories of film (chapter 4) and theories of the camera and medium (chapter 5).

Barthes's reevaluation of the word "author" and its place in literary theory may be understood in relation to vertical and horizontal methodologies. I believe that the older way of thinking about the author that Barthes asserts is now dead was a 'vertical' method in which an analyst peered through the 'surface' of a text into its 'depths' searching for the core or seed that had generated the text — *the* author. Barthes argues, in effect, that a 'horizontal' method is more productive — one that expands outward from a purported instance of authorial intervention (e.g., the appearance in a text of an authorial 'I' or a phrase that suggests a 'comment' or an 'attitude'). Thinking 'horizontally' leads an analyst toward a series of intersections and transitions within, as Barthes says, a vast "tissue of quotations drawn from the innumerable centres of culture."[22] Barthes argues that analysis should be a movement that spreads outward from a text along radial lines and circles, not downward to an essential center. He refers to the work of horizontal analysis as searching for what must be *disentangled* as opposed to what is *deciphered* by a vertical analysis.[23] While vertical 'deciphering' concentrates on synecdoche and causality in reducing a thing to its essentials so as to make a precise generalization, horizontal 'disentangling' relies on metaphors, associations, puns, and the 'flow' of reading to bridge gaps and locate connections. 'Disentangling' and finding intersections will be my goal, not 'deciphering' and dissecting.

Modern literary and film theories often have recourse to notions of "construction" and "deconstruction." The perceiver's "constructivist" activity is said to be subject to "deconstruction" by the analyst. Still, the question to ask is whether the analyst's labor is one of disentangling or deciphering. Similarly ambiguous is the call for a "piecemeal" theory of film: Are these "pieces" to be conceived as (horizontally) connected, contingent, historically relative, and linked to forms of life, or is each piece to become a single part within some grand and permanent, logical whole — a final, objective theory of film and the film medium that awaits only our ability to decipher the illusory surfaces of things?[24] The problem with a method of vertical dissection is that it assumes that relevant facts are definite and near at hand, even if presently unknown, much as an object blocks what lies behind. Furthermore, in the case of film, vertical dissection fosters a misguided drive to see more visible details, and closer, as if all differences in an image matter for all purposes.

In rethinking the place of an "author," Barthes is concerned not only with literary texts but also with "the world as text."[25] Putting this concern in terms of Wittgenstein's theory, one might say that in moving horizontally through the meanings attributed to a given world, we are actually tracing one or many of the special vocabularies or language-games that have been adopted by groups of people as a guide to one or several forms of life. A camera, too, may become a guide for us, but only after we have specified how *its* movements connect to *our* movements — to our moves — within a particular language-game. In finding, disentangling, and making connections we give a camera life.

APERÇU: THINGS TO COME

I would like to preview the chapters to come and mention some
of my basic assumptions. Each of the next four chapters takes a
different view of the nature of a "camera" and of a camera's act of
"framing." Since each chapter examines a camera in a new context,
the chapters may to some extent be read in any order. Chapter 1
introduces the issue of "analysis" ("reduction" or "vertical dissection" versus "connection" or "horizontal intersection") and argues
that a camera should be analyzed not as an identifiable *center* for
a film (the private instrument of an Author) but, instead, as a dispersed and depersonalized (impersonal) effect of watching a film.
A camera comes into being — we are able to *place* it — as we discuss and appraise our reactions to a film. A camera will appear in
many places, not just in the place occupied by the physical camera.
Furthermore, I have argued that our talk should be understood in
relation to moves within diverse language-games; that is, within selected vocabularies tied to the ways we speak about and construct,
for example, critical practices, aesthetic discourses, film theories,
narrative theories, folk theories, values, and everyday discourses.
To frame a camera, we must understand the formal or informal
language we use to see it.

The context for chapter 2 is the filmic system. Here I inventory
some of the typical ways in which we talk about the internal structure of a film. I will argue that an analyst employs such terms
as "motivation," "anthropomorphism," "point of view," and
"movement" to invoke a camera's presence or, rather, to extract
certain properties from a filmic system that may then be linked
to the "existence" of a camera. These and other terms express an
interface between our cognitive activities and a filmic system — for
example, our movement of attention while watching a film. An
important goal for a film theory is to give an account of our contact with film through a filmic system.

The context for chapter 3 is the discourse of film theory. I will
examine how various film theorists have sought to create models for
the film medium in order to justify the use of specific analytical terms
and methods. I will outline eight general approaches to constructing

a film theory derived from eight approaches to the nature of meaning. I will delve into theories of meaning generally and will argue that seeing a "camera" is one of the ways we discuss meanings in films. Moreover, cameras and meanings should be seen as relative to the needs and values of a community. I believe that a "camera," like language, is tied to a form of life and thus is "local" rather than being something possessed of a universal essence that makes it a mere physical object, logical form, or all-purpose eye.

The context for chapter 4 is the discourse of meta-theory: how do we formulate comparisons among film theories? Here I will suggest some general constraints that should be imposed on the language we choose when stating the ideas of a given film theory. These constraints on language emerge from a "mild realism" (Daniel Dennett) or "moderate constructivism" (David Bordwell), which is characteristic of any approach based on "motivated conventions" (George Lakoff) or "ecological conventions" (Torben Grodal). Accordingly, I will explore such concepts as embodiment, basic-level categorization, radial meanings, top-down and bottom-up cognitive processing, image schemata, and metaphorical projections. I will attempt to make clear the impact of such concepts on the way we talk about film theories and on the ways we create film theories, and, thus, the effects that these concepts will have on our ideas about the "image," "editing," and "narration." I will illustrate these effects by tracing the different "language-games" being played by writers who seek to advance theories of "suture" in film.

I will argue that a given film theory should be interpreted as being:

- *Grammatical* (i.e., a film theory should be seen as nothing more than the grammar of an ensemble of such words as "frame," "shot," "camera," "editing," "sound," "style," "realism," "auteur," "performance," "spectatorship," and "medium specificity")
- *Intersubjective* (i.e., a film theory should not be conceived as a set of fixed, objective, or universal propositions about film but, rather, should be tied to social practices, values, and

a community consensus about, for example, the present and past boundaries of the medium)

- *Fragmentary* (i.e., once we have given up the idea that a film theory is objective and unified — and that a film theory provides us with a comprehensive overview of film from an ideal point of view — then we will come to see theoretical descriptions of film as being partial, provisional, and relative to historical forces)
- *Figurative* (i.e., the "abstractions" of a film theory are often metaphorical projections or displacements based on bodily experiences, embodied concepts, heuristics, scenarios, and image schemata; a "camera" is an instance of just such a projection)
- *Connected* (i.e., the complex parts of a film theory should not be understood as composed of simpler and simpler constituents as if they could be dissected and arranged into a hierarchy — as if to explain film were a matter of penetrating a surface to discover the most basic and essential elements; instead, the parts of a film theory should be seen as spreading outward in ever-wider lines and curves, connecting and jumping to parts in new systems to make a network or heterarchy)
- *Impure* (i.e., qualities like those just listed suggest that a film theory should not be considered as a Theory specific to film or as itself pure and autonomous; there is no Medium of film, no film Specificity)[26]

In chapter 4 I will illustrate some of the problems of meta-theory through analyzing the notion of the "frame." What is a frame? What is framing in film? I will examine how frame lines on the screen figure for a mind or, rather, how the mind figures frame lines for a space — the space of an image, a scene, a narrative, as well as many other, more abstract "spaces" that we routinely construct in the process of comprehension. I do not believe that there is a common denominator or set of necessary and sufficient conditions that defines all varieties of the "frame." Instead, there are interlinking metaphors for the frame, a sequence of conceptions that carry the weight of a spectator's assertions from moment to moment. I will argue that the meaning of "frame" exists within the stream of a spectator's interpretation; as one breaks up the stream in various ways, one finds various "frames." Thus, to understand how a given frame functions, one must analyze not only the screen, but also how the spectator *speaks about* what the film is being taken to say.

In examining frame lines, chapter 4 will pursue an important link between film and language. This link is manifest in the way we use language to talk (endlessly) about film, including presenting conference papers and writing books. Though we may highlight a lecture with a film clip, we seldom (never?) make our arguments or discuss a film's effects by displaying images. The common ground for film and language is in the mind where *knowledge* is being represented, manipulated, and revised (as displayed in the phonological loop of short-term memory). Once we reject the idea that "meanings" exist in the world, hidden inside objects and texts, the focus of inquiry will shift to the cognitive activities of a spectator: how we see objects *under descriptions* and how *interpretations* are made, how we "connect" and "go on." A film "text" then becomes a (loose) collection of descriptions of an artifact. In addition, we will see in chapter 4 that meaning and knowledge have a basis in the body.

Jan Simons nicely sums up one of my basic assumptions concerning the relation of film and language:

> [O]nce one sees *verbalizations* of filmic representations as possible linguistic descriptions of filmic images, a more relaxed attitude towards the relationship of language and cinema becomes possible, which might prove to be more productive than either an obstinate pursuit of the study of film with linguistic concepts or a firm rejection of any linguistically inspired approach, since the place where film and language meet is not some external space where autonomous semiotic systems correlate, but the mind of a human subject, where they interact at some conceptual level.[27]

The context for chapter 5 is "language" and, specifically, the ordinary use of language in fashioning descriptions and interpretations. I will be concerned with descriptions of such states of affairs as "causation," "fiction," "fictional truth," "rightness," and even "everyday reality," a prototypical state of affairs. In particular, I will look quite closely at descriptions of "movement." We will need to understand the psychophysical details of the kinds of movements that may be encountered in watching a film. What assumptions do we make, for example, when we describe a camera movement in terms of panning, tilting, dollying, or tracking? What language-game are we playing?

The spirit of chapter 5 is that of Aristotle's "second philosophy," physics, which is an account of the mobility of things. We will discover, however, that many important movements of things are routine projections from a psychophysics into less tangible and less visible realms, for example, the motion and change that we experience when we follow an argument (moving from point to point), read, listen, narrativize, feel, remember, or entertain thoughts. Although Aristotle's "first philosophy," metaphysics, is an account of *that which makes a thing move* while being itself "free from movement" and "unmovable," I will draw instead on Wittgenstein's philosophy to argue that the "unmovable" is relative and merely an effect of our use of language — that is, a product of language-games. In connection with the "unmovable," we will investigate what is meant by "sustaining" causation. This is not to say that a given language-game may not be useful, justified, important, or part of an entrenched system of ideas (e.g., the entrenched idea that "the world was not created 100 years ago"); it is only to turn away from metaphysical absolutes toward pragmatic circumstances, toward the flow of life. Our use of language tells us about the goals we pursue and the circumstances we face. Language tells us how we have chosen to act, think, and adapt to changing circumstances.

If Béla Balázs is correct that a close-up in film performs a kind of analysis and that what is seen framed close-up in a film is only "our own selves,"[28] then it may be equally true that when we look at a film close-up in analysis, we should be re-finding what is human — that is, making connections to our interests, values, and manner of looking. To look in this manner would be to avoid

22

reducing a phenomenon to its smallest piece as if seen through a microscope: one would not be forced to decide which qualities of a thing would count as the most fundamental for all occasions. Instead, one would seek out vital links with the ways we choose to look and speak about a thing in relation to other things on a given occasion; indeed, one would discover what it means to choose.

Chapter 2: **A Camera-in-the-Text**

ANAL

Y S I S

— Intertitle from *Weekend*
(Jean-Luc Godard, 1967)

"How disturbed we should be, were there some machine that would allow us to follow the strange progress of a story as it winds its way through the thousand brains in a cinema! ... What Jules de Noailles said (recounted by Liszt), is true: 'You will see one day that it is hard to speak about anything with anyone.'"[1]

— Jean Cocteau

MOTIVATION [I]: CAMERA MOVEMENT AND TIME

When a camera is considered as a feature embedded within a text, it acquires some of the properties of the text, much like a particular aspect of a design in a tapestry can be used to talk about the tapestry. In this chapter I will review several major analytical concepts that help to bring out the features of a camera-in-the-text. I will be concerned primarily with four large-scale concepts that are used to delineate a camera: "motivation," degree of "anthropomorphism," "point of view," and "movement." My purpose in this chapter is to provide a systematic account of some of the ordinary critical language that is used to discover a camera situated-in-the-text. Later chapters will undertake to find the sources of this language, where they lead, and what sorts of cameras are brought into existence.

The concept of *motivation* takes several forms. One form measures the *time* of a narrative, that is, the development or movement of a narrative. A camera movement (or camera position, angle, focus, or some other feature) may be said to be motivated if it performs any one of the following narrative functions; otherwise, it is *un*motivated:

1. Establishes scenographic space
2. Closely follows or anticipates movement by a character or significant object
3. Continues to hold or center a character or significant object in frame (i.e., continuously reframes)
4. Moves away from, and *refuses to follow or reframe*, a movement by a character or object for reasons of narrative suspense, mystery, surprise, or good taste or censorship (e.g., a pan away from graphic violence or sexuality)
5. Follows or discovers a glance
6. Selects a narratively significant detail (e.g., an inserted dolly shot of a facial expression or important object)
7. Reveals character subjectivity

In analyzing the motivation of a camera, one must always be sensitive to the *amount of plot time* devoted to any one of the above functions in relation to its importance in the story, as well as to the *amount of screen time* consumed in relation to its importance in the plot. If one devotes too little or too much time to the function, then the camera movement (or position, angle, etc.) will be *un*motivated. For example, if a camera movement is too fast, is interrupted, or is prolonged in performing one of the above functions, then it will to some degree fail, outrun, or exceed its narrative motivation — that is, it will become unmotivated. A camera movement that is motivated by the narrative is relatively "invisible" as an element of style with the result that plot and story are foregrounded for a spectator. By contrast, an unmotivated camera movement draws attention to itself in relation to plot and story; or rather, it will seem to a spectator that there has been some kind of disturbance in the plot — a mysterious ellipsis, pause, expansion, digression, break, or obscurity. These effects are important even if a camera movement is later partially motivated or motivated retrospectively.

Examples of an unmotivated camera movement include a camera that lags behind the action and loses track of events, as in *Vampyr* (Carl Dreyer, 1932), or independently searches out information, as in *Weekend* (Jean-Luc Godard, 1967), *Sunrise* (F. W. Murnau, 1927), and *Y Tu Mamá También* (Alfonso Cuarón, 2001). An unmotivated camera may be ahead of the action (for example, waiting in an empty, darkened room for a specific character to appear) or seem to be interrupted (as in "incomplete" camera movements in certain Nicholas Ray films[2]) or unbearably prolonged as in *Weekend*, *Wavelength* (Michael Snow, 1967), *Stalker* (Andrei Tarkovsky, 1979), *Sátántangó* (Béla Tarr, 1994), *The Bridegroom, the Comedienne, and the Pimp* (Jean-Marie Straub and Danièle Huillet, 1968), *Last Year in Marienbad* (Alain Resnais, 1961), *Gertrud* (Carl Dreyer, 1964), *The Element of Crime* (Lars von Trier, 1984), *La Salamandre* (Alain Tanner, 1971), *Tom, Tom, the Piper's Son* (Ken Jacobs, 1969, revised 1971), and films by James Benning. These instances of unmotivated camera movement suggest that such movements have a wide range of aesthetic uses.[3]

Jean Mitry sets forth an aesthetic principle of film by further circumscribing a camera's motivation in relation to the time of narrative events:

> The most important thing, in all cases, is that camera movement should be justified [i.e., motivated] — physically, dramatically, or psychologically. Whether it is being used to track or is static, the camera must *follow* the action of a scene and not *anticipate* it. This law (to which we have already alluded) is basic in the sense that it is a function of the psychology of the spectacle and the expression. It does not legislate over any particular style or genre but over the whole area of expression: *something cannot be described unless it already exists.* To do so is to reveal the artificiality of the spectacle and thereby negate or destroy the fantasy it is trying to create. The camera anticipating an event is like the actor telegraphing a scene in the theater.[4]

27

I believe that Victor Perkins finds an example of Mitry's aesthetic principle in Otto Preminger's *River of No Return* (1954):

> Preminger reveals significance by a dramatic structuring of events which his camera seems only to follow — never to anticipate. Moreover, the image appears to attempt always to accommodate the entire field of action so that it is the spectator's interest which defines the area of concentration.[5]

Mitry places great stress on the idea that "something cannot be described unless it already exists." What does Mitry mean by "already exists"? In what sense do we come to believe that a fictional object exists — an object in a fictional film? Is Mitry thinking of the theory, or theories, of André Bazin that stress a preexistent reality that should be respected by a camera (i.e., respected by a 'physical' camera)? Possible rationales for this approach to film aesthetics, which rejects unmotivated camera movements and restricts motivated camera movements, will be considered in greater detail in the next two chapters. We will also need to consider the relationship that a 'physical' camera has to a spectator's experience of film and whether other kinds of cameras might exist.

MOTIVATION [II]: CAMERA MOVEMENT AND CAUSALITY

A second way of measuring the "motivation" of a camera is to assess a camera's movement as it relates to narrative causality, that is, to the movement from cause to effect within a narrative text. A camera movement (or camera position) may be said to be motivated if it functions in tandem with a cause-effect chain. More specifically, a camera is motivated when it acts to reveal *any one* of the basic elements of a narrative with respect to *any one* of the causal lines within the plot — without devoting too little or too much screen time to the element. Most narratives possess two main causal lines (e.g., a crime story interwoven with a romance story). Here are the basic elements of a classic narrative:[6]

1. An *abstract* is an implicit title or compact summary of the situation that is to follow (in the scene, sequence, or plot). Psychologists refer to an abstract or précis more generally as an "advance-organizer." It creates a framework (a propaedeutic) for perception. Occasionally the abstract may be made explicit, as in the title of a film or commentary by a voice-over narrator. An abstract primes the spectator by creating a set of expectations; it may appear as a written title, a sound, or an image. If an abstract is expanded, it becomes a *prologue*. The title of a film is an abstract; foreboding music is an abstract; an establishing shot may be an abstract; and a line of dialogue may be an abstract when, for example, it sets the "tone" for a scene.

2. An *orientation* is a description of the present state of affairs (place, time, and characters in the scene, sequence, or plot) while an *exposition* (the back story) gives information about past events that bear on the present. Exposition may be, for example, preliminary or delayed, concentrated or distributed, or continuous.

3. The first event of the story that is shown in the plot is the *point of attack*. An *initiating event* (which may or may not be the first event shown) alters the present state of affairs. A narrative that delays orientation and exposition and begins with an initiating event as its point of attack, or begins with a complicating action as its point of attack, is said to begin *in medias res*.[7]

4. A *goal* is a statement of intention or an emotional response to an initiating event (usually embodied in a protagonist).

5. A *complicating action* (usually linked to an antagonist) arises as a consequence of the initiating event and presents an obstacle to the attainment of the goal. In pursuit of the goal, the protagonist undergoes a number of arduous trials and sometimes capture and punishment by the antagonist. After a series of complicating actions, dilemmas, reactions, new initiating events, revised goals, and so on, a critical event — the *turning point* (sometimes called the "moment of truth") — leads directly toward the climax.

6. The *climax* is the action that brings to a decisive end the conflict between goals and obstacles. This is followed by the *dénouement*, that is, the outcome of the climactic action, and by the *resolution* that explains the various enigmas (flaunted or suppressed, focused or diffuse) that have been raised through previous events. The disclosure of the resolution then leads to the establishment of a new equilibrium or state of affairs that in some respects is similar to, or symmetrical with, the beginning state of affairs (creating *closure*, which ensures that the end is also a conclusion). By contrast, an *anticlimax* frustrates our expectations for a decisive end to the series of conflicts by emphasizing an action that seems only to be a digression or else is banal, irrelevant, unmotivated, or much less important than the preceding actions (e.g., a deus ex machina or ending with a display of nature). In an anticlimax, previous conflicts in the narrative seem to have been suddenly forgotten or to dissolve, rather than to resolve. This means that the narrative may have a *false resolution*; but, of course, a false resolution *may be* the point of the story (as in Antonioni's *L'Eclisse*, 1962).

7. The *epilogue* is the moral lesson implicit in the history of these events and may include explicit character reactions to the resolution. In some genres, especially the thriller, the epilogue may be followed by an *after-ending*, a new and surprising twist to the story (as in Brian De Palma's *Carrie*, 1976; John McNaughton's *Wild Things*, 1998; and René Clair's *Entr'acte*, 1924).

8. The *narration* of a story is constantly at work seeking to justify implicitly or explicitly (i) why the (often-tacit) narrator is competent and credible in arranging and reporting these events and (ii) why the events are unusual, strange, or worthy of attention. In other words, the narration of a story addresses the question of how it is possible for a spectator to possess knowledge about the story world and characters, and why it should be possessed. From another

perspective, narration may be defined as the overall regulation and distribution of knowledge in a text that determines *how and when* a spectator acquires knowledge — that is, *how* a spectator is able to know *what* he or she comes to know at a given moment (cf. *foreshadowing*). In general, several narrations will be operating simultaneously with varying degrees of explicitness and compatibility.

The narration of a story may also be viewed exclusively from the standpoint of a spectator. Here narration would be something like the "answer" that a spectator gives to his or her own "question" about *how and when* (as well as *why*) knowledge becomes available. In this view, narration does not arise simply from what is on the screen but rather includes the presuppositions and routines followed by a spectator in making sense. From this perspective, narration has an unavoidable subjective component and will seem to "fluctuate" according to a spectator's interests, background, and attention.

The above eight-part pattern may be found at both small and large scales in a narrative text — at the level of an individual shot, a sequence of shots, a scene, a sequence of scenes, a segment, as well as the film as a whole. The reason is that narrative patterns are recursive. But this does not imply that a given device must have the same narrative function at every level of a text's organization. Obviously, whatever is an "abstract" or "initiating event," and so on, at the level of a shot will not necessarily function in the same way as an "abstract" or "initiating event," and so on, when placed in the context of *other* temporal frames. In analyzing narrative causality it is important to keep in mind the *scale* at which the text is being examined: analyzing the global development of the first one third of a film, which will map clusters of actions into a developing pattern, may be quite different from analyzing the causal significance of a single gesture of a character, which may be indicative of an intention, goal, feeling, preparation to act, reaction, or something else. That is, a single gesture of a character may have a narrative function within a scene that is different from the narrative function of the scene as it relates to the next scene. Thus, an act, object, or film device may have different narrative functions when considered at different scales of the text as well as different functions at different times.[8]

In general, the basic elements of narrative are not to be found on the screen, as if they had been tacked up on a bulletin board, but instead are inside us as a way of thinking, as a way of projecting an explanation for our experiences, including the experiences we have of our Self.[9] As a cognitive activity, narrative appears in the form of a process or procedure (a procedural schema) that organizes data into a special pattern that seeks to represent both *causal structure* (i.e., to show what may follow what on local and global scales) and *causal efficacy* (i.e., to trace the possibilities for the being/becoming of an object). One of the purposes of seeing and perceiving narratively is to weigh how certain effects that are desired may be achieved, how desire is linked to possibilities for being, how events may proceed. In this way, perceiving narratively operates to draw the future into desires expressed in the present as well as demonstrates how the present was caused by the past and how the present may have effects in the future.

One should keep in mind that narrative texts include many kinds of causation. Narrative thinking is not limited to physical causation — that is, to so-called push-pull causality, where, for example, an automobile hits a vegetable stand, crushing the turnips, brussels sprouts, and asparagus spears. Causation extends to voluntary and involuntary acts by agents that may bring about or prevent an event or produce unintended consequences, as well as to the many effects of cultural products and social prescriptions that specify which actions are (un)*acceptable* as belonging together and hence (un)*likely* to occur together. Also playing a role are large-scale complicated effects, such as the causes of falling in love, unemployment, or war. Finally, the relationship between cause and effect may be depicted in a variety of ways in film; for example, a cause and its effect may be shown together, separately, in either order, with a delay, implicitly, repeatedly, or in a misleading way, or not shown at all, and there are still other possibilities. Thus, there is much work to be done when we encounter the world or a fiction and narrativize some experience in an effort to understand how things go together.

MOTIVATION [III]: CAMERA MOVEMENT AND SCALE

Another dimension of "motivation" relates a given camera movement (or camera placement, angle, etc.) to the *scale* of a shot. In classical narrative the scale of shots in a scene often varies according to a pyramid structure or a sawtooth design where one begins with distant shots — "abstract" and "orientation" — and proceeds upward toward the "point" of the pyramid, to the close-up shot which is the apex or "climax" of the scene, before falling off toward a temporary "resolution," which is usually a more distant shot confirming that a new state of affairs has been reached as compared with the beginning of the scene. Thus, an edited sequence of shots that follows this pattern of "rising" and "falling" action and tension — or else a camera movement that *changes* the scale of a shot in this way — will be narratively *motivated*.

For example, most of the lengthy camera movements in Hitchcock's *Rope* (1948) perfectly illustrate this narrativization of shot scale. According to André Bazin:

> *Rope* . . . is said to be the apex of the revolution in film directing, as the director filmed it in only ten shots. . . . The result? Certainly an interesting one and less boring than *The Lady in the Lake* (Robert Montgomery, 1946). . . . But Hitchcock's cutting in fact refers to classical cutting. Each time we are struck by his effectiveness, it is because he has managed, at the cost of a thousand resolved hardships, to create the impression of shot and reverse shot or a close-up where it would have been easy to use a single [brief] take like everyone else. This directing through continuous traveling shots — which is simply an endless succession of reframings — is completely different from Wyler's [long held]

'stationary shot' or from Welles, who managed to integrate into a single frame many moments of a virtual editing.[10]

Here is the general pattern for how shot scales may be narrativized from the beginning of a scene to its conclusion:

1. Establishing shot (provides an "orientation" for the scene; a major variant is to first show an important detail of the scene, then pull back or cut to the establishing shot, which amounts to a small-scale version of *in medias res*)
2. Long shot (i.e., master shot)
3. Medium two-shot
4. Shot/reverse shot (i.e., over-the-shoulder shots)
5. Alternating medium close-ups (sometimes point-of-view shots)
6. Cut-away (or insert shot)
7. Alternating medium close-ups
8. Close-up (or, reaction shot; the "climax")
9. Alternating medium close-ups (a mini-resolution and epilogue)
10. Re-establishing shot (provides "re-orientation," usually a reverse angle or two-shot; also used to end the scene)

Note that the visual metaphor of a "pyramid" or "sawtooth" design also sums up a strategy for narrative *movement* in a classic scene. Action and tension usually "rise" to a climax (often presented as a close-up) and then quickly "fall off" (a reaction shot followed by a long shot and transition to the next scene). Also, as the scene moves toward its climax, its range of knowledge becomes more restrictive (i.e., "narrows" toward an apex), its depth of knowledge more subjective (e.g., through the use of external and internal focalizations and the use of more animated character dialogue and facial expressions), and its communicativeness more focused and flaunted (i.e., what we come to know "narrows" to reveal a dramatic "point"). After the climax, the narration becomes less restrictive, less subjective, less focused, and more diffuse and suppressive.[11] That is, after the climax the narration "widens out": the text fosters a degree of mystery and suspense, the spectator wonders what will happen next, and the greater range of knowledge and "objectivity" facilitates a transition, or dramatic "hook," to the next important plot event, which then must be progressively established, explained, and clarified anew to the spectator in a new pyramid or sawtooth design.

Herb Lightman describes the relation between camera motivation and shot scale in terms of an aesthetic principle:

> A sound psychology underlies the use of the mobile camera. Movement purely for the sake of movement is an abuse of an otherwise forceful technique. The intelligent director or cinematographer moves the camera only when the demands of the filmic situation motivate that movement. Correctly used, the mobile camera produces a fluid continuity — a smoothly-flowing interplay of changing compositions within the individual scene. These compositions change and vary from extreme long shots to extreme close-ups without the harshness of a direct cut. Thus the audience's attention is held without mechanical interruption to the subject-matter of the scene.[12]

Both Mitry (quoted in the first section above) and Lightman are using the concept of camera "motivation" to accomplish two, merged objectives. They are *describing* an aspect of a camera in order to *evaluate* its aesthetic worth; specifically, a camera should not be *un*motivated because such a camera is not aesthetically pleasing. Consider in the argument above how Lightman enlists the following words for evaluative purposes: "abuse," "forceful," "intelligent," "correctly," "smoothly-flowing," "harshness," and, "mechanical interruption." For Lightman, an "interruption," per se, is not necessarily bad: What is bad is an interruption that is "mechanical," that is, one that draws the spectator's attention away from the smoothly flowing human drama toward the artifice of filming the drama.

Both Lightman and Mitry tacitly draw on film theories to support their claims. Lightman relies on the theory of V. I. Pudovkin[13] and Mitry on the theories of André Bazin and Sergei Eisenstein. Theories of film have been built on a wide variety of formal and

Projecting a Camera

informal theories of psychology. Thus it is no surprise that beliefs about the human body, subjectivity, and modes of attention have been projected onto a camera.

ANTHROPOMORPHISM: CAMERA MOVEMENT AND THE HUMAN BODY

A camera may be said to be more or less "anthropomorphic" in various ways. Anthropomorphism assigns human or personal attributes to an object that is not human. Although a camera is not human, we often experience some aspect of a camera — its angle of view, position, or way of moving, its "attention" to objects — in relation to a human trait. Such talk about a camera may be more than a convenience or empty rhetoric; there may be deep reasons for personifying a camera. I believe that important structures of our thought emerge from the nature of our bodies and that so-called embodied, "basic-level" categories and folk theories constitute a crucial way of understanding and acting in the world, including interacting with a film while, and after, watching it.[14] This remains true when we analyze texts. It seems to me that an important goal in designing a set of analytical terms should be their use in uncovering articulations of the human. Analytical terms, I believe, should be justified by a film theory that builds on the physical and psychological realities of spectators.

For Vivian Sobchack, the camera is more than "anthropomorphic" — it has its own body and mind. Sobchack argues that the spectator experiences the camera moving through an "anthropological" space (as if the spectator is saying, "I can . . ." or 'I have the feeling that I can . . .') *prior* to the camera directing our reflective abstractions ("I think that . . ."). Our later, reflective abstractions are based on objectified, "geometric," and theoretical spaces.[15] Sobchack asserts:

> [T]he moving camera is originally perceived by us in experience as an 'other" who is animate, conscious, and experiences and intends toward the world or toward its own conscious activity as we do.

36

She also writes:

> The moving camera is not only a mechanical instrument, an object of visual and kinetic perception; it is also a subject that sees and moves and expresses perception. It participates in the consciousness of its own animate, intentional, and embodied existence in the world.[16]

Anthropomorphism, as an analytic category, measures the degree to which a camera is being used to simulate some feature of human embodiment. One property of a camera, for example, that may be described as being analogous to a human property is based on the *position* of the camera in diegetic space: Is such a position in space a possible or usual place of viewing that a human observer might or would take in order to see a particular thing? Does the camera have a view and act in a way comparable to what we might imagine for a human observer? Also relevant are the height and angle of the camera, and the focal length of the lens (and perhaps also focus, film stock, and filters). In addition, if the camera is moving, then its speed, rhythm, and acceleration will be relevant if its movement is to be matched to a human movement, such as the movement of a person's eyes or body.

When assessing the anthropomorphism of a camera at a particular moment, a key question is the following: Which of the many qualities of a camera are being related, if any, to a typical way of human viewing or moving (or thinking and feeling), and to what degree? That is, how is a camera being narrativized with one or more human traits? If some of these traits are localized in a character, then it will be said that the camera is "subjective" or depicts in some fashion, to some degree, the subjective experience of the character.

Here is an example of speaking about a camera anthropomorphically, though not in relation to a character. Raymond Durgnat comments that in a pair of films René Clair's camera

> moved along the outside walls of apartment houses, often in *company* with some bitter-sweet tune, *peeping in* through windows

and *sidling round* chimney-stacks, *glancing in* at little vignettes of human privacy and loneliness, and *smiling ironically* [!] before moving on to the next, like a 'God's-*eye*-view' of urban man.[17]

The italicized portions of Durgnat's sentence reflect the anthropomorphisms. Note that in his description even God is anthropomorphized. Moreover, if the camera is an "eye," as is so often said, then the camera must be seeing the world upside down because the image on the film emulsion has been inverted (and reversed left and right) by the lens unless, and until, the image is returned to an upright position by the camera's 'brain' in order to be experienced. Evidently, when some metaphors (e.g., the camera's "eye") are made too literal, the truth and appropriateness of using them are lost. It is good to keep in mind that a metaphor is meant to reach a different domain than its literal reference.

Forrest Williams describes a camera movement from Max Ophuls' *Letter From an Unknown Woman* (1948) using anthropomorphic language.

> The supper scene — with its simply but tastefully laid table, the two diners framed on either side by curtains, and the camera slowly approaching in a frontal shot — is taste so pure that it becomes high imagination. The rate of approach of the camera is curiously important and affecting. . . . There had to be no sense of intrusion, but no sense of hanging back apologetically. It is not so much a tone, as a certain quarter-tone, that had to be suggested.[18]

Williams' use of the word "taste" in different senses (a "tastefully laid table," a tasteful camera movement) speaks to the broader context he invokes in order to more fully situate the camera. A slow, precise rhythm of character development is matched to the careful unfolding of an event. The anthropomorphism here is holistic and meant to suggest how the camera exhibits a discrete but straightforward view ("a frontal shot"), setting an exquisitely measured "tone" for the scene that guides a spectator's feelings toward "pure," rarefied "high imagination."

Obvious examples of a *non*-anthropomorphic camera — which might be called a disembodied, symbolic, or ethereal camera — are provided by eccentric angles, swish pans, impossible camera positions (e.g., from within a fireplace or refrigerator, from underneath a train, from inside a small box), and impossible movements (e.g., through walls or keyholes, as in David Fincher's *Panic Room*, 2002, or Brian De Palma's *Snake Eyes*, 1998). One might even imagine varieties of non-anthropomorphic cameras. For example, the anthropomorphic camera may be visualized as being intermediate between a "materialistic" or "analytical" camera at one extreme (Godard's *Weekend*, 1967) and an "ethereal, ghostly" camera at the other (Kenji Mizoguchi's *Ugetsu*, 1953).

One should emphasize that there is no necessary connection between a camera's degree of motivation (as outlined in the first three sections above) and its degree of anthropomorphism. For example, there may be a clear narrative motivation for moving impossibly through a wall or keyhole in order to see what's in the new space, though such a movement is non-anthropomorphic. An anthropomorphic camera may be either motivated or unmotivated, and a non-anthropomorphic camera may be either motivated or unmotivated. As the above example from Williams illustrates (where the camera is said to be neither intrusive nor reticent), the degree of anthropomorphism we imagine is connected both to our embodiment in a world and to our feelings of involvement with characters in their world.

POINT OF VIEW: CAMERA MOVEMENT
AND SUBJECTIVITY

A camera may appear more or less subjective, more or less objective. This aspect of a camera raises the issue of "point of view," one of the most difficult problems of narrative theory. To begin with, there is little agreement on which aspects of subjectivity need to be analyzed. For example, is point of view primarily a matter of sense perception (as in the point-of-view shot), or is it more a matter of belief, ideology, tone, mood, self-consciousness, emotion, psychology, and/or identification? Béla Balázs opts for "identification":

> In the cinema the camera carries the spectator into the film picture itself. We are seeing everything from the inside as it were and are surrounded by the characters of the film. They need not tell us what they feel, for we see what they see and see it as they see it. . . . We walk amid crowds, ride, fly or fall with the hero and if one character looks into the other's eyes, he looks into our eyes from the screen, for, our eyes are in the camera and become identical with the gaze of the characters. They see with our eyes. Herein lies the psychological act of "identification." . . . Nothing like this "identification" has ever occurred as the effect of any other system of art and it is here that the film manifests its absolute artistic novelty.[19]

Note how strong this form of "identification" is for Balázs, because he says of the characters, "They see with *our* eyes."

Another possibility is that point of view is a matter of analyzing "power" or "authority," so that the relevant question would be: To what degree, and at what times, does a camera appear to be omnipotent, omniscient, omnipresent, and/or omni-temporal? Furthermore, *whose* point of view needs to be analyzed as being embodied in a camera: the author, implied author, tacit narrator, explicit narrator, invisible observer, character, ideal spectator, or actual spectator, to name a few possibilities? With the question of subjectivity, the nature of camera movement shifts from investigating "motion," "motive," "motivation," and "motive force" toward explicit notions of agency, intention, purpose, and the use of a suitable rhetoric designed to move a spectator.

Needless to say, literary theorists have proposed many schemes for analyzing narrative point of view (see figures 2.1–2.3),[20] and since the 1980s numerous attempts have been made to analyze filmic point of view (see figures 2.4–2.11). What follows is my attempt to list the major categories of eleven schemes that have been constructed to analyze point of view. I hope to suggest through these figures the wide range of issues that may arise in deciding the relative degree of a camera's subjectivity or objectivity. Each of the major categories within a given method should be applied to a camera in order to measure the point of view at any moment. Point of view is not simply defined by a camera's location. A close-up, for example,

FIGURE 2.1   Norman Friedman's Theory of Literary Point of View

Friedman's theory moves from forms of "telling" (1) to forms of "showing" (8) by measuring the "subjectivity" of an author (1, 2), a narrator (3, 4), or internal states of a character (5, 6), or else, by measuring the disappearance of subjectivity in favor of an external presentation that provides a cameralike objectification of states of the world (7, 8).

---

1. Editorial Omniscience:

   the active presence of an author in the form of intrusive commentary and generalizations about life, manners, and morals, which are frequently given in the first person but may, or may not, be explicitly related to the story

2. Neutral Omniscience:

   editorial omniscience with the author speaking in the third person

3. "I" as Witness-Narrator:

   first-person narration by a minor character within the story

4. "I" as Protagonist:

   first-person narration by a central character

5. Multiple Selective Omniscience:

   direct presentation of the mental states of several characters (with no explicit narrator)

6. Selective Omniscience:

   internal states, as in multiple selective omniscience (above), but limited to a single character; the representation of the internal states may be more or less articulate depending on the "level" of consciousness being explored (cf. works by Henry James, Virginia Woolf, and James Joyce)

7. The Dramatic Mode:

   external description only of characters and action (with no explicit narrator)

8. The Camera:

   details are presented without apparent selection or arrangement as if randomly exhibiting a "slice of life" (with no explicit narrator)

The following categories apply in various degrees to each of the above eight types of point of view:

1. Who speaks to the reader?

   the author (first or third person), a character (first person), or ostensibly no one

2. From what distance?

   near, far, or shifting

FIGURE 2.1 (*Continued*)

3. From what position?

above (godlike), periphery, center (in the middle of the action), front (as if from third row center at a stage play), or shifting

4. Through what channels?

words, thoughts, perceptions, feelings, or actions[21]

may point out an important object in the plot for viewing, disclose a detail, suggest a character's mental state, or be emblematic, but it may also be emphatic, empathic, ironic, misleading, ideological, cathartic, or an omen. Note especially that the major categories in each scheme allow a camera's point of view to change *during* the course of a shot or not change at all across several shots. A camera's point of view may also change during a static shot or not change at all during a moving shot. It is even possible for several (perhaps incompatible) points of view to be expressed simultaneously. In sum, the selection of an analytical method will entail weighing each of the method's major categories against something (e.g., a camera) that will then be said to have acquired a certain "point of view."

The point-of-view schemes shown in figures 2.1–2.11 do not confront the "deep" subjectivity of a spectator. That is, they do not address a purported "medium" (or media) located within the mind itself where non-conscious feelings and impulses intersect and compete against one another *prior* to the appearance of conscious thought, emotion, and action. Nevertheless, using certain theories of the psyche, a camera may be defined in relation to non-conscious states. Presumably, such a camera would not simply elicit a definite psychic state in a spectator but, rather, would interact with many sorts of (non-conscious) predispositions in a spectator. I would like to illustrate the new kinds of issues that will arise in analyzing a "deep" subjectivity (point of view) by briefly sketching the approach of Slavoj Žižek.

Žižek, following Freud, identifies three important psychic stages related to libidinal development: the oral, anal, and phallic stages. Žižek argues that *motivated* camera movements have traditionally

FIGURE 2.2 Wayne Booth's Theory of Literary Point of View

Booth's theory measures the qualities of point of view by measuring the mental states and activities of a narrator.

1. Author as a Real Person

2. Implied Author (the author's "second self" in the text)

3. First or Third Person Narrator

4. Narrator

   a. Undramatized

   b. Dramatized

      i. mere observer

      ii. narrator-agent (narrator as actor)

5. Mode of Presentation by a Narrator:

   a. scene (showing)

   b. summary (telling)

6. Silent or Commenting Narrator

   a. amount and kind of commentary provided in a scene or summary by a narrator, where the kind of commentary is measured, for instance, as being relatively ornamental, rhetorical, or dramatically necessary

7. Self-conscious, Conscious, or Unconscious Narrator

8. Degree of Distance between the following (where the degree ranges from identification to alienation):

   a. implied author

   b. narrator (of any type)

   c. character

   d. reader

9. Kind of Distance between the following (where the kind ranges from deep personal concern to disapproving and includes bland, mildly amused, ironic, and merely curious detachment):

   a. implied author

   b. narrator (of any type)

   c. character

   d. reader

FIGURE 2.2 *(Continued)*

10. Change of Distance between the following (where change is measured along such axes as moral, intellectual, emotional, aesthetic, physical, spatial, temporal, social class, and conventions of speech and dress):

   a. implied author

   b. narrator (of any type)

   c. character

   d. reader

11. Reliable or Unreliable Narrator (as to the *norms* of the implied author):

   a. isolated

   b. supported or corrected by another narrator (from a position either external or internal to the action)

12. Privileged (omniscient) or Limited (to realistic vision) Narrator

   a. degree and kind of privilege

13. Outside or Inside View by a Narrator (i.e., external or internal to a character's mind; note that an inside view makes the character into a temporary narrator)

   a. depth and axis (moral, psychological . . .) of inside view[22]

functioned within one of six stylistic paradigms that evoke one or more psychic states by recalling the three psychic stages:

0. Zero-Degree Filmmaking, where montage is invisible and the camera is "neutral," resulting in the illusion of a homogeneous reality, as in silent, slapstick film;

1. Classic Analytic Montage, i.e., Pudovkin's montage [cf. the third section above on 'motivation'], as well as parallel montage, i.e., Griffith's cross-cutting montage;

2. Eisenstein's Intellectual Montage;

3. Welles's Inner/Interior Montage;

4. Rossellini's Anti-Montage, based on "the 'miracle' of fortuitous encounters"; and,

5. Hitchcock's Blot, where "the 'true' action is repressed, internalised, subjectivised" into "the domain of what is *prohibited*."[34]

FIGURE 2.3 Gérard Genette's Theory of Literary Point of View

Genette's theory measures point of view by assessing features of "mood" and "voice" using ideas from structural linguistics and classical rhetoric. The articulation of time for Genette, however, is distinct from point of view and is measured in terms of "tense" by weighing the qualities of "order," "frequency" (i.e., "aspect"), and "duration." Genette's approach to time is not outlined below.

I. Mood is composed of "distance" and "perspective":
1. Distance is measured according to:
   a. "mimesis," in which there is a maximum of information with minimal signs of the presence of a narrator (but because there is always a narrator, there can never be a pure mimesis, only the "illusion" of mimesis)
   b. "diegesis," in which there is a minimum of information with many explicit signs of the presence of a narrator
   c. type of character speech (whether uttered or inner speech):
      i. the most distant (and hence diegetic) is "narratized" or "narrated" speech where a character becomes a narrator, e.g., "I decided to marry Albertine."
      ii. at an intermediate distance is "transposed" speech, which appears in either "indirect" or "free indirect" mode
      iii. the closest (and hence most mimetic) is "reported" speech, which appears as either dialogue (in a scene) or interior monologue ("immediate" speech)
2. Perspective (degree of restriction) is measured according to whether:
   a. the narrator knows more than a character (zero focalization)
   b. the narrator knows only what a character knows (internal focalization):
      i. the narrative may be focalized through a single character (fixed focalization), several characters in succession (variable focalization), or several characters seeing the same event (multiple focalization)
   c. the narrator knows less than what a character knows (external focalization)
   d. more than one of these three types of focalization (a., b., and c.) may be present at a given moment in the text (double or triple focalization) and some perceptions of an event (e.g., what is visible) may be differently focalized than other perceptions of the same event (e.g., feelings aroused by the event); a triple focalization (as in work by Proust) is a "polymodal" discourse *intermediate* between, on the one hand, an open state of no conventions and, on the other hand, either "simple omniscience" and/or defined instances of "alterations" (see next)
   e. minor changes in focalization, or momentary or isolated changes, are "alterations" or "infractions"; for example:
      i. paralipsis: giving less information than is required by a given focalization

45

FIGURE 2.3 *(Continued)*

---

    ii. paralepsis: giving more information than is authorized by a given focalization

    iii. modalizing locutions: a narrator uses words such as "perhaps," "undoubtedly," "as if," "seem," and "appear" to say hypothetically what could not otherwise be asserted without stepping outside an internal focalization

II. Voice is composed of "person," the "time of narrating," and "narrative level":

  1. Person is not measured according to "first person" or "third person" but, rather, measured according to the narrator's relationship to the story:

    a. heterodiegetic: the character tells the story

    b. homodiegetic: the narrator tells the story either as the hero (autodiegesis) or as a witness

  2. Time of Narrating is measured according to its occurrence with respect to the time of the story:

    a. subsequent (i.e., the story is past)

    b. simultaneous (which may lead to extreme forms of subjectivity or objectivity)

    c. prior (e.g., dreams or prophesy)

    d. interpolated (the narrating time occurs between the actions or scenes of the story)

  3. Narrative Level is measured according to the 'world' (i.e., the spatial, temporal, and causal coordinates) in which a given event occurs.

    a. Any recounted event is at a diegetic level (i.e., in a 'world') immediately *higher* than the level at which the narrating act producing this narrative event is placed. For four levels, from top to bottom:

       i. meta-metadiegesis (third-degree narrative)

       ii. metadiegesis (a story within a story)

       iii. diegesis (= intradiegesis)

       iv. extradiegesis (the original narrating instance)

    b. A normal transition between two levels (e.g., between the metadiegesis and diegesis) may take the form of:

       i. direct causality (e.g., the metadiegesis is invoked to explain the diegesis)

       ii. thematic relationships (e.g., through similarity, contrast, mise-en-abîme, and exemplum)

       iii. distraction or obstruction

    c. A transgression between two levels is a "narrative metalepsis,"[23] and it is related to:

       i. pseudo-diegesis: a metadiegetic telling that is reduced to the diegetic, i.e., told *as if* it were diegetic; perhaps an example in film might be a character flashback told through 'objective' images

       ii. prolepsis (e.g., a flashforward)

FIGURE 2.3 *(Continued)*

---

iii. analepsis (e.g., a flashback); prolepsis and analepsis are examples of anachrony — a general discordance (of which there are many types) between the order of events in the story and the order given in the telling of the story; in addition, there are many types of "ellipses" affecting order and duration

iv. paralepsis (see above on focalization)

v. paralipsis (see above on focalization), especially in its temporal form as a "lateral ellipsis," should probably also be included here as potentially a metalepsis

vi. syllepsis: certain kinds of lists or groupings of events in defiance of chronology, including iterative and pseudo-iterative narrative, both of which involve a single narrative utterance that does *not stand for* all of the others (which would make it merely a paradigmatic use of singulative narrative) but, rather, is an utterance that *condenses* several occurrences (or purports to do so); e.g., "Every day last week. . . . " and "For a long time I used to go to bed early. Sometimes, when I had put out my candle. . . . " Perhaps a notion of 'pseudo-singulative' should be defined and also be included here as a syllepsis.

vii. isodiegesis: no change in narrative level though there may appear to have been a change

viii. digression: embedding a story at the same level

Five important functions of the narrator:

1. Narrative Function: the narrator's act of narrating the story
2. Directing Function: the narrator's meta-narrative remarks about the narrative text
3. Communicative Function: the dynamics of the narrating situation, and the kind of contact achieved between the narrator and narratee (who may be present, absent, or implied)
4. Testimonial Function: the narrator's affective, moral, and intellectual relationship to the story being told
5. Ideological Function: the narrator's didactic commentary, direct or indirect, on the action of the story[24]

The six stylistic paradigms (0–5) are coordinated with the psychic states as follows: oral (0), anal (1), excessively anal (2–4), and phallic (5).[35] Žižek links the oral with metonymy, the anal with metaphor, and the phallic with a "signifier without a signified" — with "total ambiguity" — as well as with a hallucinatory desire, dread, and compulsion linked to the uncanny.[36]

FIGURE 2.4 David Bordwell's Theory of Filmic Point of View

Bordwell's theory measures a camera's range and depth of knowledge, communicativeness, self-consciousness, and judgmental tone.

1. Range of Knowledge (degree of restriction or access to knowledge about the fictional world)

2. Depth of Knowledge (degree of character subjectivity)

3. Communicativeness with respect to a given range and depth (e.g., degrees of flaunted or suppressed gaps, diffuse or focused gaps, temporary or permanent gaps); a "gap" is a question or problem of perception and may appear in various forms, such as gaps that are spatial, temporal, causal, or intentional (for instance, an unknown character motive is a gap in the character's behavior that a spectator attempts to 'close' by risking a hypothesis)

4. Self-Consciousness (degree of acknowledgement of the audience)

5. Judgmental Tone (ranging from mockery to compassion)[25]

FIGURE 2.5 Seymour Chatman's Theory of Filmic Point of View

Chatman's theory measures a camera's relation to: a character's perception, the cause-effect chain, an attitude, and the reader's interest-focus.

1. Filter (the depiction of a character's perception)

2. Centrality (the relationship and importance of a character to the cause-effect chain)

3. Slant (the depiction of an attitude)

4. Reader's Interest-Focus[26]

With respect to the phallic blot, Žižek argues that Hitchcock creates in a character and in the audience a (i) *feeling* of menace, threat, horror, anxiety, strangeness, hidden or double meanings, or a feeling for the uncanny, by (ii) *embedding* a small anomalous feature, an incongruous detail, something that does not belong, that is out of place, that sticks out (sticks up! — namely, the *phallic blot*, the appearance of *power*, analogous to a penile erection) into the (iii) natural, familiar, ordinary, even idyllic landscape of our lives.[37] For Žižek the phallic blot functions as a "double framing": first, the blot frames a "hole" in the fabric of the real world, of normality, but only

FIGURE 2.6 George Wilson's Theory of Filmic Point of View

Wilson's theory measures a camera's relation to: the spectator's perceived epistemic distance, the spectator's assessment of reliability, and the spectator's access to authoritative knowledge.

1. Relative Epistemic *Distance* from our usual habits of perception and common-sense beliefs (including our knowledge of film conventions)

2. Degree of Epistemic *Reliability* or justification for the inferences that we draw from the "visual manifolds" of film

3. Epistemic *Authority* or degree of alignment between audience knowledge and character knowledge (or other source of knowledge)[27]

FIGURE 2.7 Jacques Aumont's Theory of Filmic Point of View

Aumont's theory measures the (mis)alignment of four basic types of "gaze" linked to: a camera's position, the spatial perspective of the image, narrative perspective, and the narrator's attitudes.

1. Position of the Camera

2. Perspectival System employed to depict space (e.g., central perspective)

3. "Narrative" Point of View of:

   a. character

   b. auteur

   c. spectator

4. Mental Attitude of the Narrator: its intellectual, moral, and political judgments[28]

after it has been recognized and "removed" as anomalous (leaving behind the "hole" as a 'window' onto the unseen, the forbidden, the repressed). Secondly, the newly created "hole," in turn, acts to frame the "whole," the rest of the real, from the inside out(ward) — ultimately out toward the spectator and into the spectator's psyche to open up the repressed of the unconscious (a 'window onto the soul').[38]

As examples of the Hitchcockian anomalous feature, i.e., the uncanny detail or stain that functions as a phallic blot, Žižek mentions the following:

a windmill that rotates against the direction of the wind in the idyllic Dutch countryside (*Foreign Correspondent*, 1940); a dead body in the idyllic Vermont countryside (*The Trouble with Harry*, 1955); a murder concealed by a festive cocktail party (*Rope*, 1948); an ordinary key to an apartment that points to a murderer (*Dial M for Murder*, 1954); friendly Uncle Charlie who is a pathological murderer embedded in his sister's happy family in a small American town (*Shadow of a Doubt*, 1943); the hero himself (James Stewart) whose suspicious gaze, while on the way to visit a taxidermist, turns an ordinary London street into a sinister place (*The Man Who Knew Too Much*, 1956); the hero himself (James Stewart) whose probing, obsessive gaze finds a murderous neighbor living in an ordinary apartment house who is able to realize and enact the hero's desire, his "fantasy figurations of what could happen to him and Grace Kelly" (*Rear Window*, 1954); and, in Hitchcock's "final irony," nature itself in the form of birds becomes the 'anomalous feature,' "the 'unnatural' element that disturbs everyday life" (*The Birds*, 1963).[39]

Using Žižek's method, I believe that one may also search for phallic blots on a smaller scale in Hitchcock's films in order to explain the fascination and terror that move the spectator from moment to moment through a scene. For example, in the opening scene of *Rope*, it would seem that the following ordinary objects function as 'mini-blots': the curtains on the window (as seen from outside the apartment *after* we hear the scream from inside); the rope hanging out of the wooden chest containing the body that was strangled with the rope; the wooden chest itself as a table for food and drink for the cocktail party; and, especially, the candles atop the wooden chest.[40]

According to Žižek, Hitchcock's prototypical *tracking shot* appears in four guises and all four are tied to the phallic stage:[41]

0. The zero degree of tracking is an obsessive, drawn-out time of indulgence and deferral where the camera advances 'on/to a phallic blot,' moving slowly from a large-scale view to a close-up of the blot[42]; Žižek refers to the "blot" as the "meaningless stain" and the "demented stain,"[43] as in, one supposes, a stain of se/men-semantics.

FIGURE 2.8   Francesco Casetti's Theory of Filmic Point of View

Casetti's theory measures the communicative intersection of a camera's "gaze" (sender/origin) with an implied observer's "gaze" (receiver/destination), which together generate a convergence of three "points" (see below) that delineate a textual configuration (a context or frame) that anchors the flux of images and sounds to a single type of "point of view" within a discourse.

The two basic "gazes" that form a scene:

1. Camera's Location during filming

2. Ideal Position of an Observer witnessing what is projected on the screen

The convergence of lines from three "points" to make a "point of view":

1. Point through which one shows (the Enunciator; 1 above)

2. Point from which one observes (the Enunciatee, or "anti-subject"; 2 above)

3. Point which is seen (the Énoncé; the discourse through which 1 and 2 operate)

Four canonical configurations of "point of view":

1. Objective View: A scene is presented "anonymously," adhering to either a theatrical or realist conception of mise-en-scène where all the elements are clearly placed, but without anyone's gaze determining their placement: "I gaze at something and make you gaze, too." This configuration involves an exhaustive *seeing* (perceptive point of view), a diegetic *knowing* (cognitive or informational point of view), and a solid *believing* (the degree of faith or epistemic or emotive point of view).

2. Impossible Objective View: By using incongruous camera angles, colors, etc., a scene is configured in a way that does not allow the view to be attributed to any human character. The work of the technical apparatus here is obvious; the camera blatantly presents its own functioning. The enunciator's gaze is figurativized in the camera itself: "What you see, is thanks to me." This configuration involves a total *seeing*, a metadiscursive *knowing*, and an absolute *believing*.

3. Interpellation: A scene is staged in order to recognize someone outside the text to whom the film makes a direct appeal, "hailing" this "you" in the form of an aside. The enunciator, in the form of a narrator, a voice-over, titles, etc., directly addresses the spectator. Interpellation can be considered a gaze without effect because it addresses an offscreen space that can never be made visible. This configuration involves a partial *seeing*, a discursive *knowing*, and a relative *believing*.

4. Subjective View: A scene is structured so that we see a character who gazes, and then we see what is seen through that character's eyes. Along with the character, we see only what we are shown, with the sense that the course of action has been decided in advance: "I gaze, and make you gaze at the one who gazes; I am making the character see what I make you see; you and the character see what I show you." Thus, the viewer in the subjective configuration produces a gaze without intention. This configuration involves a limited *seeing*, an intradiegetic *knowing*, and a transitory *believing*.[29]

FIGURE 2.9   Douglas Pye's Theory of Filmic Point of View

Pye's theory measures a camera's relation to five dimensions: space, time, cognition, evaluation, and ideology.

---

1. Spatial Axis
2. Temporal Axis
3. Cognitive Axis
4. Evaluative Axis
5. Ideological Axis[30]

---

1. The reverse of the zero degree of tracking, i.e., moving slowly back from a blot to a larger view.
2. The precipitous, hysterical tracking shot which may employ jump cuts in revealing a blot.
3. The immobile tracking shot where the camera is frozen, locked in place, and not able to move while some "heterogeneous object," i.e., the blot, 'penetrates' the "frame" of the shot.

Notice, in particular, that many critics would not characterize the last two versions of the Hitchcockian tracking shot as a "tracking shot" or "camera movement" because the motion appearing on the screen has come from editing or mise-en-scène. Žižek would probably reply that he is not interested in such a 'formalism' — in those effects perceived by the spectator to be merely on the screen, merely motion. For Žižek the real 'camera movements' are in the mind of the spectator. Žižek relies on the theories of Freud and Lacan to make these 'camera movements' visible to us rather than drawing on, say, the theories of Bazin and Pudovkin, as do Mitry and Lightman (see the first and third sections above).

Žižek's 'unmoving moving' camera movements raise a general question about what is to count as 'movement.' Are there various 'kinds' of movements in film and, if so, which ones belong to a camera, or, at least, which ones may be 'borrowed' by, or attributed to, a camera?

FIGURE 2.10   Edward Branigan's Theory of Filmic Point of View

My two theories measure the way in which a camera is embedded in the matrix of a case grammar and/or the way a camera is functioning with respect to one or more levels of narration.

---

1. A particular point of view is a set of specific values of the six general elements (functions) of a generative "case grammar": origin, vision, time, frame, object, and mind; and/or

2. Point of view is the relationship between any pair of the eight basic "levels of narration": historical author, extra-fictional narrator, nondiegetic narrator, diegetic narrator, nonfocalized (character) narration, external focalization, surface internal focalization, and deep internal focalization.[31]

   "Levels of narration" may be further described with respect to the following properties:

   a. the temporal relationship between any two levels (e.g., simultaneous, partially overlapping [compressed, contractionary, expansionary, diffuse], continuous, elliptical, intermittent [flashed], discontinuous, or isolated)

   b. the degree of compatibility between any two levels (e.g., independent [unrelated], parallel, compatible, subordinate [embedded], inconsistent, conflictual, or contradictory)

   c. the degree of perceptibility of a level (e.g., flaunted, explicit, circumstantial [based on background conditions], implicit, suppressed [obscured], or repressed [denied])

   d. the degree of stability or reliability of a level (e.g., uncorrected [omniscient, prospective], retrospective, ambiguous, enigmatic, restrictive, deceptive, false, or unpredictable)

   e. the degree to which a perceived level is identifiable (e.g., highly detailed, definite, partially specified, sketchy [elastic, vague], indefinite [underdetermined, undetermined], or indeterminable)[32]

   f. the degree of narrativity of the levels, i.e., the type of discourse produced by a "weaving" of the levels within a particular time span (e.g., a heap [omnium-gatherum], catalogue, description, permutation [repetition and variation], lyrical association, episode [incident, interlude, digression, pause], unfocused chain, focused chain [i.e., a series of causes and effects with a continuing center, usually a character], simple narrative [i.e., a series of episodes collected as a focused chain], complex narrative, meta-narrative, or admixture)

FIGURE 2.11 Bruce Kawin's Theory of Filmic Point of View

Kawin's theory measures the extent to which a camera is speaking in first-, second-, or third-person mode.

---

1. First Person:
   a. voice-over
   b. subjective sound
   c. subjective camera
   d. mindscreen of a character, author, author's persona, or the text itself (a "mindscreen" is the presentation of what someone is thinking rather than, as above, what someone is saying, hearing, or seeing)
   e. first-person self-consciousness of either an author or the text itself
2. Second Person (films that tell "you" what to think and do, e.g., propaganda films)
3. Third Person (i.e., where there is no apparent narrator):
   a. third-person unself-consciousness
   b. third-person self-consciousness of either an author or the text itself
   c. third-person unself-conscious "point of view" of a character (third-person "point of view" refers to a special technique of "subjectivizing the objective")
   d. third-person self-conscious "point of view" of either an author or the text itself[33]

SOME KINDS OF MOVEMENTS: CAMERA MOVEMENT AND SPACE

Žižek's theory of subjectivity raises a basic question about the nature of motion on the screen. Depending on the occasion, some or many kinds of motions may be lumped together and strictly or (very) loosely called "camera movements." Critics may, of course, draw whatever distinctions they deem necessary for their arguments and evaluations. The criteria they employ for making distinctions, however, are not neutral but lead inevitably to other assumptions. Let me suggest a tentative list of some kinds of movements that produce "motion" on the screen.[44]

1. Psychic Focus: A "static" image may elicit certain kinds of mental or psychic movements in a spectator that the spectator then projects back into the image, animating it, perhaps in unexpected ways (as in Žižek's psychoanalytic theory above).

2. Deep Focus: A static shot of deep space in deep focus may allow the spectator's *eye* (attention? inner eye?) to "move" through diegetic space, tracing through foreground, middle ground, and background (as in Bazin's film theory).[45]

3. Rack Focus: The focus of the camera lens "moves" among foreground, middle ground, and background (while pictorial perspective remains unchanged).

4. Zoom: The focal length of the camera's lens changes to enlarge or shrink the space seen by the spectator (by zooming in or out), i.e., an object seen in the image changes its size while *pictorial perspective remains unchanged* and the camera itself does not move.[46]

5. Pan, Tilt, or Rotation: The camera stays in place but alters its orientation by panning, tilting, or rotating, i.e., turning left/right, pointing up/down, or rotating clockwise/counterclockwise (while pictorial perspective remains unchanged).

6. Dolly, Track, or Boom (Crane): The camera itself moves through a locale by dollying, tracking, or craning, i.e., moving forward/back, left/right, or up/down; this kind of movement *changes* pictorial perspective, generating a sensation of "kinetic depth" for a spectator, i.e., planes at different distances from the camera will be seen by the spectator to be moving at different velocities with respect to the camera's position.[47]

7. Active Follow: The camera moves (in one of the ways above) in order to *follow* alongside an object (usually a character) that is moving in the foreground so as to hold it steady against a changing *background*; or, as in a camera movement that traces a curved path or arc, the *foreground* changes while the object, moving in precise coordination with the camera but at a slower speed in the background, is held steady;[48] I propose to call this an *active* follow shot.

8. Passive Follow: Neither the camera nor an object in the foreground (usually a character) is moving but both are being carried through space (for example, both camera and character are in a car) so that the camera *follows* the object which is held steady while the *background* is continually changing; or, as in

the case of two trains that are moving on parallel tracks (as in Lars von Trier's *Zentropa*, 1992), neither the camera nor its object in the second train is itself moving though both are being separately carried so that the camera and object are not in motion relative to each other but the *foreground* is continually changing; I propose to call this a *passive* follow shot.[49]

9. Reframe: The camera moves to *reframe* a character or object, i.e., to continue to follow something by holding it steady in the center of the frame during or after its movement; or else, the camera moves *just before* a character or object by anticipating the speed and direction of its movement. Usually the object being reframed moves only short distances, such as a character sitting at a table who occasionally shifts his or her body in a medium close-up shot.

10. Rear or Front Projection: The foreground and background of the image are split apart so that a film may be projected onto one of these planes (the projected film will be seen as a second-generation image in the composite image); either the foreground or background or both may contain various kinds of "movements."

11. Optical Printer: The camera of the optical printer may create moving effects by rephotographing one or more other films to create, for example, fades, dissolves, wipes, spirals, superimpositions, and an optical "pan and scan" of a widescreen film (cf. a superimposition with the devices of deep focus and shot/reverse shot; cf. a "pan and scan" with a pan).

12. Special Effects: Numerous "special effects" in film create distinct impressions of movement (animation, morphing, etc.).

13. Subjective Effects: Any of the preceding kinds of movements (including, for example, expressive decor or ways of seeing decor as in 1 and 2 above) may be attributed to a character and thus be seen in some fashion, partially or wholly, as a movement of a character's body or else a movement of a character's mind (attention, curiosity, desire, dizziness, anxiety, fantasy, memory, psychosis . . .). Subjective movements resemble a fiction within a fiction.

Which of the above kinds of movements should count as a "camera movement"? Which movements are common and why are some disfavored?[50] When only one kind of movement is used systematically in a film, quite subtle effects may be achieved, unless the film is only movement.[51]

A critic, of course, may legislate rules for these kinds of movements. For example, in relation to non-follow movements, Herb Lightman says:

> Except in a travelogue, it is not considered effective technique to *pan* a static object — although many film-makers have done so in an effort to force action into an otherwise dead scene. At best this is a forced technique and should be avoided except where inserted for special effect. Mere movement of the camera can never compensate for a lack of action within the scene.[52]

What does Lightman mean by "action"? Which kinds of motion should appear onscreen and which ones are distractions? Jean Mitry argues, for example, that only some kinds of subjective movements should be represented onscreen and other kinds are inappropriate for the medium of film.[53]

One of the general lessons here is that when we try to confine the definition of a camera to its physical manifestation as an apparatus/object or try to confine a text to its physical manifestation, the many kinds of movements we wish to talk about (summarized at the end of chapter 1) will begin to undermine such restrictive definitions.

WHEN THINGS CHANGE: CAMERA MOVEMENT AND ATTENTION

By way of conclusion, I wish to offer some refinements to the preceding analytical terms and suggest a few additional issues involving camera movement and the movement of our attention. I have defined a *motivated* camera in relation to its narrative function within a film's articulation of time, in relation to elements of classical narrative causality, and in relation to a narrative sequence of changing shot scales. A camera has also been defined according to its perceived degree of *anthropomorphism* (relative embodiment), its degree of *subjectivity/objectivity* (point of view), and, finally, its *movement* arising from *motion* on the screen and *fictional movement* in the diegesis.

Judgments involving a camera's degree of motivation, anthropomorphism, and subjectivity are ultimately tied up with general theories of narrative that may lead to conflicting characterizations of the nature of classical narrative. Stephen Heath, for example, proposes a theory of classical narrative and then proceeds to raise serious questions about how one should use such terms as motivation, anthropomorphism, and subjectivity when talking about a camera.[54] In analyzing camera movement, one soon becomes entangled in various theories of narrative, theories of point of view, and theories of film. Problems about a camera that concern ontology, epistemology, aesthetics, technique, kinds of movements, ideology, realism, history, and technology soon lead into larger, integrated theories that propose one or more contexts that are required in order to understand the concept of a "camera." In the chapters to follow we will examine some of these contexts and the effects they have on how we use the word "camera."

It is important to keep in mind that a camera may fit a specific description when it is first seen (i.e., prospectively) but suddenly seem different, or "change," when it is reconsidered in the next shot or later in the film or after the film has ended (i.e., retrospectively). A camera's qualities may change for mysterious reasons. David Bordwell observes that "even in ordinary films, the camera's position changes in ways that *cannot* be attributed to a shift in a spectator's attention."[55] Nevertheless, a camera's old position, its change to a new position, as well as the new position may all be *motivated*. The reason is that we are not able to anticipate everything that happens in a narrative; indeed, the narrative process depends on our knowledge being incomplete. We expect the occasional and abrupt, "revelatory" moment. Thus, we cannot always shift our attention in synchrony with a camera. This raises the general issue of how a camera's activity is related to various shifts in our interest and attention with respect to actions seen in the diegesis. Does a camera always follow an action or does it sometimes lead or stalk? Or mislead? Or wander?! Does a camera have an unconscious (Žižek)? The notions of a "stalking," "unreliable," or "wandering" camera, and of "unconscious optics," of course, raise questions about anthropomorphism and point of view.[56]

Dudley Andrew finds a stalking camera in F. W. Murnau's *Sunrise* (1927):

> Later, the man, back to us, wanders toward the marsh, and the camera, full of our desire, initiates one of the most complex and thrilling movements in all of cinema. It crosses the fence at its own spot, turns on the man who in his stupor passes by it and makes for the vamp. But the camera finds its own, more direct path, pushing past bushes until she is revealed in the moonlight. When the man reenters screen left we are doubly startled, having forgotten that we had abandoned him. Indeed, we are perhaps ashamed to have reached the vamp before him in our driving impatience. This shame is intensified at the end of the sequence when the camera, nose in mud, sniffs after the retreating sinners. It is a daring, highly unconventional shot, and it delivers its image of guilt not only by its content (high-heel shoes oozing with mud, while the marsh refuses to give up the imprint of the shoe), but by making us feel guilty as we literally track the couple down.[57]

André Bazin offers an example of a wandering camera:

> Throughout the entire last part of *The Rules of the Game* [Jean Renoir, 1939] the camera acts like an invisible guest wandering about the salon and the corridors with a certain curiosity, but without any more advantage than its invisibility. The camera is not noticeably any more mobile than a man would be (if one grants that people run about quite a bit in this château). And the camera even gets trapped in a corner, where it is forced to watch the action from a fixed position, unable to move without revealing its presence and inhibiting the protagonists. This sort of personification of the camera accounts for the extraordinary

quality of this long sequence. It is not striking because of the script or the acting, but as a result of Renoir's half amused, half anxious way of observing the action.[58]

Does it also make sense to talk about a "postwandered" camera — a wandering that has already taken place and is inferred after the fact? Consider these examples, the first two based on Antonioni's *Red Desert* (1964), the last on Godard's *Weekend* (1967):

(i) Cut to a shot of a wall; hold, then the head of a character slowly enters through the bottom of the frame; the camera tilts down to reframe the character in a closer shot.

(ii) Cut to a shot containing an out-of-focus background; hold, then a character enters the foreground already in focus.

(iii) Fade in on a shot of a path that leads out of a forest to a highway with a wall in the distance, accompanied by nondiegetic music; hold, then fade out; we see three seconds of black screen while the music continues; fade in again on the same shot while the music continues, hold; a character walks into view in the distance, turns, sees something, and comes down the path toward the camera, which tilts down to reframe the character in a closer shot as the character says, "Hello."

Note that the literal camera movements in (i) and (iii) are only reframe movements, and there is no camera movement at all in (ii). The "wandering" part of the *movement* has apparently occurred prior to the beginning of each of the shots, that is, somewhere "between" the end of the previous shot and the beginning of (i), (ii), and (iii). To put it another way, the "wandering movement" has already been incorporated in the choice of the initial camera position. One might extend this reasoning to include unbalanced or awkward compositions, unusual camera angles, obstructed views, and character movement in the mise-en-scène that is mismatched to a camera's view. Furthermore, despite the similarities, there is a subtle difference between the three cases above related to point of view. Although all three are "ahead" of the action, the first has "imperfect" knowledge of what will happen, while the second and third have "perfect" knowledge.

If the above analysis of a "postwandered" camera is accepted, then are the distinctions among camera movement, editing, and mise-en-scène becoming blurred? Specifically, what constitutes an unseen camera movement that occurs "between" two shots that, moreover, has somehow "missed" the dramatic mise-en-scène? Surely a camera movement "between" the shots can occur and may be inferred from the shots on the screen, at least in special cases (e.g., an "interrupted" tracking shot). But at what point, then, does camera movement "between" the shots end and "editing" begin? The problem here is that such concepts as "camera," "movement," "editing," and even "shot" cannot be defined without considering how the mind works while watching.

The present chapter has dealt with relatively concrete aspects of a camera by surveying analytical concepts directed at movements such as a change of focus, zoom, and dolly back or forward to enlarge or concentrate the field of view (for example, items 3, 4, 6, and 9 on my list above of kinds of movements). The exact nature of a camera — what it really "is" all by itself — has been left (for now) somewhat vague in favor of talking about how we may choose to think about the properties of a film text. When we focus on one or more of these properties, we have begun the process of marking out the boundaries for the use of the concept "camera" in our thinking. Is it possible that an even more fundamental connection between camera and mind exists?

I believe it is significant that psychologists who study the processes of *attention* — through which our awareness of things undergoes a change — have recourse to the metaphors of *zoom lenses*, *moving spotlights*, and *close-ups* in explaining what attention is and does.[59] Whereas our eyes may move three or four times a second, attention may shift 10 or 15 times a second or more. It takes 120 milliseconds to move our eyes to a new location but only 30 to 40 milliseconds to shift our visual attention. Psychologists describe attention as a mechanism that creates a smaller or larger viewing area or causes a viewing area to shift (e.g., by a "zoom" in or back, or a "pan" left or right). This area (over which attention may move) is a *continuous perceptual or conceptual domain* that offers a mental representation of a geometrical space or else is a mental map of an abstract "space." Attention is at work making what is "blurry" or "ambiguous" at a specific point in the space clearer and more vivid while making the rest of the space temporarily less distinct or not visible. There would seem to be an interesting connection here between a movement of attention and the appearance or disappearance of "ambiguity." This does not mean, however, that what is made clear and distinct is thereby "true" or that the goal of "analysis" is to make *ideas* clear and distinct.[60]

At any given moment our perception of the world, and of a film, is incomplete because of limitations of mental capacity and of cognitive processing (especially memory). In addition, the movement of our attention limits knowledge because we are unable to consciously perceive or recognize a thing without the mediation of attention, and attention can be focused on only one or two things at a time. If it is true that the operation of attention is in some ways analogous to a zoom lens, a moving spotlight, or a close-up shot, then it may be possible to extend the analogy to cover passive, or involuntary, forms of attention (e.g., when a sudden noise or movement instantly draws our attention) by drawing an analogy with passive non-movements of a camera (e.g., the Hitchcockian immobile camera described by Žižek that refuses to move or suddenly moves) in relation to directed movements of a camera (for example, movements that evoke intentions or expectations).[61]

Despite the intriguing analogies between a camera and attention, a large gap remains between a zoom lens on a camera and the metaphorical application of zooming in or out to describe human attention. It is my belief that one of the objectives of film theory should be to bridge this gap. A given film theory should seek to develop a set of intermediate concepts that show the connection between, say, a camera movement and a movement of the mind — that show not just the different ways a piece of equipment can move, but how a camera *registers* with us. Hence, many other cognitive activities besides attention will become relevant in explaining a camera's activities. (Recall Bordwell's point above that not all changes in a camera's position can be attributed simply to shifts in our attention.) Such a film theory would result in a new way of thinking about a camera. We would come to see a camera as an entity that is spread out, or dispersed, across several domains rather than seeing a camera confined to a single frame as a thing that is, say, either physical or mental.

The chapters to follow will attempt to bridge the gap between the peripatetic movements of a camera as a piece of equipment and the "meanings" we take and make from its many movements in film. The next chapter will examine various camera techniques (e.g., deep focus, kinetic depth, motivation, anthropomorphism, and subjectivity) in order to uncover a variety of narrative and film theories that offer competing explanations of the nature and role of a camera. The final two chapters will look further into issues of "meaning" and "movement" in order to suggest how an interlocked set of concepts might bridge the gap between material and mind, world and film language. We will discover that a camera is fixed to movements of our mind and to the ways we talk about the meanings of a film. Many relevant (intermediate) concepts will emerge in the final two chapters from such notions as the following: embodiment, basic-level categorization, radial meanings, top-down and bottom-up cognitive processing, image schemata, heuristics, ordinary language, metaphorical projections, fictions (counterfactual conditionals), causal laws, sustaining causes, language-games, objects under description, and "rightness" of rendering as a standard of judgment, rather than "truth." The goal of the next three chapters is not to "close" the gap between the camera as a physical object and the camera as a discursive object. Nor is the goal to eliminate the gap by reducing one kind of camera-object to the other, but simply to mind the gap — to fill in some of the links, and to show why and when a camera has a life in more than one place.

Chapter 3: **What Is a Camera?**

"The camera therefore stands metaphorically for everything one can possibly shoot. It is but another word for language. Speaking like Heidegger, one could say that the camera is the little dark house of being."[1]

— Jean-Pierre Geuens

REWORKING THE QUESTION

What is a camera? At first glance, the answer seems obvious. We know perfectly well what a camera is. But then again, perhaps the confidence with which we answer should cause us to hesitate. One of the lessons Noam Chomsky teaches (with respect to the concept of "grammatical") is that some of the most important things to analyze and explicate are precisely our intuitions — those beliefs that appear self-evident and certain.

The question "What is a camera?" resembles André Bazin's famous question "What is cinema?"[2] Both questions seem to call for a special kind of definition that seeks to isolate an inherent quality, an essence, shared by all instances of "camera" or "cinema" while being absent from all things not a camera or not cinema. In this approach an object's unique existence is defined by a set of individually necessary and jointly sufficient conditions. One problem that has arisen in asking this kind of general question, however, is that the relationship that an object has to one or more *contexts* is not given adequate importance in defining the object. In thinking about the nature of an object, we should keep in mind that a thing is not defined simply by its intrinsic properties (e.g., material and shape) but also by its placement within various *causal* sequences as well as its *relationships* to other things (other contexts, other states of being). For example, a "sofa chair" may be characterized by saying that it belongs in the context of a "living room" and is used to lounge on rather than merely sit on. It may also be contrasted with other pieces of furniture and related to, for example, being a "possession," a "gift," a "mat for a cat," an "entity," a "home for coins fallen from pockets," and an "example" in an essay. The "sofa chair" will have a different status depending on the context and the degree of generality one wants to achieve.

Thus, our first task will be to reformulate the question "What is a camera?" by avoiding the ontological verb form "is" and by incorporating some important contexts. (The word "is," of course, derives from the infinitive "to be," whose gerund form, "being," suggests an inquiry into the fundamental and irreducible nature of an entity apart from any context or else imagined in an "ideal" context.) I propose instead to ask how the *word* "camera" functions in the language we use to talk about cinema. What do we do with the word "camera"? In what contexts does the word function?

Before tackling this question, however, let us briefly consider a parallel question concerning a photograph. Is a photograph always used as a statement of fact, as in "Here is the eagle that I saw in the tree"?[3] I believe that a photograph has many modes of being. Depending on the context, a photograph of an eagle may be used in any of the following ways (and doubtless in additional ways):

1. To identify a physical feature of a (singular) thing: "Here is *the* eagle that *I* saw in *the* tree with *the* clouds" (an eagle as *the* eagle; *I* as *the* person who took *the* photograph)
2. To be a sample of a thing: an eagle as a *typical* eagle (not all eagles will be typical, for example, a baby eagle; furthermore, some samples may serve as prototypes in a schema — an eagle may be typical of a diurnal bird of prey but not typical of a "bird," for which a sparrow would be a better exemplar, say, in parts of the United States)
3. To be a type of (general) thing: an eagle as a *vertebrate* like a fish or human

4. To be an emblem: a quality of an eagle, such as its purported strength, is *transferred* and altered to fit another object such as a nation (an eagle as a symbol for a nation)
5. To be a memento or fetish: a feeling or a quality of another object is *transferred* and altered to fit an eagle (an eagle as a souvenir or a thing of superstition)
6. To reveal a feeling: an eagle as (apparently) *alert* or vigilant
7. To make an impression: an eagle as a vivid *form* embodying sensory qualities, such as brightness, texture, and aerodynamic balance
8. To reify an intangible thing: an eagle's view from above as embodying an ideal point of overview, thus standing for the attainment of objective or transcendent *knowledge* (an eagle's-eye view)[4]
9. To fictionalize: an eagle as a *mythic* creature like a gryphon (and, of course, not all fictions will be false, just as not all metaphors are false)
10. To narrativize: an eagle as a *villain* or ally in a plot, such as the Eaglet and the Gryphon who interact with Alice during her adventures in Wonderland

The depiction of an object's physical features (see 1 above) may be said to be literally "in" a photograph when there is a context that directs us to look in that direction. "Is that bird in the photograph an eagle or an osprey?" Other uses are not as much in the photograph as "in" a context through which the photograph does something or acts in a certain way. The *context* is not itself photographed: We do not see the context that makes the eagle *be* a specific eagle, or be typical, a vertebrate, a nation, a fetish, alert, a form, a way of seeing, a gryphon, or a villain. A photograph of an eagle has many ways of appearing to us, and of being. That is, one cannot know the meaning of a photograph — what a photograph is *of* — simply by looking at the photograph without at least assuming a context. To further complicate matters, a film text may bring several contexts (several kinds of knowledge) to bear on a single image.

It is no answer to say that the photograph, *first of all*, is of an eagle and that various "meanings" are then attached to the eagle like lacquer applied to an object. The reason is that one may begin anywhere in thinking about an object; there is no single, causal arrow that produces thought step by step. For instance, a person looking at the photograph of an eagle, given the proper context, may at first see an example of a *typical* eagle or a *typical* bird of prey (say, when looking at the photograph in a dictionary) or may at first see a *vertebrate* (when looking at the photograph in a biology textbook). Later the person may come to see a *specific* eagle in *the* tree or perhaps not see the specific eagle at all. Furthermore, meanings are not like layers of lacquer. In the same way that a given photograph cannot be distinguished from the fact that it is "of" something, so an object cannot be separated from its "meaning." An object is bound to meaning because there are always one or more contexts in which it appears or is described or is imagined; one cannot hope to scrape off various meanings and be left with an object pure and simple for a disinterested perception.[5] Similarly, one cannot scrape away the "objects" in a photograph and be left with only a photograph.

I believe that the above considerations concerning the nature of a photograph and its meanings hold true for the nature of a "camera." Here are the questions I wish to address in this chapter: How do we discuss a "camera"? In what contexts? What does "camera" mean as a term used by critics? How has the idea of a "camera" become meaningful to us within a cinematic institution? What do we do with the word "camera" when it functions in a description? I believe that the word has many uses and consequently refers to many sorts of cameras. Moreover, these many uses may harbor deeply incompatible conceptions of what a camera is said to be, and, for that matter, what cinema is said to be.[6]

The introduction above of such words as "meaning," "use," "function," and "description" in questions about the "camera" suggests that we must inquire into the general nature of signification. What do we mean by "meaning"?[7] I will assume that a theory of meaning, in its most general formulation, seeks to elaborate the relationship between an entity *present* to our senses and another entity *absent* from our senses; that is, when we experience one thing, something *else* might also come to mind. The present entity may be, for example, an alphabetic shape drawn in ink or a shape registered through the chemicals of a film emulsion, while the absent entity may be, for example, an "idea," a "category," a "quality," a "hypothesis," a "feeling," an "association," a "memory," or an object elsewhere in the world. It may also be the case that the absent entity is brought to mind but is *not* conscious. (A simple example: It has been established that when reading a sentence that contains an ambiguous word, a person is often not aware of the ambiguity because alternative interpretations of the word, including interpretations of words not in the sentence but with merely the same initial phoneme, were evaluated in a preconscious buffer and all but one were blocked from consciousness.) How is it, then, that a present entity, A, *stands for* (or stands in for) something else, B, which is absent? The answer as to what constitutes "presence" and "absence" and how these are to be related to a person's mental state can be located only within a specific theory of how meaning is said to be made.

Not surprisingly, many processes have been advanced by theoreticians in an attempt to explain the overall movement from presence to absence, and additional distinctions have been made concerning preliminary, intermediate, and subsequent stages of meaning. Most important, the "movement" from presence to absence may not be unidirectional. What is "absent," "possible," or "expected" (to become present) may actually operate to bring something *into* being, to make us notice a new thing of the relevant type when we look. For example, after learning the distinction between "attached" and "cast" shadows, we will be able to notice these types of shadows (and the differences in their color temperatures) in the world around us and in the films we watch. We will also come to appreciate their different effects, even though the shadows were seemingly "always there." The same is true for more abstract categories, such as "dénouement" or "alienation." Thus, in the widest sense, analyzing the "meaning" of something is simply a way of talking about how a person is *reacting* to the thing as well as talking about a person's *predisposition* to react to that type of thing and hence the *effect* of having reacted. What type of thing it may be cannot be determined by material and shape alone, but only by judging the thing relative to a context. Some of these "contexts" exist in the way a person has of looking at the thing or acting toward it. I am tempted here to say that a context is simply a "frame" for seeing and acting, but, as we shall discover in the next chapter, the word "frame" leads to a set of new and difficult issues even though the word has a useful, literal sense when referring to a "film frame." ("Here is *the* frame that I saw when I held the celluloid strip to the light.") The literal sense is quickly lost, however, and a maze of interconnected possibilities is opened when we begin to speak about a "frame" in other senses, such as a "camera framing."

To sum up: The concept of meaning encompasses both the seeing of a thing (sensing, recognizing) as well as the influence of the categories being applied to the thing (understanding, interpretation). Although a thing, such as a written word, may be said to possess a meaning, and although that meaning may be explained to someone by using a series of words, the meaning itself is not to be found in any one or more of the words that are used but, rather, in the perceiver's *response* taken as a whole. How and why a perceiver responds is the central question.[8] A person's "lived physical existence" (ordinary routines, familiar skills, expectations, memory, growth, and change) is obviously an important source for generating meanings together with a person's metaphorical projections of his or her "lived physical existence" into new, less familiar domains (producing new kinds of expectations and responses). Still, one should not forget — and here I am anticipating the conclusion of this chapter — that making use of words is already an important and fundamental way of responding to the world and hence primary evidence of meaning or, we might say, demonstrates meaning in action. I am trying here to avoid asking an ontological question about "meaning" in favor of concentrating on what *happens* when meaning is said to be present. Could we not say that "things happen" and we give as *reasons* for those happenings our belief in the presence of "meanings"? In this way of thinking, "reasons" and "responses" exist, but "meanings," although a convenient shorthand for a process of responding, have no independent existence as tangible or intangible things; that is, a "meaning" is neither something physical like lacquer on a vase nor is it a special type of mental representation or distinctive type of feeling or experience.

I believe that the notion of a "camera" is inextricably bound up with the above sorts of questions about meaning and response. A critic's statement about some aspect of camerawork is ultimately a claim about what meanings and emotions are generated in a spectator and what a spectator will take a film — and its camerawork — to be. This suggests that quite a number of cameras are possible in accord with various theories of meaning (purported contexts) and that one critic's camera is not necessarily that of another critic. I wish to examine some of these different usages of the word "camera" by focusing on films with a narrative structure. The result is that the sort of camera a critic postulates will also depend upon the *value* assigned to narrative by his or her society; that is, narrativity is not something private and individual but, rather, like competence in a language, functions within a particular, standard framework for organizing causal descriptions.[9] The usefulness of narrative for thinking about the world is relative to the needs of a specific community and the ability to express those needs within the framework. Consequently, the type of *history* we write about narrative will be a summation of our beliefs as to what counts as narrative, what it is used for, and what it ought to be.[10] Thus, I will argue that our notion of the camera, finally, is governed both by our assumptions about the process of meaning within narrative structure and by the value of narrative to society, or, rather, we might say that our theory of meaning itself has a social value and responds to our deepest beliefs about society and its workings.

I will now survey eight major conceptions of the camera in order to demonstrate for each camera at least one connection to a narrative theory and social value. The eight cameras are not meant to be exhaustive, but merely illustrative. If this enables us to rethink the concept of camera — or at least to gain some distance from it — then the way will be open to reformulating our ideas about narrative comprehension and to rewriting the history of narrative. I want to emphasize at the outset that I will not be arguing for a grand, new camera as the sum of all the old ones, for that would be a peculiarly unwieldy one and would merely recapitulate the histories already written about narrative cinema.[11] My goal is simply to unwind the beliefs to which we are committed when we employ the word "camera" in discussing certain responses we may have to a film. I will conclude by suggesting what areas of research have been opened by the most recent theories of the camera.

FOUR CAMERAS: FROM MACHINE TO SUBJECT

I will begin with the visual stimulus that appears on the screen and the role that is claimed for a camera in the production of the stimulus. In this context a camera is simply a "box" holding an all-important light-sensitive film emulsion that will become the source of a projected image. (Of course, not all images on the screen have come from the film emulsion; for instance, an image may have been painted or created through a "special effect" or made out of computer code or sensed by pixels in a charge-coupled device.) The presence of this "boxlike" camera may be made even more conspicuous by allowing it to *move* during the act of filming. (And, of course, not all motion on the screen has come from a movement of the camera-as-box.) What is known as the *kinetic depth effect*, or monocular movement parallax, explains how certain camera movements are able to produce a striking effect on the screen. I am employing the kinetic depth effect to serve as an illustration of how the camera-as-box becomes a machine-at-work.

Consider the following situation: A beam of light illuminates an object and throws the object's shadow onto a screen. A perceiver views the shadow from the opposite side of the screen (see figure 3.1).[12] The shadow is strictly two-dimensional; however, if a motor rotates the object, the perceiver will immediately see a three-dimensional shape on the screen even though the moving shadows remain two-dimensional. The kinetic depth effect relies on the fact that the human perceptual system is able to use the *motion* of the shadows to *mentally construct* a three-dimensional entity that is not itself

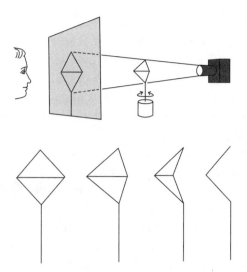

FIGURE 3.1 Kinetic Depth Effect

The kinetic depth effect shows how movement can endow perceived objects with three-dimensional shape. The shadow of a bent wire form (shown at the bottom in four different orientations) looks as flat as the screen on which it is cast as long as the form remains stationary. When it is swiveled back and forth, the changing shadow is seen as a rigid rotating object with the appropriate three-dimensionality. The direction of the rotation remains ambiguous. Illustration copyright © 1968 by Estate of Bunji Tagawa. All rights reserved.

directly visible (since the object is on the opposite side of the screen). Applying this experiment to cinema, we can say that the motor that rotates the object is analogous to the motion-picture camera that gently turns the world for our inspection. Here the "camera," like the motor, becomes the unifying principle of a sensory display. The movement of a camera becomes the simplest inference that we can make about a changing set of stimuli on-screen that gives volume to a space existing elsewhere. Through a camera's agency, two-dimensional shadows are transformed into three-dimensional objects.[13]

In this approach to defining a camera, meaning is a *percept* that can be studied through the methods of sensory psychology. The camera becomes part of a complex perceptual process linking sensations present on a screen to something absent or beyond the screen, just out of sight (an object, a camera). A focus on sensory processes — especially on their failure to *guarantee* an exact match between percept and object — forms the basis of an *illusion* theory of meaning.[14] (For example, in the above case of the moving shadows onscreen, the *direction* of the object's movement behind the screen remains ambiguous; the object appears to be moving alternately clockwise and counterclockwise.) Plato's famous application of the concept of illusion to art is explicitly recalled in such modern theories as those of E. H. Gombrich and, for film, Jean-Louis Baudry.[15] Noël Burch spells out the consequences for a camera in such a theory by arguing that certain camera techniques can *break* the spell of illusion that normally holds a spectator captive to imperfect or ambiguous appearances that are a (poor) substitute for unseen objects. Burch, for example, argues for "surface" over "depth" effects and for "gratuitous" camera movements.[16] Histories of narrative can then be written that trace the degree to which cinema succumbs to, or escapes from, perceptual illusion. Thus, one might oppose the filmmakers who supposedly promoted illusion, such as Edison, Porter, Dickson, Raff and Gammon, Smith, Ince, Griffith, and De Mille, to those who have viewed cinema as a toy or as science, such as Méliès, Lumière, Marey, Muybridge, Warhol, Godard, Snow, and O'Neill.[17] According to one writer, "The experimental film is not just an experiment in the scientific sense, but it does resemble science in that each of its films are stages in the study of the Being of the Camera."[18]

It is not enough, however, in writing a history of narrative forms, to understand the details of various theories of perceptual illusion. One also needs to understand why the theories were popular, that is, how the concept of illusion might operate within a given historical setting to articulate the needs and issues of a community. For instance, in Renaissance Italy the Catholic Church decided that the positive values of a heightened illusion of reality in paintings based on Biblical narratives (fostered principally by the development of linear perspective) outweighed — although just barely — its dangers (idolatry).[19] One might also argue that illusionism expressed the interests of a rising merchant class and that realistic depictions aimed at another economic stratum, possessing a different collection of interests, would need to take a different form. The point here is that a term such as "camera" assumes its place within a larger theory of narrative production (in this case, as building on, or struggling against, illusion) as well as within, or against, the values assigned to that production by a particular society.

So far we have considered the camera as the origin of an illusory sensation (e.g., of kinetic depth), but a second approach would hold that it is simply a sensation — a sensory *material* to be experienced in its own right apart from its immediate source. This approach, typified by Noël Burch's early work, takes as its starting point a complete inventory of the possible forms and types of sensation.[20] The effects produced by a camera become one of many groups of "parameters" to be manipulated and varied across the film as a whole in order to build up a new kind of 'picture,' or way of looking, independent of looking *at* what caused the sensation. The goal is to select sensory materials that will force themselves on a spectator's attention by breaking with his or her habitual and practical, everyday experience. Thus, the spectator becomes a site for shock effects: discontinuity, provocation, disorientation. The key criterion for the camera is a demand to make the world unfamiliar, strange, new, and better. Forms that are present to our senses onscreen are said to be capable of bringing absent, unnoticed entities to our attention through a process of "defamiliarization."[21]

What is unfamiliar depends on what is familiar, which, in turn, depends on the dominant forms of realism in a particular historical setting. In this approach "realism" is merely a style, method, or strategy of representing a consensus or community perception of the real through the use of an art medium. Hence, a camera's effects are defined and described against a historical standard and shift with the times to maintain an adversarial position and an ability to defamiliarize. The result is that the history of film is conceived in terms of an avant-garde whose mission is to refuse the dominant practice and explore frontiers.[22] A camera ideally becomes active, even obtrusive; in Sergei Eisenstein's phrase, the camera should be "hewing out a piece of actuality with the ax of the lens."[23]

When we abandon the notion of a camera as an adversary to the world, though, and instead place the accent on its "natural" connection to the world, we reach another, more orthodox version of a camera. This approach stresses the necessary, scientific links among objects, light rays, and film emulsion. Across this (one-way) bridge, reality passes into the film and its reproductions. A camera escapes being the product of mere sensation (shadows) and becomes the bearer of tokens from the world. A photograph is then interpreted as a strict *map* of the landscape in front of a camera's lens. What is present on the screen is causally related, in the manner of a fingerprint, asserts Bazin, to absent entities.[24] Not only objects can be recorded in this manner but, as Arthur Danto notes, the camera itself, especially through its movements, makes the "mode of recording part of the record"; that is, the camera, too, may leave a photographic mark frozen on a loop of time.[25]

Nevertheless, the resulting conception of a camera and its movements is decidedly static and narrow. Is a photograph always employed as a map of a landscape? (Recall that my answer was no when earlier I listed ten uses of a photograph of an eagle.) A camera in the orthodox view is reduced to a form of deixis, a gesture pointing toward objects and occasionally toward itself as an object. The camera seems to say, 'Look *here* at *this*.' In addition, the camera becomes the anchor point for 'motion' appearing on the screen, as in a pan left: 'Look over *here* to the *left*.' The film's chemical emulsion is also deictic: 'Look *now* at what was actually *there* (*then*).' On the basis of this deictic logic of the emulsion, one may conclude that an image seen *here* and *now* on the screen points to the specific time that existed *there* and *then*. Furthermore, when one considers under- and overexposure, the film's emulsion actually points to a range of time: The blackened image of underexposure shows the time that existed *before* the thing would have been there-then in optimal exposure, while the whitened image of overexposure shows the time *after* the thing would have been there-then in optimal exposure — that is, we are being shown a time too soon or too late to see perfectly. Extending this logic, certain optical effects such as fades and dissolves may be said to signal greater time shifts. In sum, the camera sees and remembers.

For the above reasons, some writers have held that photography is simply too real in picturing space and time, and allows the photographer too little creative control, to be a genuine art form.[26] As Roger Scruton believes:

> The history of the art of photography is the history of successive attempts to break the causal chain by which the photographer is imprisoned, to impose a human intention between [an object] and [its] appearance [in a photograph] so that the [object] can be both defined by that intention and seen in terms of it.[27]

If Scruton's "human intention" were to be added to a camera's deictic act, then the camera's function could be described as follows: '*You* will later see what *I* see now (because *I* am pointing the camera for a reason).' The two uses of the word "see" in this description are ambiguous and may span a wide range of mental events from sensing, recognizing, and exploring to arguing, explaining, narrating, and interpreting. (Cf. 'I see what you mean.') A number of aesthetic theories will emerge from this sort of formulation as different restrictions are placed on the (proper) use of the word "see."

The remarkable subtlety of André Bazin's film theory is due in large measure to a powerful synthesis of two conceptions of a camera. The first — just mentioned — compels a camera through physical law to record a *profilmic*, or pro-photographic, reality. At the same time, however, a second causal force binds the camera to a *postfilmic*, or post-photographic, reality. This second component of the camera is the reality of a spectator's *viewing situation*, which is controlled by perceptual law and general psychological principles. Realism in the cinema, according to Bazin, is due not merely to the scientific basis of the photographic image but is also, he insists, based on "those conditions which respect certain physiological or mental facts of natural perception or, more exactly, in rediscovering *equivalents* for them."[28] Bazin asserts that a "universal psychological experience" underlies the many devices of film. He declares, "Our legs and neck didn't wait for the cinema to invent the tracking shot and the pan, nor our attention to contrive the close-up."[29] Note that the effect of this type of comparison is twofold: The turn of a spectator's head acquires a mechanical component (which may be simulated by a machine) while, simultaneously, a camera becomes more human.

Bazin is not alone in emphasizing a spectator's viewing situation and in searching for filmic equivalents to human perception, attention, and interest. Karel Reisz, Gavin Millar, and Ernest Lindgren likewise employ psychological premises, although they reach different conclusions. In fact, these writers effectively reverse Bazin's prejudice in favor of the long take and instead posit editing as the essence of cinema.[30] Camera movement for them becomes simply another method of transferring the spectator's attention (analogous to eye movement, according to Lindgren)[31] and is therefore treated as a subcategory of editing.[32] In the present context, I am less interested in the particular conclusions drawn from these psychological premises than in the logic employed: In each instance a specific film technique is traced back to a putative "normal mental mechanism by which we alter our attention from object to object in real life."[33] What is fundamental for Reisz, Millar, and Lindgren is editing, while for Bazin it is the duration of the image and the movement of a camera. The methods of reasoning, however, are identical.

For Bazin, a camera, acted upon by reality, must react in place of an absent spectator, but only in ways that are homologous with the laws of human perception. Two of the cinematic techniques championed by Bazin are "deep focus" in onscreen space and "lateral depth of field" in the activation of offscreen space.[34] The two techniques complement one another and serve to unite the two main strands in Bazin's work dealing with profilmic and postfilmic realities beyond the image. Deep focus, for him, means 'non-selective' focus and hence a gain in the perceiver's ability to select freely what is important in the image. At the same time, certain kinds of lateral camera movements increase the perceiver's confidence in his or her independence: the freedom not only to scan an image in depth but to predict or wonder what *will or could* be shown at its edges at any moment.[35] The overall aim is to ensure that the perceiver sees present entities on the screen in the exact way he or she *would see* absent entities beyond the screen, including absent entities that are off-screen and perhaps *never* shown![36] Combining this postfilmic rationale ('would see') with the profilmic rationale (seeing what was there-then, what 'once was') yields the Bazinian idea that the perceiver sees present entities on the screen in the exact way he or she *would have seen* absent entities if he or she could have been present. In such a theory of meaning, the value of narrativity for society lies in releasing documentary reality and disclosing real conditions of viewing and vision.[37] 'Comments' by an author or manipulations of plot may obscure but cannot finally defeat such Bazinian properties of the (real) world as ambiguity, multiplicity, chance, independence, continuity, density, detail, and even mystery. For Bazin, a neorealist documentary lies hidden within every narrative.

Realism for Bazin, then, is a complex interaction between conditions forced on a camera by both the profilmic and the post-filmic. Realism is rooted in the real and is not simply a matter of an arbitrary (or familiar) style, method, or strategy. Bazin's notion of realism is opposed by the (arbitrary) conventions of narrative and by "expressionism," which constitute all those tricks of the trade — the artifice of art — that a filmmaker can summon to stimulate and guide a spectator's attention, principally through plot, montage, and character psychology. Realism versus expressionism, however, quickly becomes a brutal dichotomy perpetuated in many histories of film narrative by opposing the work of Louis Lumière and Georges Méliès. In addition, this dichotomy is reflected in the most common and durable refrain in all of orthodox criticism, whether applied to film or any of the other arts, namely, that a spectator must never become aware of the actual techniques employed by an artwork, for that reveals not reality and truth but rather the contrivance and biases of an individual — the artist. A camera serves external reality; it cannot photograph an intention or what is inside the mind. Thus, camerawork must never be 'self-indulgent,' 'obvious,' or, worse, become 'obtrusive.'[38]

Narrative, too, is subject to the 'unobtrusiveness' principle. The history of narrative is interpreted as an evolution in search of a satisfying accommodation between the extremes of realism and expressionism — of vulgar naturalism and crude artifice.[39] It should be said that although Bazin remains within this orthodox tradition, he emphasizes not so much an "evolution" as a "dialectical" interaction between the extremes that generates successive states of vibrant equilibrium.[40] He maintains that the favored techniques (e.g., deep focus and lateral depth of field) are neither necessary nor sufficient to reveal reality; one also needs an artist's insights and (careful) contrivances.[41] These ideas add nuance and power to Bazin's theory without compromising central principles.

FOUR MORE CAMERAS: FROM PSYCHE TO SOCIETY

With Bazin's theory we have reached a point where a camera is being defined in relation to a postfilmic viewing situation. If this context is broadened to include the psychology of other persons and entities (e.g., authors, narrators, and characters), we arrive at a new conception of a camera. This new camera is meant to disclose human consciousness wherever it may be found in its full range of feelings and motives, not just in a spectator's basic ways of looking and perceiving. The underlying process is termed *expression*, a word that derives from Latin and means literally "to press out," namely, to force outward that which is concealed within. What is present on the screen for our inspection is now the residue of some other person's or entity's private state of consciousness. For example, the so-called subjective camera can be used to elicit the feeling and viewpoint of a character who is seated, walking, drunk, dizzy, fearful, desirous, dreaming, remembering, and so forth. Other, more "neutral" or objective shots are still based on this model; it is simply more difficult to ascertain *whose* consciousness (and what state of consciousness) is being portrayed. The so-called "perfect view" shot,[42] for example, may be said to depict the attention of an invisible, ideal observer.[43] Ultimately, our task as spectators in an expressionist theory is to reconstruct through "empathy" the hidden emotions and imagination not only of characters, but also of various narrators and observers whose presence may be explicit, implicit, contradictory, disguised, remote, or invisible.

A special target of expressionist theories is the author — the so-called original and First Cause. In this context empathy functions as the inverse of intention. We are to look within ourselves to understand the feelings being pressed into the design of the story through intentional acts of an author. Empathy and intention complement one another because they draw on a presumed universal psychology of human beings, at least as to basic emotions and behavior. Thus, what begins as a spectator's inspection of the externalized states of a fictional character or other persona concludes with the spectator's decisive look inward, accompanied by heightened feelings of recognition and revelation.

Expression theories grew from the Romantic movement of the first half of the nineteenth century and stressed the creative sensibilities of a lone individual.[44] The artwork is said to achieve congruence with an artist's internal state by means of simple reflection,[45] the operation of innate brain fields,[46] or sheer willpower — the irresistible intention of an auteur who forces us to recognize ourselves. According to the last, the director of a film wields a camera as a pen or paintbrush for our benefit.[47] A history of narrative film written on this basis becomes essentially a random (but evocative) collection of anecdotes about individuals who, touched by genius, have triumphed over all obstacles and become great teachers about the human condition. The resulting film history is little more than Andrew Sarris' "Directorial Chronology 1915–1967."[48]

A new sort of camera emerges, however, to the extent that a spectator is assigned a more central, cognitive role in the production of ideas. If we interpret the expression of an author as something other than an involuntary reflex, or self-serving display of consciousness to be absorbed and imitated by a spectator, and instead emphasize that the author has engaged in a purposeful *communication*, we arrive at the idea that an apparent *transmission of information* has occurred for someone's benefit. In a communication theory of narrative, the narration of a story assumes a literal sense: An author translates *knowing* into *telling* followed by a spectator who reconverts the telling into knowing.[49] The attitude or viewpoint of the author, or at least some species of narrator, is transmitted with minimal resistance (lessened by the critic) to the spectator. The outcome of this quasi-conversation is knowledge about reality, inflected by the author's or narrator's view of it. The precise nature of the causal connection between sender and receiver — which is rooted in the mathematics of information theory — must be carefully adjusted as a communication model is applied to language in general, to literature, and to film.[50]

The function of a camera in such a scheme is, I believe, analogous to what Roman Jakobson describes as the *phatic* element in language.[51] The camera provides the physical and psychological *channel* by which we enter and remain in communication. One could perhaps go further and define certain camera maneuvers analogous to the ritualized formulas of the phatic that seek to establish, prolong, scrutinize, and break off communication: "Shall we start? Do you see? Watch this! Are you still interested?" In general, the camera allows us to remain in (imperfect) contact with a variety of implied authors, narrators, observers, and characters, all willing to speak to us and provide information. Our primary task is to discover with whom we are in contact — that is, whose "voice" is being heard in the narrative through the channel provided by the camera. In Nick Browne's words, we must search for the "narrating agency or authority which can be taken to rationalize the presentation of shots" and, one assumes, to rationalize the presentation of shot transitions, camera movements, mise-en-scène, exposition, tension, momentum, surprise, close-ups, ellipses, metaphors, sounds, and so on.[52] Discovering the identity of a narrating agency allows a spectator to anticipate what might be learned from a source of information and to evaluate the credibility of the source. Critics have described an amazing array of narrators in films, including the "collective" consciousness of a village and of Paris as well as the "central" consciousness of characters, a donkey, God, and even inanimate objects.[53]

It is no wonder that a camera itself can be awakened to consciousness within a communication theory and so described in blatantly anthropomorphic terms. A pan is again like the turn of someone's head but no longer that of a character in the story or of the Bazinian spectator. The camera acquires a mind of its own. Accordingly, critics have described the camera as impulsive, bold, curious, lewd, tactful, disorderly, exhibiting a sense of smell, and even "smiling ironically."[54] One assumes, as well, that it has an ear for conversation. Anything that stands out as 'unrealistic,' 'garish,' 'intrusive,' or 'disruptive' in a film can be conveniently reinterpreted as a commentary, message, rebellion, digression, or (in the case of *temps mort*) a reflective pause by a camera or narrator. In Jean-Luc Godard's *Vivre sa vie* (*My Life to Live*, 1962), a camera's mental states are said to be especially prominent:

> It [the camera] stares wide-eyed through the window, like a prehistoric animal.

> [T]he camera moves more quickly than Nana does, its anticipation of her action suggesting both foreknowledge and narrative impatience. The camera could even be said to spy upon and to trap Nana, since its vantage point and its high-angle pans associate it with a surveillance apparatus.

> The camera can't wait for Nana to live through the remaining hours or days before she fully accedes to a life of prostitution. It demands that she begin immediately.

And in Godard's *Le Mépris* (*Contempt*, 1963):

> But if Paul and Camille relate to Italy existentially rather than via painting or sketching, the camera remains a nineteenth-century tourist. It still needs to make images.

> The camera seems to want to show us how distant it is from him [Paul], in every sense of the word.

> [In answer to the question, "Is Godard's camera faithful to Camille only by betraying her?"] It seems to me that it is. In a way, the film never says 'Camille,' no matter how the camera lingers on the image of her body. It [the film, the camera] says: "Eve," "Penelope," "Bardot."[55]

The 'unobtrusiveness' principle, characteristic of profilmic theories of the camera, is here effectively reversed so that it is now laudable when a camera becomes self-conscious and reflexive, ambivalent and elusive, meditates upon film theories, and flaunts the artifice of a film's construction ("the camera can't wait . . ."; "the camera seems to want . . ."). At this point communication begins to slide back toward an expressive theory of meaning and the reconstruction of intentional and empathic states.

Communication theories, with their stress on rhetoric and commentary, are particularly adept at dealing with complex and "difficult" films such as those of the art cinema. A history of narrative can be based on the increasing exploitation and awareness of authorial forms of address: overt commentary, indignation, irony, melancholy, ambiguity, paradox, playfulness, lyricism, enigmatic presentations, unreliability, and so on.[56] Unusual camera movements become the very mark of conspicuous narration. An insistence on framing and reframing through a wandering point of view exposes a degree of self-doubt mixed with the compulsion to tell, which surpasses a merely photographic simulacrum of the world.

However, if one dissects the notion of communication — the compulsion to tell and the compulsion to absorb a telling — one may find at the core of these two impulses repressed desires and wish-fulfillment rather than simple messages. This leads to a new type of camera where the notion of transmitting a message from one person to the next is replaced by a theory of what it means *to be* a person who can know and tell as well as experience a telling and have a telling experience. In this approach film becomes a phantasy that is mutually sustained by an author and spectator, each of whom forms an *identity* with and against the other through the mediation of fictional characters. "Unconscious desire" replaces "conscious intention," but otherwise the basic structure of narrative discourse remains unchanged: desire-path-obstacle-resolution-return (of) to desire.

Psychoanalytic theory holds that an individual is split into conscious and unconscious strata. Film reflects this split by possessing both manifest and latent textual levels. The manifest level is plot and style; the latent level is that which is denied, displaced, censored, sublimated, or repressed by the phantasy narrative. Meaning for an individual depends on a movement from secondary to primary processes of the psychical apparatus: a descent from present, manifest sensation appearing on the screen, which is governed by the reality principle and the "daily residue," toward what is absent from, merely latent in, consciousness — for example, instinctual energy and pleasure, cathexis, deferred revision, narcissism, ambivalence, anxiety, parapraxis, masochism, trauma, and dread.[57] "For the cinephile, there is a moment in a film," reports Paul Willemen, "when cinema, in showing you one thing, allows you to glimpse something else that you are not meant to see."[58] Psychoanalysis seeks to explain this movement from manifest to latent meaning. Because psychoanalytic theory encourages a degree of skepticism about conscious meaning (communication, the secondary process), it is not surprising that many writers employing this methodology view cinema as an illusory presentation; that is, what is present on the screen is viewed as merely a nexus of symptoms and defense mechanisms or else a means of regression toward earlier (primal) stages of libidinal development.[59] In this way a "camera" can be dismissed as a purely secondary, surface manifestation of film.

Alternatively, it might be argued that a camera has an important task in facilitating unconscious dream-thought. The reason is that unconscious impulses, no matter how abstract, must be transformed into visual images in order to appear in dream. The nature of dream means that thoughts that admit of visual representation will be preferred, while others will be displaced toward pictorial substitutes.[60] In the framework of film-as-a-dream, a camera accomplishes this visualization and other related tasks (e.g., condensation, elaboration, and censorship) in ways that often escape our notice, so that one might properly speak of at least two cameras within the psychoanalytic mode: a manifest camera and a repressed camera. Paul Willemen has provided some examples from the work of Max Ophuls. Willemen shows how a verbal metaphor may be transformed quite literally into a camera movement that *at the same time* reveals the repression that the original word had sought to mask.[61]

It is apparent that the unconscious mechanisms studied by psychoanalysis outrun the usual historical categories applied to narrative, such as style, genre, period, nation, director, writer, and studio. Psychoanalysis shares with illusionist theories of narrative the need for principles of grouping based on various psychological effects on, or drives arising from, a spectator. An appropriate historical category might be "mode of discourse," which is to say a broad group of films of differing styles and genres that enact a limited matrix of preoccupations and resolutions (i.e., a class of films in search of a particular libidinal economy). Instead of focusing on the psychopathology of an author or character, or searching for "Freudian symbols," the "mode of discourse" approach envisions film as a set of "symptoms" under continual (psycho)analysis by the spectator. The film's symptoms unfold a "phantasy scenario" that permits the spectator to adopt a succession of multiple, contradictory roles as the "analyst." Thus far, study has centered principally on the so-called classical narrative. Within this mode of discourse, it has been argued that a camera embarks the spectator on a "motionless voyage" of "imaginary presence" that repeats phallic aggression while giving visual form to the unconscious of a patriarchal society.[62]

Here is Laura Mulvey's celebrated formulation of the patriarchal unconscious:

> The male unconscious has two avenues of escape from . . . castration anxiety: preoccupation with the re-enactment of the original trauma (investigating the woman, demystifying her mystery), counterbalanced by the devaluation, punishment or saving of the guilty object (an avenue typified by the concerns of the film noir); or else complete disavowal of castration by the substitution of a fetish object or turning the represented figure itself into a fetish so that it becomes reassuring rather than dangerous (hence overvaluation, the cult of the female star).

This second avenue, fetishistic scopophilia, builds up the physical beauty of the object, transforming it into something satisfying in itself. The first avenue, voyeurism, on the contrary, has associations with sadism: pleasure lies in ascertaining guilt (immediately associated with castration), asserting control and subjugating the guilty person through punishment or forgiveness. This sadistic side fits in well with narrative. Sadism demands a story, depends on making something happen, forcing a change in another person, a battle of will and strength, victory/defeat, all occurring in a linear time with a beginning and an end. Fetishistic scopophilia, on the other hand, can exist outside linear time as the erotic instinct is focused on the look alone. These contradictions and ambiguities can be illustrated more simply by using works by Hitchcock and Sternberg, both of whom take the look almost as the content or subject matter of many of their films.[63]

Nonetheless, "one does not dream in languages one does not know." For this reason Christian Metz argues that an understanding of the primary process of the unconscious also requires a careful analysis of the secondary process through the disciplines of semiology, linguistics, symbolic logic, phenomenology, and other "close relations."[64] The result is that cinema is conceived as a language in which meaning is symbolic.[65] That is, present entities refer to absent entities through the operation of *rules* shared by a community, for example, the rule that governs a specific denotation ('cat,' 'mat') or the rule that converts a sentence from passive to active. Furthermore, the act of 'following rules' presupposes the existence of 'regular practices.' Thus, in order to understand the rules, one will need to pursue the following activities according to Metz: "the direct study of societies, historical criticism, the examination of infrastructures," as well as "political economy."[66] In short, one must study the regular practices of which the rules are evidence. Bazin's postfilmic 'viewing situation' has been considerably expanded to now include a spectator's 'habits' and 'preferences' in watching. What is at stake is the study of a way of life.

In such a scheme a camera would no longer be conceived as a real, physical object moving around in a profilmic or postfilmic reality in order to show the choices being made by an invisible observer (where a pan is a turn of the head) or else to relay no one's point of view (i.e., the world objectified). Instead, film is rid of misleading and reductive anthropomorphisms.[67] 'Humanism' is relocated within a larger process whereby society fabricates meaning for itself according to prescribed conventions of behavior, canons of interpretation, and accepted practices.[68] The qualities that count as 'human' would be defined through a given social system and not by an immutable, a priori conception of 'human nature.' Thus, instead of seeking residual traces of human narrators who have somehow been mapped into film, the 'symbolic' approach would concentrate on various rules and procedures through which symbols are manipulated by a community to create texts with nominal speakers and narrators.

Metz believes that a camera does not stand in by default for an absent observer but, rather, is embedded in the text as a "purely cinematographic" signifier linked through community rules to a narrative signified.[69] What interests me, however, is a slightly different formulation that begins with a spectator and then asks how a camera *may be of use while watching a film*. What place does a camera occupy in the account of our comprehension that we render, often implicitly, to ourselves? How do we use the term "camera" to tell ourselves a story about our accumulation of thoughts, memories, anticipations, feelings, and beliefs? The answer, I suggest, is that the term "camera" becomes a reading hypothesis or heuristic aimed at comprehending fictional space and time — a way of applying to a text various *labels* that are being generated by ongoing acts of interpretation while watching, or while remembering having watched. This formulation attempts to capture a viewer's activity in processing sets of narrativized images. Such a sequence of narrativized, fictional images and sounds provides a new and very different context for the term "camera" than does a single frame on celluloid, or multiple frames, which were captured by a thing that recorded the physical features of other things such as actors and props while simultaneously excluding sound, narrative, and fiction. I believe that when viewers and critics normally talk about the "camera" in a film, they are not referring to something physical that was pushed around on a set. Instead, the word "camera" functions as an abbreviated way of referring to those "analytical or heuristic procedures" that are imagined as motivating a viewer's interpretive behavior ("now I see . . .," "I should have seen . . .," "I see what the character is saying . . .").

When one focuses on a spectator's interpretive behavior as a starting point for thinking about a camera, a film 'as it appears on the screen' loses its status as a purely objective phenomenon and the sole determining factor in elucidating meanings. Accordingly, the nature of film analysis undergoes a change: The goal is no longer to uncover an interpretation that is certain and definite (even if 'open' meanings or several interpretations are located), but, rather, the goal is to delineate an indefinite series of interpretations that are relative to particular issues, problems, or social contexts, including relations to other films. In this approach an 'analytical method' offers neither discovery nor proof but is merely a tool of convenience in generating a plausible interpretation within a relevant context. In such an approach, the camera also becomes a tool of convenience.

Metz states his new idea about the nature of film and film analysis in the following way:

> But I no longer believe that each film has *a* textual system (the one I suggested . . . for a film of Griffith's, *Intolerance*, is only one of the systems possible, a stage in the work of interpretation . . .), nor even . . . a fixed number of quite distinct textual systems (several "readings" of the same film). In this (or these) system(s), I now see [merely] *working conveniences* . . . — sorts of "blocks of interpretation" already foreseen or established by the analysis, sectors of signification . . . that the analysis has already *selected* at different moments in its in fact interminable movement from the *indefinite* thickness of the textual system as I now see it, that is, [I now see analysis] as this perpetual possibility of a finer,

> or else less apparent structuration, of a grouping of the elements into a new configuration, of the registration of a new *significatory pressure* which does not annul the preceding ones . . . , but complements or in other cases distorts and complicates them, at any rate points in a slightly different direction, a little to one side (a little or more than a little). . . . [A]t present I feel that this [significatory] pressure [created by analysis], this "activity," comes into play not only inside a textual system but for any one film between each and the next one to be discovered; or, if it is thought that there is only one such [textual] system in all, then the analyst will never complete his exploration of it and should not seek any "end."[70]

I believe that a 'camera' may be thought of as a 'tool' in the kind of analysis sketched by Metz. A camera may become part of a mental procedure employed by a spectator to solve interpretive problems. Of course, when the question being addressed is not interpretive, then the nature of a camera will change. For example, if one were to ask what kind of camera Griffith employed to make *Intolerance* in 1916 or how a Technicolor camera in 1932 was designed to render color in a special way utilizing a prism and three film stocks, then the answers would involve historical and technical details, and the resulting cameras would be quite unlike the one that is imagined during a spectator's comprehension of a given film narrative.

Those who speak confidently of *the* camera seem to have in mind only a prototypical instance in which an object is shown on the screen through a straight-on angle and in focus with a normal focal-length lens. Consider, by contrast, the non-physical "camera" a spectator projects while watching the following:

> animation; optical effects (which are especially prominent in 15- and 30-second television commercials); superimposition (in which two images become ghostly together and shift luminance values lighter with double exposure or darker with bi-pack exposure); a split screen showing two images (how many cameras are seen: one,

two, *or* three?); films built up from stop motion photography (i.e., pixillation effects: how many cameras?); swish pans; nonhuman acrobatic movements as in Snow's *La Région centrale* (1971); the vertiginous staircase shot in Hitchcock's *Vertigo* (1958); a continuous camera movement that represents discontinuous time; a nondiegetic insert (a new camera?); and such special effects as a tracking shot through a miniature of a village in Borzage's *Secrets* (1924) and past a spacecraft in Lucas' *Star Wars* (1977).[71]

In the last example we may simply see a spacecraft that moves instead of a camera that moves, and we will certainly be in a different relation to the object than that of the camera employed in original photography. Indeed, we can ask the same kinds of questions about how we hear a sound while watching a film: Do we imagine several microphones roaming throughout fictional space in search of sounds? When we hear nondiegetic music, do we imagine an unseen concert hall or a tape deck in a recording studio? Is it an "illusion" that we hear the voice of a character as well as an actor? Once we give up the idea that a physical camera and physical microphone are at the root of all seeing and hearing — measuring our every activity when we watch and listen, as an hourglass holds its sand — then the film experience will be seen to depend not only upon the single causal process of recording image and sound, but will be seen to emerge naturally from the diversity of our lives and a multiplicity of kinds of causatives. Meaning, interpretation, and fictiveness will appear less mysterious, less like arbitrary encrustations on a film and more a part of what we do when we think and negotiate daily life.

MENTAL MODELS AND GRAVITY

If we do not see through a profilmic camera, then how exactly are we seeing? Raymond Durgnat describes a shot from Hitchcock's *Psycho* (1960) in which a camera follows water moving along the bottom of a bathtub to a drain; when the camera reaches the drain, it moves forward until the drain and swirling water completely fill the screen. Durgnat then reflects on the words that he chose to describe the shot:

> One writes "the camera closes on it [the bathtub drain]," and some spectators will register this happening, but the phrase is really a form of words for a less definable effect: our gaze approaches the enlarging object, which, filling our field of vision, monopolises our attention (and, perhaps, presents new aspects). Before it was a, maybe poignant, *detail*, now it, and *its* details, acquires a new *poetic force*. The rule of thumb would be, that, whether or not we briefly think about what the invisible, irrationally present camera is doing, it's what's on screen that predominates in our perceptions and our minds. It's to do, not with "illusionism," "mystification"; it's a case of "out of sight, out of mind" (and it's reversible, depending on context and other factors). The mention of the camera in this popular form of words reminds us how aware spectators are that a film is "only" a film, a "construction" and that they don't normally confuse diegesis with reality. A special interest in camera movements is entirely justified, but it can get out of hand, as when formalists suppose that spectators "think" scenes as if they were being watched by a camera, or that the camera corresponds to an invisible watcher-narrator (who may even verge on being an "unacknowledged character in the drama"). Moreover, no camera observes a scene; it only records it. But all that's another essay.[72]

In this passage Durgnat argues that the word "camera," as it appears within a "popular form of words," is misleading. He says that a spectator does not watch a scene *through* a profilmic camera nor think about a scene by picturing a camera that is watching the scene nor imagine a camera to be an invisible narrator or invisible character. Instead, there is "a less definable effect" related to "our attention" and to the "new aspects" (thoughts, feelings) that may come to us from "what's on screen." For Durgnat the mind works with, and upon, material from the screen; the mind does not envision some kind of camera-entity — a machine, organism, or agent — and then wonder what the thing is seeing. The camera is not a spectator's alter ego or an *Other*. The use of the word "camera" by a spectator shows only that he or she knows a film is a construction that should not be confused with reality. The important point that Durgnat makes is that when a spectator uses the word "camera" in a description of a shot, the word should not be understood in isolation from its context so as to be mistaken for the name of a concrete entity, a *substantive*; rather, the word must remain embedded within the description as a whole so that it is clear that what is being talked about by using the word are a spectator's *movements of attention* together with other processes of mind while reacting to the screen.

What is the spectator doing while looking at the screen? I believe that he or she is continually experimenting with patterns by attempting to piece together possible and likely *mental models* that will give shape to events on the screen. The viewer is thus in a different place, so to speak, than the profilmic camera (and microphone). Consider, for example, how the viewer constructs the overall space of a scene. He or she mentally joins fragments of shots and sounds into a tentative, ordered whole, makes conjectures, and fills in what is missing. The so-called illusion of three-dimensionality created by the classical film is complete not when a profilmic camera has shown everything in a room — which, anyway, is usually prohibited by the 180-degree rule — but when the viewer is able to imagine himself or herself in numerous places *apart from* the immediate optical view. To fully understand the space of a scene, one must be able to project new spaces from new angles. The viewer can demonstrate this ability by imagining being in the scene and moving about to assume new angles, or by making a drawing that reveals characters and objects from new angles (e.g., from overhead). Such a drawing should be understood as itself fictional, as a record of the viewer's inferences about a set of spaces, not as a reconstruction of how a profilmic camera was positioned on a set.

Besides making judgments about space, a viewer projects a stream of hypotheses about such factors as time, causality, character personality and motive, the efficacy of action, exposition, enigmas,

93

plausibility, ethics, metaphors, rhythm, point of view, and much more. In general, a viewer comes to understand scenes by making detailed *models* of events. What might be termed the "classical" camera is simply the invitation to employ certain norms or standard procedures to fashion and test one's hypotheses. A viewer attempts to see what he or she knows, expects, and desires under the generic label "camera." Here the term "camera" stands in for those procedures that have been successful in the past. When a viewer's confidence in his or her predictions is high (i.e., the viewer's constructed, mental models are well developed and reasonably supported by evidence), the film achieves a high degree of "reality." This does not mean that the viewer never makes mistakes; in fact, the art of storytelling requires that there be "surprises."

Perhaps an analogy would clarify the idea of a camera that is the construction of a spectator. Rudolf Arnheim contends that one of the ways a person understands the composition of a painting is by hypothesizing the effects of gravity.[73] By imagining a downward force acting on the graphic forms, the person is able to bring out unique features of the composition, such as symmetry, stability, balance, regularity, form, "weight," and others. Hence, rotating an abstract painting through 90-degree angles often produces a series of astonishingly distinct pictures.[74] My contention is that the "camera" is a hypothesis of this sort and can be used successfully to expose pertinent features of visual texts.[75] It may well be, however, that modes of discourse other than classical narrative demand different norms or reading procedures and thus will solicit labels other than, say, establishing shot, follow shot, reaction shot, cutaway, point-of-view shot, and so forth. This does not mean that we are all becoming more skilled and sophisticated as readers but, rather, that the rules of language — the conditions of intelligibility for a community — are sure to change and that this change will be correlated with a change in the social situation. The key question concerns what we choose to do with the word "camera," including its metaphorical extension into the other arts. Indeed, theorists speak confidently of a type of literary point of view called "the camera" and refer to a type of verbal

FIGURE 3.2   A Comparison of Eight Conceptions of the Camera

Major Conceptions of the Camera	Theory of Narrative Meaning: How Are Present Entities Related to Absent Entities?	One Favored Camera Technique	One Major Value of Narrativity for Society	One Major Principle for the Writing of a History of Narrative
1. Camera as Origin of a Sensory Display (A Machine)	Illusion (e.g., of depth)	Kinetic Depth	Hallucinatory Involvement	Edison, Griffith (vs. Lumière, Méliès)
2. Camera as Sensory (or Material) Form	Defamiliarization	Unmotivated Camera	Art as Social and Political Tool	Pressure from an Avant-garde
3. Camera as Recorder of the Profilmic (An Act of Pointing)	Casual: the Physics of Light Rays ⎫ Bazinian Theory	Deep Focus (Objective Camera)	Reproduction of Visible, Unobtrusive Reality	Lumière (vs. Méliès)
4. Camera as Agent for a Postfilmic Viewing Situation	Perceiver Sees A as He or She Would See B (subjunctive conditional) ⎭	Lateral Depth of Field	Reproduction of Human Perception at Work	Renoir, Welles; Neorealism
5. Camera as Expressive of Bodily and Mental States	Intention	Subjective Camera	Celebration of the Individual and the Inner World	The Auteur
6. Camera as Channel for Communication	Casual: Signal Transmission	Personification of the Camera (= narrator's presence objectified)	Information (and information about information = reflexivity)	Art Cinema
7. Camera as Phantasy	Unconscious Mechanisms	Visualization of Dream-Thought ("representability")	Visual Pleasure and the Dynamic of the Repressed	Classical Cinema
8. Camera as Semantic Label or Reading Hypothesis	Symbol	?	The World as Narrative Text	Types of Reference: Filmic and Nonfilmic Codes; Reading Procedures

narration as "showing."[76] If theorists such as Metz are correct that film is symbolic, rule-governed, and a language, then the camera metaphor exploited by literary theorists becomes much less contrived or metaphorical and more an important insight into how we handle information when we think.

Today the camera seems to be neither a machine nor an invisible witness recording facts of the world but, rather, an aspect of a collective subjectivity — a name for how we ourselves are talking and thinking about cinema at a particular time for a particular purpose (see summary in figure 3.2). As a collective subjectivity, the camera's status fluctuates in the twilight area between material object and interpretive subject, between world and language. According to Metz, "[T]he cinema is at once a weak and a robust mechanism: like the human body, like a precision tool, like a social institution. And the fact is that it is really all of these at the same time."[77]

The notion of a "camera," then, seems to depend finally upon how the members of a community *agree* to confront the nature of physical existence, including the materiality of the human body, through language. As a consequence, any project that attempts to recast the history of film narrative, and the social values narrativity serves, must at the same time rethink how we have used the term "camera" to cover a machine, a social institution, and the human will, all at once.

Chapter 4: How Frame Lines (and Film Theory) Figure

"I am not saying [that the word 'good'] has four or five different meanings. It is used in different contexts because there is a transition between similar things called 'good,' a transition which continues, it may be, to things which bear no similarity to earlier members of the series. We *cannot* say 'If we want to find out the meaning of "good" let's find what all cases of good have in common.' They may not have anything in common. The reason for using the word 'good' is that there is a continuous transition from one group of things called good to another."[1]

— Ludwig Wittgenstein

"Let me float a large, somewhat nebulous proposal: that the majority of essays in the humanities have as their primary methodological orientation an interest in complexity and ambiguity. A plurality of texts describe cultural locations, practices, identities, and objects as hybrid, mixed, impure, marginal, dislocated, disoriented, Creole, Pidgin, transcultural, liminal, meta-, para-, quasi-, or otherwise complex and ambiguous. The pleasure of the text is produced by the very focus on hybridity, mixture, and other kinds of irreducible complexity as much as by whatever other insights are gained into the cultural locations, practices, and so forth, that are the texts' nominal subjects.

"To the extent that this is generally true, the commonest rhetorical strategy in recent scholarship is to demonstrate a state of unexpected complexity or a pitch of ambiguity that cannot be reduced to simpler schemata."[2]

— James Elkins

"[A] realist aesthetic and an expressionist aesthetic are hard to merge. . . . The art cinema seeks to solve the problem [of merging the two aesthetics] in a sophisticated way: by the device of *ambiguity*. The art film is nonclassical in that it foregrounds deviations from the classical norm — there are certain gaps and problems. But these very deviations are *placed*, resituated as realism (in life things happen this way) or authorial commentary (the ambiguity is symbolic). Thus the art film solicits a particular reading procedure: Whenever confronted with a problem in causation, temporality, or spatiality, we first seek realistic motivation. (Is a character's mental state causing the uncertainty? Is life just leaving loose ends?) If we're thwarted, we next seek authorial motivation. (What is being 'said' here? What significance justifies the violation of the norm?) Ideally, the film hesitates, suggesting character subjectivity, life's untidiness, and author's vision. Whatever is excessive in one category must belong to another. Uncertainties persist but are understood as such, as *obvious* uncertainties, so to speak. Put crudely, the slogan of the art cinema might be, 'When in doubt, read for maximum ambiguity.'"[3]

— David Bordwell

WORLD, LANGUAGE, AMBIGUITY

Does the world dictate language or does language dictate a world? Does the real-world existence of a cat and mat motivate the words, "the cat sat on the mat," complete with definite articles? That is, does the world give rise to things we need to say? Or, instead, does a human conceptual scheme bring into existence (express) a specific sort of world, making prominent only certain kinds of actions, qualities, categories, resemblances, and relations? Do our habitual actions create a language that makes familiar a world? Consider, for example, the worlds that might be produced through conceptual schemes that contain the following words:

beauty, charmonium, number, permission, value, ennui, mnemon, hippogriff, unobtanium, absence, nondescript, freedom, estoppel, balance, possibility, beguine, combustible, phagocytes, phlogiston, normal, irony, privacy, time wasted, coalescence date, splinter bid, iatrogenic cause, spacetime foam, stream-ripping software.

Posed in this manner, the basic question does not have an answer. The alternatives, as it were, are too far apart (one world, many worlds). To make progress on this question one needs to explore the causal interactions that *mediate* between a strict realism and a strong relativism. One needs to examine in greater detail the cognitive systems and mental representations involved in fashioning *descriptions* that are intermediate between world and language comprehension. How we choose to characterize a thing has an effect on how we see the world, feel, speak, and act.

A similar quandary arises concerning the relationship of "story" and "style." Does a particular story naturally give rise to a form of expression or does expression alone create a vision that defines a unique story world? Other aesthetic oppositions that seem to be intractable in the same way include story/discourse, content/form, and material/meaning.[4] F. Elizabeth Hart has argued persuasively that there is a vast middle ground of methodologies between the extremes of realism and relativism that can illuminate aesthetic issues.[5] She argues that a second-generation cognitive science based not on logical computation or fixed structure but on figural, embodied, emotive, and ecological processes is able to address some of the intricacies of how a person thinks about self and environment in mediated, adaptive ways. In the field of film and media studies, Torben Grodal has employed this kind of approach, which he calls "ecological conventionalism," to systematically reconfigure basic problems of theory and analysis.[6] Grodal's admirable work has begun to fill in the gaps between the extremes of realism and relativism.

One aspect of "realism" is its use by critics as an *analytical concept* for isolating a particular experience of a spectator. In a careful analysis, Grodal identifies eleven types of "realism" said to be prevalent in audiovisual representations. He finds that the term "realism" is "used in many different ways, causing ambiguity or inconsistency in [its] meaning."[7] He also considers the relationship of realism to a postmodern skepticism and relativism. It is in this spirit that I would like to examine another term used by critics: "frame." The word "frame" is central to our vocabulary of viewing. It is, however, an ambiguous word and may be used in many inconsistent ways. Grodal declares, "'Frame' is a word with many meanings and functions." He reviews five main cognitive processes implicated in the word "frame."[8] This multiplicity will pose a problem for persons writing about film or those reading film criticism. Nevertheless, what I wish to concentrate on is a different side of "ambiguity": the fact that ambiguity may be convenient, disguised, and deeply constitutive of the way we are able to think and use language, and of the way we live in the world and watch film.[9]

I believe that the more closely one looks at film, the more closely one is looking at *why* one watches film[10] and how one *talks about*, and revises, the memory of what has been experienced.[11] A spectator's experience of film is much more than what is seen and heard on the screen. Watching a film requires a spectator to make judgments moment by moment and to actively construct models of locale and agency using folk knowledge, expectations, wishes, inferences, heuristics, scripts, metaphors, social schemata, and numerous forms of memory. Because film plays within the mind and not simply on the screen, the analyst must attend to the way a spectator uses language to encode his or her responses. With what vocabulary do we watch and to what purpose? I suggest that a critical vocabulary, even when systematized, is not always designed to be exact and unequivocal (a "realist" language) but sometimes is meant to be ambiguous and flexible in order to better fit the desire to watch, participate, shape, speak, commend, and transform (a "relativist" language).[12]

In what follows I want to demonstrate the ambiguity of the concept of frame as it appears in critical discourse.[13] What are the sources of its ambiguity? How is the concept of frame designed to function in our talk? What are the implications for constructing a film theory? But first, the notion of ambiguity is ambiguous!

Linguists have distinguished several kinds of ambiguity, two of which are homonymy and polysemy.[14] In the case of homonymy, two words spelled in the same way possess unrelated, or at least very distant, meanings (thus, separate lexical entries):

1. She withdrew money from the *bank*.
2. She was fishing in the river from the *bank*.

1. The dog's bite is worse than its *bark*.
2. The tree's leaves are lighter than its *bark*.

1. She *saw* a *saw* on the workbench and
   recalled the old *saw* about not putting off
   work that can be done today.

By contrast, in polysemy a word has distinct, though related, meanings, or at least meanings that are fairly close (thus, a single lexical entry):

1. She bought the *newspaper*.
2. The editor was fired by the *newspaper*.

1. He broke the *bottle* [container].
2. The baby finished the *bottle* [contents].

1. The man *ran* into the woods.
2. The road *ran* into the woods.
3. The argument *ran* into the night.
4. The voice-over *ran* into the scene.

1. Cephalus recited to Socrates the old saw of *like* to *like*.

In this book I will discuss only polysemy and will treat a polysemous word as opening onto a special type of category that George Lakoff calls a "radial" category — that is, a category in which ambiguous meanings of a word are linked, creating, as Wittgenstein says, "a continuous transition" from one group of things to another

group of things with the same name.[15] Incidentally, the word
"open" just used is dazzling in its polysemy, as is the word "figure"
in the title of this chapter, as well as the word "good" mentioned
by Wittgenstein in the epigraph (i.e., "good" may describe a film,
a breeze, a concept, a friend, a car, a road, a memory, a meal, a
conversation, a scolding, a color, a generalization, a time, a voice,
a pencil, a hand, a reason, a beginning . . .). Because the word
"open" functions in many cases as the opposite of "frame," we
should expect it to be polysemous. "Open" may apply, for example,
to a door, book, text, eyes, personality ("he is an open book"),
mind, road, country, economy, doubt, and future.

Radial meanings are important to analyze because they are
intimately connected to the way in which we confront and describe
familiar, everyday situations and solve ordinary problems. Radial
meanings help organize our memory and are part of imagination
— that is, "visualization" in the broadest sense. Although any
given situation is unique, the links among radial meanings provide
"a continuous transition" from one group of things to another based
on a set of preexisting analogies. This allows a given situation to be
described as being part of a series of past and possible future events. As
Lakoff emphasizes, however, radial meanings are neither predictable
from a core meaning (because as a whole they fail to have relevant
common properties, a collective essence) nor are they the result of
a series of arbitrary conventions, but something *in between* — a
motivated convention based on living within a community and sharing
a way of life.[16] Radial meanings are an embarrassment to Objectivist
(nonembodied, "realist") theories of meaning and rationality as well
as an embarrassment to certain philosophical tenets. According to
Mark Johnson, polysemy is one of seven fundamental challenges to
'metaphysical and epistemological' realism.[17]

SOME RADIAL MEANINGS OF "FRAME"

I will now list and briefly discuss fifteen different, though related,
ways of employing the word "frame" in discussions about film.

Although typical, these ways do not exhaust the possibilities. In the remainder of the chapter I will weigh the implications of the polysemy of "frame" for how we think generally in the cinema and how we build theories of cinema.

1. The frame is the *real edge* of an image on the screen that has resulted from limits imposed on celluloid inside a physical camera and projector so that, for example, a projected image can be said to be "in frame" or "out of frame" on the screen.[18] A spectator, however, is not really seeing an actual edge. The edge of an image onscreen is not the edge of an individual exposed frame from inside a film camera but, at least, a composite edge that is made up of a number of exposed frames, because in watching a film a spectator does not see each individual frame halted on the screen as if a series of slides were being shown.

2. The frame is the *subjective contour* or illusory border of an image that is projected by a spectator. A subjective contour is not inferred or imaginary but, rather, is an *explicit* visual feature to which specialized neurons respond in a particular cortical area of the visual system. Thus, when a dark object appears on the screen, but far from the center of the image, a spectator will see the dark object as being partially cut off at a certain point by a "straight line," which will be seen to be continuous with other, brighter straight line segments, the sum of which will form a luminous rectangle that will be said to "frame" the entire image. That is, there need not be an actual line through the dark object; a spectator's perceptual system will fill in the "line" and make it "straight" so that the dark object will be seen to be separated from the equally dark surround, which lies beyond the border of the image. Notice in this case that the "frame" of straight line segments is experienced as being *overlaid* on the image so that the image is being cut off at the sides. From this conception of framing comes the expectation that at a later time, when an object or "frame line" moves, we will be able to see *more* of what was blocked.

3. The frame is the *gestalt form* of an image that makes it appear as a rectangular whole because of principles of good continuation and closure. The "outer" frame acts to bias such internal relations as figure-ground organization and proximity groupings. Sometimes, however, the word "frame" refers not to the outer framework of edges or lines but to the entire (gestalt) "background" of the image relative to a foreground plane or object. Framework and background may become confused in this manner because for some cases the movement of either the framework or the background or both produces the identical percept (induced motion in an object).

4. The frame is the *shape* of an object or group of objects seen outlined inside an image. For example, a "vase" on a table will be seen as framed by a distinctive shape as well as by the top of the table and background curtains. Note that a framing "edge" of an object is defined simply by an abrupt perceptual change — a difference or contrast — in either the illumination or the colors of adjacent regions, whereas a framing "line," in addition to having two "edges," possesses extension (length) and thus can be used to build a figure within an image (e.g., a vase). Furthermore, since *contrast* between edges is at its greatest intensity when edges occur in the same plane, a series of frame lines that are composed on the flat screen of a film or on the canvas of a painting offers more striking contrasts than do frames dispersed in multiple planes (i.e., dispersed in three dimensions) on a theater stage or in real life.[19] Also these sorts of frame lines may be widened into a "margin" or "verge."

5. The frame is the overall *composition* of an image, its disposition and balance of figures, forms, colors, lighting, angle, perspective, focus (in several senses), movements, and subspaces. When one speaks of the "framing" or "misframing" of a shot, one has in mind the composition of the shot in relation to a convention or expectation. A simple example of "framing" in this sense would be a shot that shows an image within the frame of a mirror on a wall, or a shot that frames a doorway that frames a view (e.g., the shot that frames the land of Oz

in color through the doorway of Dorothy's dingy farmhouse), or a view over a cliff edge that frames a valley below. Much study has been devoted to various "principles" of composition in the belief that the arrangement of shape, color, and movement can clarify and intensify the meaning of an object or facial expression.[20] The composition, or some element of the composition (e.g., sharp focus, a spotlight, moving light, or distinctive color), may then be said to "frame" or bracket the object or face.[21] Note that shot composition is dependent on viewpoint, whereas, for example, the framing of a "scene" is independent of any one, or all, of the spatial viewpoints presented through the shots (cf. definition 11).

6. The frame is the *totality* of the two-dimensional *area* of an image as well as the totality of the *three-dimensional space* represented by an image (e.g., a storyboard panel or a film frame that depicts a locale).

7. The frame is the *physicality* of what surrounds an image — i.e., the materiality of a screen and perhaps the auditorium itself, like the wooden frame or museum that holds a painting.

8. The frame is the *implicit rationale* for the seeing of an image. When the rationale for the presence of an image is stated metaphorically in terms of everyday situations of viewing, one might think not of an auditorium, but of a window in a house or train or the view from an amusement park ride. If the observer is imagined to be walking, then one might think of a doorway that allows a spectator to "enter" the fictional scene or to become a strolling, nineteenth-century *flâneur* who encounters transient and haphazard, everyday situations,[22] or instead one might think of someone walking toward a destination with a definite purpose in mind, which would produce impressions of the journey quite different from those of a *flâneur*. The gestalt figure-ground of definition 3 above has been transformed into a figure now walking on ground. Moreover, if one were to replace the "glass" in the metaphorical window with other kinds of optics, one would be able to construct additional rationales for the

105

seeing of film (as film theorists have done) based on analogies with such instruments as the camera obscura, camera lucida, concave mirror, microscope, telescope, periscope, and kaleidoscope (the last of which is useful for explaining distortions and changes in a visual field).

To elaborate a few variations of the standard metaphor of a viewer in front of a window, framing in film might be likened to (i) what is witnessed *through* the frame of the "window," or to (ii) what is seen to be constrained and *shaped* by the frame of the "window" (cf. 4 above), or — when the window becomes partially fogged or else light wanes with the coming of "twilight" — to (iii) what is *reflected* in the window as a "mirror," namely, the person who tries to look and/or the world of the person who tries to look.[23] Furthermore, if the "window-as-a-mirror" is reversed so that its mirrored surface faces away from the viewer (functioning as a one-way glass to conceal the viewer from sight), then the viewer becomes a perfect voyeur who (iv) subjects everyday life to observation or close *inspection* with the result that what is seen acquires a new dimension, an 'excessive' quality or 'aura.' As Wittgenstein notes, "To observe is not the same thing as to look at or to view."[24]

Siegfried Kracauer's film theory is an example of how framing may be likened to the act of carefully observing or inspecting everyday life through, in effect, one-way glass. Kracauer argues that "physical existence" may be established through film not only by *recording* (i.e., in effect, by simply looking at or viewing something through the window) but also by *revealing* "things normally unseen," such as "the familiar" (the overlooked, the taken-for-granted) as well as "the refuse" (garbage and sewer grates, i.e., the normally lost and discarded 'details' of a shot or scene). Another "blind spot of the mind" that film framing may reveal through active inspection is what Kracauer calls "unconventional complexes": "The motion picture camera has a way of disintegrating familiar objects and bringing to the fore

— often just in moving about — previously invisible interrelationships between parts of them." Also, "normally unseen" is the "transient": "It may be anticipated that the street in the broadest sense of the word is a place where impressions of this kind are bound to occur."[25] Kracauer's invocation of the "street" in this context reminds us that the metaphor of a viewer looking through the window of a building has a radial connection to someone who is walking through town (i.e., the window, in effect, is now moving).

Kracauer's approach to "things normally unseen" is reminiscent of Walter Benjamin's notion of "unconscious optics." Benjamin begins by saying that Freud's book *The Psychopathology of Everyday Life* is relevant to film: "This book isolated and made analyzable things which had heretofore floated along unnoticed in the broad stream of perception." (Notice the metaphoric use of the verb "floated," which suggests something hidden beneath a surface while presuming also that 'time' is like a river.) In the book Freud offers an analysis of things normally unseen even though public — unseen because the behavior that is being observed appears in the guise of a simple 'mistake' in doing something that normally a person has the ability to do. Freud argued that careful inspection would show that such a 'mistake' might well be tied to unconscious processes.[26]

In all four cases of the frame as a window (i–iv above), keen judgment may be required to separate (i) what is seen through the glass (perhaps darkly) from the influence of (ii) whatever lies unseen beyond the frame as well as from (iii) what is 'partly reflected' *on* the window or from (iv) what appears on closer inspection to be only a symptom of "things normally *un*seen." That is, critical judgment may be required to interpret diverse 'hidden and mixed traces' within the window's visible display in order to discover an appropriate rationale for seeing what should be seen. The significance of what 'should be seen' may appear initially to be ambiguous, implicit, suppressed, or involuntarily repressed within the (merely) visible. The task of a critic is to teach a spectator how to perceive what is really on the screen, for the measure remains the *visible*: what is 'unseen' is still *contained within* the seen. (Shortly we will investigate the nature of a 'container' metaphor.)

Not all film theories develop analogies based on everyday situations of viewing or on container metaphors. Sergei Eisenstein insists that a spectator will experience successive images in a film as appearing not *next* to each other in a linear flow on the screen (as pieces of a larger picture) but, rather, on *top* of each other in a dialectical collision.[27] This illustrates how Eisenstein's film theory is not built upon analogies with ordinary situations of looking at (framing) something while standing, riding, walking, or using an optical instrument.

9. The frame is the *view* that is given on a fictive action from within the diegesis. Examples: a point-of-view shot that frames a character's view; an eyeline match; a dream sequence; a subjective flashback; an expressive angle or external focaliza- tion (revealing a character's "frame of mind"); and a camera reframe (recentering a character). Gerald Mast analyzes how the dynamic flux of a character's changing state of mind is conveyed in Chaplin's *Easy Street* (1917) by the character's movements toward and away from the frame edges, and concludes that "the cinema frame, like the fun house mirror, achieves its magical fun because it has edges and borders that are not so much physical boundaries as psychological limits and barriers to visual perception."[28] Jean Mitry argues that characters' movements, camera movements, and contin- ual changes of shot tend to make the spectator "forget the 'frame.'" Mitry adds, "Thus if everything contrives to make us forget the frame as such, everything contrives at the same time to make us feel its effects."[29] Mitry has it both ways, whereas Bazin would have us forget the frame in favor of a photographic and phenomenal "realism" (e.g., through con- tinuous sweeping camera movements that create a "lateral

depth of field"[30]) while Eisenstein, Arnheim, and Burch would have us remember the frame as an antidote to "realism."[31]

I would like to explore briefly a special case of framing a character's view. If the identity of the character who has the view becomes problematic in some way, or the character somehow becomes "absent" from his or her point-of-view shot, then what remains of the "subjectivity" is merely its framing, which is now seen as enigmatic, fragmented, de-centered, alienated, uncanny, liminal, or empty in some measure.[32] This produces a partially unanchored framing or "semi-disconnected" point of view within the film. The "art cinema" — as discussed by Bordwell in the epigraph — is one type of film practice that focuses precisely on these sorts of ambiguous and uncertain (character) states of being in a world.[33] These states are depicted at a remove from everyday actions that exist in a present and immediate, but fleeting time.

Torben Grodal has argued that the art cinema strives for an effect of "high art" by seeking to represent that which seems permanent and permanently out of ordinary time (something "higher," a soul, a true identity). Grodal shows how art cinema depicts oblique meaning, abstraction, possibility, recurrent memory, unusual mental states, disembodiment, and transcendence in conjunction with unmotivated dissections of perceptual flux through "difficult" stylistic exercises, obscure editing, and *temps mort*. In addition, Grodal argues that the art cinema aims to evoke negatively colored emotions cut off from familiar objects and specific situations, such as euphoric and lyrical experiences, the sublime, melancholia, nostalgia, pleasure-in-pain, ambivalence, and estrangement.[34] The various effects of such metaphysical "high art" are valued by scholars in the humanities, as Elkins contends in the epigraph. It may be that scholars are drawn to these forms of ambiguity and difficulty, even when weighing the products of visual culture generally, because of their search for a middle ground between realism and relativism, where seeing the value of an artwork demands special skills and sensibilities that lie between an uninformative realism and a self-indulgent relativism.

10. The frame is the *rhetorical figure* that interprets or bears upon a situation. Examples: a metaphorical image (for example, in the metaphor, "man is a wolf," "wolf" frames "man"),[35] a musical cue used as foreshadowing, a repeated shot used for emphasis, an eccentric camera angle or position, and an unmotivated, wandering camera.

11. The frame is the *scene* that provides an overall context for describing or encapsulating various separate actions that together make up an unfolding event. A scene represents knowledge that is always more than what appears on the screen at a given moment, and more even than the sum of all the shot-fragments relating to the event because there are always elements "off-screen" that are never shown but are presupposed by the action. Some of these unseen elements are a direct consequence of the framing onscreen.[36] Here are a few examples of how a scene frames an event for a plot: an establishing shot (frames the location of the event and, in effect, poses the question "What is important about this locale?"); a reaction shot (frames a character with an attitude toward a series of actions); a match on action (frames a movement); crosscutting (frames two related movements); a detail shot (highlights an important object within a causal chain); a retrospective match (reframes in a different light what has already been seen);[37] and sound perspective (frames the position of a sound source within a locale). Characters, too, may "make a scene," for example, a character whose emotional reaction to an event is insincere or hysterical or who "frames" a person for a crime that he or she did not commit (as in *Who Framed Roger Rabbit*, Robert Zemeckis, 1988).

12. The frame is the *narrative structure* (narrative framework) that contains or embeds various parts of a story. Examples: a prologue (frames the story to come); a frame story (a story about the story); foreshadowing (frames a future event); suspense (something we learn that a character doesn't know

frames our response to the character's actions); implied authorial commentary (frames an attitude to the story); a nonsubjective flashback (the past as a frame for the present); closure (reframes the beginning of the story); and voice-over (frames one or more scenes).

13. The frame is the *narration* or discourse that produces a story (i.e., produces a series of linked events and scenes as "evidence" for an argument about how things go together). Sometimes it is said that narration takes the form of either "showing" or "telling," or some other vaguely personified or apostrophized form, such as observing, participating, searching, or experiencing.[38] In general, the narration may be characterized by a *set of principles* (which may be implicit or inconsistent) that act, for example, to select, organize, restrict, obstruct, fragment, deform, censor, abstract, condense, magnify, revise, correct, substitute, exclude, communicate, emphasize, transpose, link, unify, and/or confer duration on elements of a plot in relation to a story.[39] Several "levels" of narration may be operating simultaneously or sequentially where each level acts to regulate (frame, restrict) a spectator's access to a kind of information. Consider, for example, the many types of character knowledge to which we may have access through different levels of narration, through different "cameras" (9 above).

Note, in particular, that when a film *excludes* something in the narration, what is being "framed" is the fact that something is *not* being framed, whether or not a spectator may notice a gap at the time. A simple example is the discreet pan away from lovers, but there are many other complex and subtle moments of framing what is not being framed. Classical narrative, for instance, makes use of *concealed* forms of foreshadowing that can be recognized only in retrospect. The narration tries to lie as little as possible so that a spectator will not blame a duplicitous narration, but only himself or herself for failing to see the truth sooner.[40]

A camera angle that provides the so-called "perfect" or "ideal" view is strictly relative to the plot (and to other angles) and is, at best, only momentary because there are many secrets that must be kept while narrating. A "perfect" or "ideal" view may be combined with certain other discursive principles and then embodied in the form of an "invisible observer." In effect, one has taken a specific kind of narration and created the invisible observer as a "downstream" metaphor (by projecting 13 onto 8 or 9). The new metaphor, however, leads some writers to begin speculating about the nature of the personality and thoughts of the invisible observer and about whether it is really possible for a spectator to see through "its invisible eyes" or to move instantly through space at each shot. But is this any way to treat a metaphor? To literalize it? Do we treat *fictions* in this manner or characters? By mistreating metaphors and frames, and striving to be ever more exact, we forget the many different ways we may speak and be, make meanings and act. Moreover, one shouldn't forget that film theories, often criticized for being remote and metaphorical, can also be too literal-minded.[41]

14. The frame is the general *psychic state* or disposition that undergirds a spectator's emotions while watching a film. Examples: identification (i.e., not just "looking at" a character, but also "looking after" him or her); narcissism and misrecognition (*méconnaissance*) that lead to the process of identification; fetishistic scopophilia; fantasy; masquerade; dream processes (e.g., Petric's claim that Tarkovsky's "elimination of the image's borders" is meant to fashion an "obfuscated peripheral vision" characteristic of dream); self-conscious and reflexive framing; emotional buffer frames (Grodal); displacement; disframing (Heath); deframing (Metz); and the double framing of the blot (Žižek).[42] For psychoanalytic theories of the psyche, explicit or conscious meanings may possess a radical *ambiguity* because they may appear in a "distorted form" in relation to their sources in the unconscious (distorted, for example, by defense mechanisms and repression).

15. The frame is the relevant subset of our *world knowledge* that is presupposed by a story and/or applied to a story by a spectator. "World knowledge" provides a context or set of background assumptions used for comprehension and interpretation. In general, a spectator is confronted at every moment by the problem of deciding *which few ones* of the countless inferences that may be drawn from an image are *relevant* for the occasion.[43] The total number of such inferences is enormous because the number of *categories* and *aspects* that may be attributed to an image, and to its placement within a sequence and context, is enormous. One might go further still to speak of the knowledge associated with *possible* worlds.[44] From the strict "realism" of definition 1, we have now arrived at a definition amenable to several versions of "relativism." How is it, exactly, that the world is to be "known" through a "frame"? Which frame? Which world?

Daniel Dennett offers a definition of frame based on 'world knowledge': "We can understand a frame to be a finite subset of data, a window on an indefinitely larger world of further data."[45] For Dennett, a frame gives rise to diverse kinds of data or information *patterns*. Dennett explores a range of patterns that may arise from a given frame, including simple visual patterns (cf. the gestalt laws of definition 3), more complex visual patterns (as suggested by his use above of the metaphor "window"; cf. definition 8), and such nonvisual patterns as a belief structure or intentional stance (cf. definitions 13, 14, and 15). Dennett shows that there is a deep connection between a frame and the many patterns of physical, symbolic, and bodily information that emerge from it. The patterns, however, are neither reducible to a single, underlying objective pattern that might be exposed through analytical dissection, nor are the patterns completely arbitrary as if they were merely a collection of different points of view. Dennett argues persuasively, I believe, for an intermediate, "mild realism" that avoids the extremes of realism and relativism.[46]

Richard Rorty argues for a description of 'world knowledge' that is somewhat more radical than Dennett's. The following is Rorty's account of how multiple contexts, and myriad kinds of world knowledge, may be used in a capricious manner by Western intellectuals:

> From an ethico-political angle, however, one can say that what is characteristic, not of the human species but merely of its most advanced, sophisticated subspecies — the well-read, tolerant, conversable inhabitant of a free society — is the desire to dream up as many new contexts as possible. This is the desire to be as polymorphous in our adjustments as possible, to recontextualize for the hell of it. This desire is manifested in art and literature more than in the natural sciences, and so I find it tempting to think of our culture as an increasingly poeticized one, and to say that we are gradually emerging from the scientism which [Charles] Taylor dislikes into something else, something better. But, as a good antiessentialist, I have no deep premises to draw on from which to infer that it is, in fact, better — nor to demonstrate our own superiority over the past, or the non-Western present. All I can do is recontextualize various developments in philosophy and elsewhere so as to make them look like stages in a story of poeticizing and progress.[47]

Rorty's 'any-context-whatever' (within the moral framework he adopts) has a strange affinity to the other extreme in which impressions are said to emanate from the world *prior* to any context or frame (cf. definition 1). As an example of the latter, consider Stan Brakhage's utopian reverie:

> Imagine an eye unruled by man-made laws of perspective, an eye unprejudiced by compositional logic, an eye which does not respond to the name of everything but which must know each object encountered in life through an adventure of perception. How many colors are there in a field of grass to the crawling baby unaware of "Green?" How many rainbows can light create for the untutored eye? How aware of variations in heat waves

can that eye be? Imagine a world alive with incomprehensible objects and shimmering with an endless variety of movement and innumerable gradations of color. Imagine a world before the "beginning was the word."[48]

Genuine art in Brakhage's view has the potential, at least momentarily, to break us free of all compartments and containers, whereas the view Rorty sketches traps us inside an endless maze of compartments. Neither the multiframe nor frameless approach can locate a privileged, unqualified frame for our 'awareness' of the world by finding an anchor in 'thought alone.' In the following sections, I will argue that a better understanding of the radial nature of 'frame' must include the 'body.' The nature of the 'body' will provide an anchor for at least some forms of thought and action.

HOW DO WE THINK IN THE CINEMA?

How do we make judgments while watching a film? Where is "interpretation" to be located? What defines the uniqueness of the film medium: Is it a material? An expression? Is the "three-dimensional" space of an image illusory? (What is real, what is not, in film?) I believe that when a critic settles on a particular radial meaning of "frame" as the most important and "literal" meaning, he or she will discover already in place a theory of film that addresses these questions along with a special rhetoric for employing the word "frame." For this reason I believe that a "theory of film" may be thought of as *the grammar of an ensemble of words*, such as frame, shot, camera, point of view, editing, style, realism, auteur, performance, spectatorship, and medium specificity, accompanied by selected radial extensions of these words. I believe that a film theory is not simply a set of objective propositions about film, because "film" — that is, the grammar (the vocabulary) of the words that describe film — is not fixed but is tied to culture, value, and a consensus about, for example, the present boundaries of the medium (i.e., the properties we select that presently interest us relating to the materials of the medium) as well as the present ideas that are used 'to clarify our experience of film.'[49] What we think of as cinema comes from the uses we make of our thinking.

As an illustration of the grammatical nature of film theory, consider the role of *intentionality* in film — that is, questions about which agents are responsible for which acts in a film (an author, narrator, character, spectator . . .). It will be found that the acts attributed to an agent depend on which of the radial meanings is chosen as a frame of reference. Consider the first meaning of frame above — that is, where the frame is defined relative to the *real edge* of an image on the screen resulting from limits imposed on celluloid inside a physical camera. Thinking in this way, the primary agent will be the cameraman (standing in for the auteur) while the spectator plays little or no role. Similarly, in the second meaning of frame above (i.e., where the frame is experienced as superimposed onto the image, blocking out parts of what can be seen), it seems natural to think that someone (an auteur) has made a decision to show one particular thing while excluding all else. These two ways of thinking emphasize the material reality of film production (a realism, a historical fact) while also connecting the frame to ideas of "planning" and "contrivance." In other uses of the word "frame," however, the spectator will assume a more significant role, ranging from ordinary ways of looking and moving (e.g., 7–9 above) to forms of narrative reasoning (e.g., 12–13) to nonconscious perceiving (a relativism, e.g., 14–15).[50] Notice that while a frame may be literally *rectangular* in definition 1, it is being projected by definitions 2–15 into numerous other "rectangular" shapes as well as non-geometric shapes.

One shouldn't think that the act of framing is confined to visible and/or visual aspects of imagery. Sound can frame. The sound track can make an object visible by directing our attention to it; a sound can portray the extent and qualities of a locale; a sound can express an aural point of view; a sound can refer to an object offscreen; a sound can summon visual experiences; a sound can rhetorically frame meanings; a sound can invoke a motive, an emotion, and world knowledge; and so forth. Furthermore, all films (including silent films) must embody an aural rationale that frames how each sound *can be heard* (for example, cf. 8).[51] A frame may be visible or audible, and either type may produce a visual or aural frame in mind.

Roughly speaking, I would say that uses of the word "frame" in ways 1–7 draw mostly upon processes of "bottom-up" perception while ways 8–15 draw mostly upon processes of "top-down" perception.[52] Uses of the word "frame" falling in the middle of the list (7, 8, 9) reflect so-called "basic-level categories" as opposed to "subordinate" and "superordinate" categories (lower- and higher-numbered definitions, respectively). Basic-level categories reflect phenomena that are experienced as concrete and "real" through bodily based processes (e.g., gestalt perception, mental imagery, and motor interaction). A basic-level category is the highest level at which a single mental image can represent an entire category. For example, an expert will be able to visualize the subordinate categories, "brown-capped chickadee," "reticulated giraffe," and "Indian paintbrush," but even an expert cannot visualize such superordinate categories as "vertebrate," which includes birds (and flightless ones like the Calayan rail), mammals, fishes, and reptiles; or "trash fish," which includes many fish species; or "plant," which includes trees, vines, shrubs, fruits, vegetables, and flowers. One may easily visualize such basic-level categories as "chair" and "car," but not the superordinate categories, "furniture" and "vehicle." Basic-level categorization of objects, actions, emotions, social groups, and so on is one of the far-reaching discoveries of a second-generation cognitive science.[53] It is also a key concept in Torben Grodal's fundamental rethinking of the nature of art cinema. Grodal argues that art cinema works to transcend online, transient body states (basic-level) in favor of permanent, higher meanings (superordinate emotions and oblique meanings). Art cinema fosters ambiguity and uncertainty by employing unusual stylistic devices to fragment the diegetic world (basic-level) into an impenetrable, subdiegetic environment (subordinate-level) that challenges and dissects basic embodied existence and points toward "higher" truths in a supra-diegetic reality (superordinate-level).[54]

It is important to realize that when the frame is conceived as a *top-down principle* (in ways 8–15), the frame will not at all be *visible* in the same manner as an edge or subjective contour of an image (as in ways 1 and 2) because cognitive activities beyond the visual system will be required in order to make the effects of the frame appear on-screen. When thinking top-down, for example, it is natural to regard the *editing* of a film as being a kind of "frame" (especially in relation to ways 10–15). Furthermore, when thinking top-down, a single, continuous camera movement may be seen as discontinuous, as representing several narrations even though diegetic time remains continuous (e.g., Alfred Hitchcock's *Rope*, 1948). By contrast, thinking bottom-up about film (in ways 1–7) makes what appears on the screen seem "concrete" and distinct, suggesting a kind of "realism" composed of precise, subordinate categorization while, at the same time, making acts of interpretation seem abstract and secondary — a collection of arbitrary, upstream metaphors. A top-down approach, however, frames a type of viewing or intelligibility for a spectator that is neither directly on the screen in the form of "cues" nor tied to the time of presentation (projector time). In top-down thinking the shapes and colors appearing on screen will seem "abstract" and secondary, merely an illusion, imitation, form, description, symptom, or downstream metaphor of some *other*, more concrete, though invisible, reality in the world. Thus, thinking top-down suggests a kind of "relativism" composed of a stream of superordinate, nonvisual categorizations. The art cinema, in particular, strives to make what is on the screen seem ambiguous, uncertain, incomplete, empty, and/or illusory so as to provoke a (top-down) awareness of unseen and felt realities that exist in a supra-diegetic reality.

Sergei Eisenstein developed ideas about film by thinking both bottom-up and top-down, though he is most famous for advocating a "language" of film that is primarily a top-down process. Eisenstein urged that to understand cinema, one should avoid analogies with the visual arts, such as theater and painting, and instead think carefully about mental processes that are nonvisual such as language and emotion.[55] In the present age, where each new form of digital media provokes a frantic search for its unique features, I believe that the lessons of Eisenstein remain pertinent. One should be cautious about focusing too quickly on physical characteristics, technology, and typical operations of a medium at the expense of radial sorts of connections to other media — connections based on higher-order mental functions and tasks that may be selectively performed by a great many "older" media. The reality status of a new medium is relative.

It would be *good* to recall Wittgenstein's admonition: "One thinks that one is tracing the outline of the thing's nature over and over again, and one is merely tracing round the frame through which we look at it."[56] We often seem to find a new thing's nature only by forgetting how familiar are the methods and criteria used to define a particular kind of newness.

A ROLE FOR THE BODY — THE CONTAINER SCHEMA

I would now like to outline the nature of "frame" in terms of how we look at it as a mental procedure. This will point in a new direction toward the role the body plays in forming conceptual schemes that frame our "awareness" of the world. Gilles Deleuze asserts that the body's diverse reactions to an everyday world, including dreams, are crucial in fashioning the categories that we use to speak about and describe the world.

> "Give me a body then": this is the formula of philosophical reversal. The body is no longer the obstacle that separates thought from itself, that which [thought] has to overcome to reach thinking. [The body] is on the contrary that which [thought] plunges into or must plunge into, in order to reach the unthought, that is life. Not that the body thinks, but, obstinate and stubborn, it forces us to think, and forces us to think what is concealed from thought, life. Life will no longer be made to appear before the categories of thought; thought will be thrown into the categories of life. The categories of life are precisely the attitudes of the body, its postures. "We do not even know what a body can do": in its sleep, in its drunkenness, in its efforts and resistances. To think is to learn what a non-thinking body is capable of, its capacity, its postures. It is through the body (and no longer through the intermediary of the body) that cinema forms its alliance with the spirit, with thought. "Give me a body then" is first to mount the camera on an everyday body.[57]

How can one "mount the camera on an everyday body"? What could this mean? Deleuze's answer is intricate and lengthy, as suggested by his broad characterization of what the everyday body "can do . . . in its efforts and resistances." It will not be enough, for example, that a body can stand in front of a window (as in 8 above). Deleuze contends that "to think" is to learn about all the skills, states, and possibilities of the body as well as its failures (tiredness, waiting, despair, doubt, vertigo); the body is not a transparent window for the mind. I will take a somewhat different approach to this problem based on a second-generation cognitive science. My answer will be simpler, though perhaps more limited, than the one proposed by Deleuze. My starting point for connecting a camera's framing to "an everyday body" will be a concept drawn from cognitive psychology — the *container* image schema. As we shall see, this concept weaves together frame, body, the everyday, and mental procedures.

An "image schema" is much more *diagrammatic* and abstract than the image one encounters in film studies, which tends to be a detailed sort of mental picture with quasi-photographic features. An image schema in cognitive psychology represents only general structural features of a thing, not a particular thing or memory of a thing. One type of image schema is the "container" schema. It is a template that specifies the boundary conditions that divide something into a diagrammatic "inside-boundary-outside." It is one of the most powerful and pervasive *embodied* schemas used in recognizing patterns, solving problems, reasoning, explaining, and planning. An "embodied" schema is a nonconscious kinesthetic structure arising from *physical and bodily existence* (e.g., arising from our percepts, movements, and manipulation of objects). The range of bodily experiences also includes social norms that impinge on behavior and thought.[58] Thus, embodied schemas are neither "universal" nor "arbitrary" but are based on *typical* actions and feelings of the body in *typical* situations. Most important, an embodied schema, such as the container schema, may be extended by metaphors and metonymies into other realms (e.g., to kinds of framing in the realms of painting, theater, literature, and music, and to the emotions, as in the idea that "anger is the *heat* of a fluid in a container").[59] Indeed, the reason that polysemous meanings are radial — are related to one another — is because the meanings have been projected from a specific image schema through a series of metaphors and metonymies.[60]

The container schema (embodied, kinesthetic, nonconscious, and imagistic) underlies, for example, the way in which we imagine that objects are *inside* space, parts and qualities are inside objects, beliefs and memories are inside the mind, examples are inside categories, meanings are inside films, and ideas are conveyed in words even when innuendo is in a conversation. Moreover, we imagine a chair to be *in* the corner and in view, a glass to be in our hand, and orange juice to be both inside a glass and inside our bodies as we are in our clothes and in a mood inside a room, a car, a marriage, Denmark, and the Society for Cinema and Media Studies. Consider also this sentence: "Tell me a story to figure *out*, but leave *out* the minor details." That is, a given container encloses and excludes, and may be framed by other containers. Moreover, a container may be expanded metaphorically to produce new, more abstract containers. For example, our notion of framing in film may be expanded through analogies that make new sorts of containers out of the womb, Plato's cave, and unconscious subterranean tunnels, not to mention plot events as sugar coating on a pill, icing on a cake.

As a summary, I offer figure 4.1, which is a graphic representation of an *image schema* for the notion of "radial meaning," in which each of the individual boxes frames a single category of meaning based on a container schema while the set of boxes taken as a whole represents a single lexical entry (a set of related meanings) for a polysemous word.[61] I have been arguing, of course, that the word "frame," as used in film studies, is radial in meaning and, moreover, that each meaning of "frame" may itself have radial components created through a series of local metaphors, as in 8 above, in which a spectator is imagined to be standing in front of a window, walking, riding, or using an optical device. Container schemata variously structure our thinking within the 15 domains of framing in film. Although every frame encloses like a "container," what is "inside"

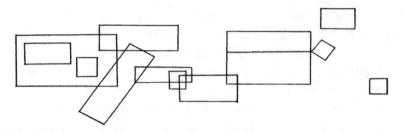

FIGURE 4.1   Radial Meaning

A graphic representation of an image schema for the notion of "radial meaning," in which each of the individual boxes frames a single category of meaning based on a container schema while the set of boxes taken as a whole represents a single lexical entry (a set of related meanings) for a polysemous word.

(the contents) and the nature of the "enclosure" (the criteria for the containing thing) are different for each of the 15 domains. The manner in which a container schema is applied to a domain will determine how inferences are drawn and conjectures made about what is framed. It also sets conditions for "breaking the frame," because one cannot mark an inside without imagining somewhere an outside.

To illustrate how the container schema may be applied to the act of framing, consider the "frame" when it is defined in terms of a "narration" (see 13 above). Figure 4.1 may then be interpreted as a distribution of narrations in a text in the form of a heterarchy rather than a hierarchy.[62] "Breaking the frame" of an individual subjective narration might then be accomplished through certain strategies of the art cinema (see discussion in 9 above). To take another example: When the "frame" is defined in terms of a "scene" composed of an edited sequence of shots (see 11 above), figure 4.1 may be interpreted as an unusual editing pattern that refuses to develop the scene as a simple hierarchy of spaces that illuminates an event at assorted scales. Nonanalytical editing schemes that generate a heterarchy have often been explored by the art cinema and demonstrate that editing, in general, need not be conceived as merely a series of embedded local juxtapositions but may include, for example, matches between shots 1 and 3, 5 and 2, 4 and 12.[63] To imagine editing as merely an immediate juxtaposition is to imagine that we have no memories other than the most recent and no schemata to frame our sight.

A final example: When the "frame" is defined in terms of an "implicit rationale" derived from ordinary situations of looking at objects during daily life (i.e., a basic-level rationale; see 8 above), the situations will become connected in a radial manner and may be metaphorically projected to create a set of linked *film theories*. The resulting film theories, however, will not probe all possible differences among spectators and situations but, rather, will assume that all spectators share certain abilities (e.g., the ability to be alert, to look with interest through a window, to ride in a vehicle, walk, or use an optical instrument). What counts as "framing" or "breaking the frame" will be determined by the metaphor that governs the prototypical viewing situation — that is, determined by the *scenario* we have imagined that brings together the appropriate activities that define a "framing" — such as imagining that we are standing in front of a window that restricts our view in one or several ways (see 8 above) so that what is "offscreen" may suddenly appear (if allowed by our scenario) and "break" the frame. Whether a character's "look at the camera," to take a much-discussed example, will act to "break" the frame depends on which "frame" is at issue, that is, *which* definition of "frame" is chosen as the context for understanding a "look at the camera."[64] Given a particular scenario that defines a framing and a breaking of the frame, the next question would be to ascertain the proper role for camera movement, film editing, sound, narrative, character development, and so on, by fitting these elements into the chosen scenario.

The previous example raises a fundamental question: Can a single, unified theory of film be constructed? Could there be, for example, a single, unified theory of "frame lines"? Perhaps a film theory, like a polysemous word, can only be constructed of dispersed but linked "pieces," each with a *distinct* logical structure defined by ecological conventions (Grodal), motivated conventions (Lakoff), moderate constructivism (Bordwell), or mild realism (Dennett). This is another way of saying that a film theory is not entirely "objective" but, instead, responds to the actual circumstances (patterns) in which it finds a past or present use; that is, a film theory operates by sanctioning a set of living analogies (what Deleuze calls "categories of life") through which it may be applied to objects such as cameras and films, spectators and worlds.[65] Thus, I believe that more than "logic" and constituent "analysis" will be required in order to assess a film theory, because entrenched within the theory are important wide-ranging metaphors, working schemas, and scenarios connected to a way of life. A film theory cannot adequately be evaluated by testing only its internal consistency or its examples. ("Faulty" examples are easily converted to "hypothetical" ones, because film theory is not a species of film history or criticism.[66]) The key problem remains to discover the proper parts and relations of a film theory. Not all of these relations, however, will be internal to films, and not all of these relations can be encompassed (contained) by a single schema, metaphor, or logic.

Consider, again, the container schema. If one focuses on the "boundary" of the "inside-boundary-outside" of the schema, one creates a "surface-depth" metaphor along with associated ideas of "transparency," "invisibility," and "shadowiness" (semi-obscurity) as well as the limit cases of "opaqueness" and "mirroring" in which the "depths" are completely obscured. In relation to the surface-depth metaphor, a surface that is "tinted" may be said to complement or interfere with the "real" color that lies beyond/below, whereas it may be thought that when looking into a mirror, you see only you and nothing beyond/beneath — as if there were you only and the only you is there complete. (Here it is the psyche that is said to have a deeper, concealed level that impinges on the surface — the unconscious as a container within a container.) The surface-depth metaphor leads to the general idea that the surface, border, or present "frame" of something must be "broken" in order to reveal the real or to allow the emergence of new insights or to enter (reflect) a liminal region out beyond.[67] The "breaking" of the boundary, however, does not always come from the "outside"; for example, in Freud's notions of the "uncanny" and of "projection," something that should have remained hidden (beneath the mirrored surface) has broken to, and through, the surface. The container schema, with its dynamism of both "containing" and "breaking free," provides an opportune breeding ground for the ideas of convention (surface) and subterfuge (depth): a durable metaphor, certainly, for the way many people view reality.

The camera can be made to fit the surface-depth metaphor in a variety of ways by asserting, for example, that the camera only shows us the world through a window, only shows us the surface of the world, or only shows us a reflection of the world. *Film theory*, too, can be made to fit this metaphor of surface and depth. According to some writers, the purpose of film theory is simply to reveal what is hidden beneath film generally and/or hidden beneath films as if there were an "objective logic" of grouping all the hidden elements together at a certain "depth" below the appearance of phenomena. Although a single schema, logic, or metaphor may capture something important about a phenomenon or about a set of explanations being offered by a film theory, its usefulness is limited to the way in which we have formulated the initial question. And we formulate a question with a purpose in mind when faced with circumstances. The "answering" schema or metaphor is thus relative to criteria, not absolute.

As an analogy to assessing the validity of a film theory — to assessing the logic of how a film theory groups its key elements — consider the statement that "the camera tracks left." Does this "analysis" into the constituent parts of a shot begin to isolate the nature of a "camera," or is it rather a false simplification that elides the metaphors and schemas through which we were able to conceive of a camera as being *in* a scene in the first place? Notice how the statement "the camera tracks left" creates a mental picture of a camera as a simple physical (objective) object that must obey certain "laws":

> What is *it* that can "track"? Even when not tracking, shouldn't *it* still be a thing *capable* of tracking? What other types of movements are *like* tracking? What types of things might be found to the "left"? Is the "left" an adjacent place in time and space? (If we track left, then right, would we "return" to our starting point? How much time would elapse?) What defines the things to be found to the left? Would we expect to find the camera itself to the left? If not, then is the camera somehow "outside" of film — a *cause* of film?

A film theory will attempt to yoke together a series of mental pictures of its major concepts: "Lighting" is in a shot, a "camera" makes a shot, two shots make "editing," and so on. The question remains: Where have the mental pictures come from and do they speak to the appropriate "categories of life?"

I believe that a productive approach to the nature of the "camera" would be to examine the sorts of pictorial metaphors we routinely entertain thinking about it. What are the implicit scenarios that make different cameras become present in our mental imagery? For example, we may think of the camera as a machine, an instrument (like a paintbrush or pen), a technique, a rational principle, an idea, or a part of nature. Is it movable, anthropomorphic, observant, or inanimate? What sort of camera has a "point of view"? We can easily imagine scenarios for these many sorts of cameras because of their connection to daily life. Do specialized contexts exist that create still more cameras? In deciding which scenario might be appropriate for a given occasion, the claims of film history and criticism will be relevant.

A complete description of framing in film from a cognitive standpoint (i.e., from *within* a cognitive frame . . .) would involve, besides pictorial metaphors and the container schema, such schemas as the source-path-goal schema, which addresses the framing of a *time* span (i.e., a time frame, as in a long-held shot) as well as judgment heuristics, such as "anchoring and adjustment," which begin to address the dynamics of a person's attention.[68] Indeed, the movement of attention suggests an alternative to the "surface-depth" metaphor. This new "attention" metaphor would be based on a flat domain that is being traversed by a moving spotlight or zoom lens. Analyzing an "object" would involve a choice of scale and being sensitive to part-whole and adjacency relations (as in a heterarchy) rather than searching for what is hidden in/by the depths of an object.[69] The "attention" metaphor treats an object as part of an archipelago, not as the entrance to a mine shaft.

This larger perspective on "framing" is a reminder that framing cannot be limited to techniques or technology, nor to "film aesthetics," "general aesthetics," or simple conceptions of the "camera," because schemas and reasoning procedures play a vital role in many different areas of community life. Thus, figure 4.1 may also be interpreted as a distribution of mental models in a population that, taken as a whole, characterize a culture. Particular mental models, of course, may appear in several cultures. Nothing within a cognitive approach suggests that there is *purity* to be accorded to image, motion, sound, or language. Nor do the components of working memory and attention (i.e., a specialized language processor, phonological rehearsal loop, visuo-spatial sketchpad, general workspace (consciousness, short-term memory), executive functions, and sensory buffers) suggest that a particular cognitive function holds priority over others, even if functions are arrayed differently for different tasks. Indeed, the complexity (impurity) of even simple cognitive tasks suggests the pertinence of a remark by Edgar, the film director, in Godard's *Éloge de l'amour* (*In Praise of Love*, 2001): "When I think about something, I'm really thinking about something else."

COLOR AS CONTAINER

I would like to illustrate how basic-level, embodied thinking can provide an answer to a specific problem in film aesthetics involving the appearance of color. Recall that Stan Brakhage asks us to imagine what the perception of "green" might be like prior to its association with the *word* "Green" (see 15 above). Presumably, the word "Green" acts to subtract something greenish from the world of sensations, leaving behind a colorless abstraction. Furthermore, I believe that when the problem of color is considered more closely, we will discover a lesson about the nature of film "framing" as well as a lesson about the nature of the "framing" undertaken by a film theory.

Tinting is a process of coloring an image with a uniform wash of a single hue by dyeing the celluloid base. Tinting results in the lighter areas of an image being colored in the chosen hue while the darker areas remain unchanged. On the other hand, *toning* is a process that colors the darker areas of an image while the lighter

127

areas remain unchanged. Toning is achieved by employing a metal compound to color the exposed (blackened) silver in an emulsion after a positive print has been made (yielding, for example, an iron blue-green, uranium red-orange, or sulfur warm brown-sepia). A toning-like effect may also be achieved by printing a black-and-white negative onto color stock with a filter interposed. William Johnson remarks, "Toning usually has a more delicate effect than tinting."[70] Though Johnson doesn't explain his reasoning, one may speculate as to why toning might appear "more delicate."

Tinting acts to color the lighter areas of an image. These areas tend to depict the action of *light* on sky, air, and space. As a form of energy, light is naturally mutable, that is, changeable and *without* a definite, solid shape. We expect light to be subject to frequent changes according to natural conditions and to assume various colors, for example: the perceived blue of distance and sky; the whitish glow of beams of light in a forest; the purple clouds and the pinks of sunrise and sunset; the flickering yellow-orange of firelight; the morning fog that mutes color; the reflected light from an object that takes on a complimentary hue; and the heightened purity of hues on an overcast day when the clouds have blocked infrared wavelengths and diffused the sunlight, making the grass a more vivid green on our side of the fence. Light does not "move" in the way that material objects do, and we do not "control" its movement as we usually control the movement of objects (even if we may switch room lights on and off). Light feels less substantial and more "remote" to us. Therefore, light is more often thought of as a kind of "background" for the substantial parts of daily life represented by material objects and persons in movement.

Toning acts to color the darker areas of an image. These areas tend to depict objects, persons, and landscapes. In contrast to the ephemeral quality of ambient light, material objects and persons appear solid and close: We touch, hear, and move them; we travel a landscape. These objects and persons are not supposed to "change" their color. Indeed, the human perceptual system works to hold color constant over a broad range of illumination. There is survival value for humans in maintaining an object's hue because hue usually connects to the *nature of the material* of the object; a "greenish" banana, for example, will be seen to be unripe under many lighting conditions. Thus, when the dark areas of an image are toned, objects in the image appear to *shift* slightly in their basic color, suggesting a slight overall change in our kind of world rather than merely a slight change in the changeable lighting on our familiar world. Toning seems to connect to the very fabric of the world, while tinting seems to be just a change in illumination. Put another way, toning alters our sense of the familiar hue of an object while preserving the object's intrinsic gray scale, whereas tinting alters the hue of light falling on the object while preserving a uniform lightness for the light.

Nevertheless, it is not strictly true that tinting produces no gray scale. If one looks closely at a small area of an image, one will see the surface color take on different values — darker here, but lighter there. For example, a tint will appear darker over a region showing a distant mountain but lighter over sky or snow. However, this is true only when one "forgets" about the mountain so that the darkness of the mountain becomes separated from the mountain in order to give the tint a darker value than elsewhere in the image. On the other hand, if one does *not* forget about the mountain, and instead sees a scene with objects arrayed at different distances, then one will perceive a uniform tint overlaid on mountain, sky, and snow. In this way of looking, it is the mountain that will appear to possess a gray scale, not the light falling on the mountain. Furthermore, all of the hues in the scene will appear equally shifted by the tint. This effect — well known to painters — is called "color transparency."[71] It is an experience of seeing one color as "semi-transparent" in relation to another color so that *two* colors are being seen, one behind the other: a dark mountain with a gray scale seen *as if* through an unchanging, tinted *glass*. When a person experiences a single color, he or she is observing (bottom-up) what is physically present on a two-dimensional surface — namely, a gray-scale variation of a single hue as well as what is strictly present on the retina (because there can be only a single color and intensity at each point on a surface and on the retina). By contrast, when a person sees two colors occupying the same place on a two-dimensional surface (e.g., on a painting or photograph), an embodied, higher-order (top-down) mental process has constructed a locale containing either two objects at different distances (i.e., a distant thing seen through colored glass) or one object lit by colored light.

Technology reinforces the perceived difference between tinting and toning — that is, between the flatness, fixity, and transparency of tinting, and the materiality and delicate gray scale of toning. Tinting can be achieved by simply coloring light, such as by attaching a filter to a light source, camera, or projector, as in Kinemacolor. But colored light in this sense is seen to be merely *arbitrary* coloring, much as when one says, "His words were colored by anger" or "The event was colored by his recounting" or "Her actions were placed in a bad light," meaning that the "coloring" and "lighting" is superficial, transitory, and biased.[72] Toning, however, has a quite different effect: It creates a finely graded hue that seems to emanate from the very materiality of an object, as if the object were glowing with some new essence independently of ambient lighting and context.[73] Toning makes the colors on a film screen appear to come from the world itself, to be a discovered "inner glow" of things, to somehow be in touch with the (hidden) spirit of things. This puts toning on the side of art — an Art that has the power to reveal the objective nature of things (*in* an image, *in* the world) — while tinting is merely technique (to be put *on* or *over* an image, to be added *to* an image like a highlight on an object). In short, for a viewer, toning appears to be a matter of ontology and tinting a matter of decoration (or of "explanation" or of "rhetoric" . . .).

I believe that the perceived difference between tinting and toning can be tied to the larger problem of how we perceive "framing." If tinting seems to decorate an image, then it will appear to a viewer as if the tinted color were on some kind of separate, transparent surface, that is, as if the tint were somehow part of a *container* for objects and persons. Tinting will appear to *frame* toning because we believe light is (like) a canvas displaying the objects of our everyday world that we see, hear, touch, and put into motion. In this scheme the camera would be imagined as the *physical frame* for the "canvas of light" (i.e., the camera will hold in place, or contain, light and lit-up objects; cf. 7 above), or else the camera would be imagined to be (like) the *window* of its viewfinder, lens, or shutter (i.e., the camera will be a mobile window; cf. 8 above), or else the camera would be a fictive view on an action from *within* the diegesis (i.e., the transparent camera-window will be an invisible moving "eye"; cf. 9 above). In all three cases, the camera becomes, like tinting, a frame *for* an embodied, basic-level world — a framed world in which we take enormous interest and in which we believe there lie secrets to be revealed, not merely recorded, just as toning goes beyond mere tinting (i.e., with toning the "world" is shown to exceed the "glass" through which we look). The fact that the camera is conceived as being a "support" for a window or as holding up a "window" to a world or as becoming simply a window-eye (7, 8, 9) means that the values to be sought in the corresponding forms of film art will include such *values* as restraint, unobtrusiveness, proportion, balance, unity, and clarity (i.e., when the camera is conceived as being a "support" for something, it must bear the "weight" equally so as to produce "proportion" and "balance" — and a "window" is rectilinear and so evinces "proportion, balance, unity"; and both camera and "window" are designed to serve and support the world and hence must be "unobtrusive"). One needs only to conceive of the window glass (8) as being *tinted* (or to conceive of the spectator as wearing tinted glasses) to see the significance of the distinctions between tinting and toning, between technique and valuable insight, between manipulating light through a camera-glass and revealing the true colors of the world, between camera framing and genuine Art, and, finally, between, as Stan Brakhage might have said, a Name and a multitude of percepts, Green and green.

In this section I have not been attempting to discover the essence of tinting and toning — what they really are. They are different in some circumstances and alike in others.[74] Rather, I have been attempting to mark how they function in an aesthetic practice when our way of looking becomes enmeshed in a nexus of commitments, overlapping metaphors, and embodied imagery. I have been examining the status of framing within a specific set of film theories (7, 8, 9) that draw upon an embodied set of root metaphors, schemas, and scenarios. For this group of film theories, tinting may be subtly distinguished from toning. Moreover, when film is conceived in terms of embodied mental imagery (7, 8, 9), it seems natural to conclude that the defining features of the medium will be visual and that the correct theory of film will provide us with a single picture of the nature of film rather than provide a list of dispersed but linked "pieces" subject to change (as in a heterarchy; cf. fig. 4.1). That is, one can construct a single picture of the nature of film that amounts to a kind of window through which one views film. The question would then arise: If film theory is like a transparent or tinted glass, why do we need a window to look through to the window of film? Is anything truly explained by such a system, apart from the arbitrary tints added by the theorist? Some of the detractors of film theory and its study have a mental image of film theory as simply another window overlaid on the window of film.

As we have seen, there are many ways of conceiving framing other than through ordinary ways of looking and moving or watching through a "tinted window," and, indeed, some of these ways cannot be conveniently pictured (e.g., the superordinate categories in 10–15), while other ways provide only specialized, fragmentary pictures (e.g., the subordinate categories in 1–6). In general, nonembodied, nonbasic-level approaches will open toward vastly different conceptions of the camera, film, art, and, of course, the human body and thought.[75] Ambiguity, uncertainty, incompleteness, anomaly, and aura become important qualities to find in films and to theorize. What kind of film and film theory, Deleuze might wonder, could respond more fully to a body's resistances, hesitancies, anxieties, and failures — to a body's disembodiment and disempowerment? For an answer, Deleuze turns to films of ambiguity and difficulty — to art cinema and to experimental, independent, and political cinemas: Antonioni, Rivette, Warhol, Cassavetes, Godard, Rocha, Akerman, and Straub/Huillet.[76] Deleuze believes that such films will provide clues for constructing a film theory that, in effect, reveals 'tones' in the medium of film, not just 'tints.'

CAESURA AND SUTURE

"We must, moreover, distinguish between *figuration* and *representation*.

"Figuration is the way in which the erotic body appears (to whatever degree and in whatever form that may be) in the profile of the text. For example: the author may appear in his text (Genet, Proust), but not in the guise of direct biography (which would exceed the body, give a meaning to life, forge a destiny). Or again: one can feel desire for a character in a novel (in fleeting impulses). Or finally: the text itself, a diagrammatic and not an imitative structure, can reveal itself in the form of a body, split into fetish objects, into erotic sites. All these *movements* attest to a *figure* of the text, necessary to the bliss of reading. Similarly, and even more than the text, the film will *always* be figurative (which is why films are still worth making) — even if it represents nothing.

"Representation, on the other hand, is *embarrassed figuration*, encumbered with other meanings than that of desire: a space of alibis (reality, morality, likelihood, readability, truth, etc.). . . . Of course, it very often happens that representation takes desire itself as an object of imitation; but then, such desire *never leaves the frame*, the picture; it circulates among the characters; if it has a recipient, that recipient remains interior to the fiction (consequently, we can say that any semiotics that keeps desire within the configuration of those upon whom it acts, however new it may be, is a semiotics of representation. That is what representation is: when nothing emerges, when *nothing leaps out of the frame*: of the picture, the book, the screen)."[77]

— Roland Barthes

I would like to examine an influential theory of framing in film based on superordinate categories — the Lacanian psychoanalytic theory of "suture." The theory of suture attempts to explain how a separation between various framed parts in a film is overcome in order to articulate a coherent, unified filmic expression. We will discover several lessons here about how framing is used to manage various forms of "discontinuity": difference, split, edge, break, breaking the frame, punctuation, and otherness. We will also discover again the importance of embodied schemata. Deleuze's emphasis on the body echoes Barthes's notion (above) of the erotic body of a text, "figuration," which, Barthes says, "leaves the frame," even "leaps out of the frame." As we shall see, suture is a theory about how 'figuration' in certain pairs of shots is able to 'break' the frame and then sew it back together. More generally, "suture" is said to operate not just in film but throughout social practice: "As a concomitant of every act of signification, suture in some form or other accompanies all linguistic and social practices."[78]

Jean-Pierre Oudart illustrates the concept of suture with an example from Buster Keaton's Civil War story, *The General* (1926). In the film, a battle at Rock River begins with a high-angle, extreme long shot of a large number of Union troops in the distance moving toward the camera and beginning to ford the river. Oudart says that "at this stage, the spectator does not yet perceive either the framing, or the distance, or the camera's position; the image is still for the spectator only a moving and animated photograph." After nine seconds, however, a new stage of the shot emerges:

> Suddenly the enemy soldiers [the Confederates] rise in the frame at the bottom of the image, inordinately larger than the others. The spectator takes a moment to realise, like the Poe character who sees a butterfly as large as a ship, that the [Confederate] soldiers have occupied a rise above the river, which was hidden by the position of the camera. Then the spectator experiences with vertiginous delight the unreal space separating the two groups; he himself is fluid, elastic, and expanding: he is at the cinema. A moment later, he retreats; he has discovered the framing. Suddenly, he senses the space he cannot see, hidden by the camera, and wonders, in retrospect, why such a framing

was used. . . . [The protagonists] no longer have the innocent "being-there-ness" of a moment ago, but instead have a "being–there–for-ness." Why? In order to represent an Absent One, and to signify the absence of the character [Keaton's character, Johnnie Gray] which the spectator's imagination puts in place of the camera. At the same time, or rather in the meantime, the filmic field, dilated by the spectator's reverie, has been tightened up. Its objects (the two armies, the slope, and the river) now form a signifying Sum, closed upon itself like the indivisible signification of a kind of absolute event. Yet the haunting presence of the other field and of the Absent One remains.[79]

For the purpose of analysis, I will list what I take to be nine stages of Oudart's description of a spectator's changing attention during this shot from *The General.* A spectator's awareness would seem to alternate between pure, sensory 'experience' and intellectual 'discovery.'

1. The spectator experiences an animated photograph, "prior to cinema,"[80] not a genuine cinematic field. The spectator does not perceive the framing, the distance, or the camera's position, but only the photograph's lively and energetic appearance due to the movements of the Union soldiers.
2. The spectator discovers that he or she is at the cinema when Confederate soldiers suddenly rise up through the bottom frame line. (The Confederates had been "hidden" by the camera.[81])
3. The spectator experiences a "vertiginous delight" in an "unreal" filmic space and its depth of field. (The spectator is "fluid, elastic, and expanding.")
4. The spectator discovers the "framing" when he or she suddenly understands that an unseen space has been "hidden" by the camera.[82] Why was such a framing used? What is its purpose? Objects present in the image no longer have the "innocent 'being-there-ness' of a moment ago, but instead have a 'being-there-for-ness.'"[83]

5. The spectator experiences (imagines) an Absent One located "in place of the camera" in the unseen, hidden space.

6. The spectator discovers a "signifying Sum," the meaning(s) of the filmed event; he or she discovers that cinema is a closed discourse.

7. The spectator experiences the "haunting presence" of the Absent One within the unseen, hidden space in relation to the image.

8. The spectator discovers the Absent One in the *next* shot (a reverse field showing the previously unseen space).[84] The new shot provides a *suture* that closes the gap with the previous shot through "the abolition of the Absent One and its resurrection in someone [a character?]."[85]

9. The spectator experiences in the new shot what was anticipated by the previous shot while, at the same time, he or she remembers what used to be present in the previous shot. That is, the spectator senses time as *simultaneously* prospective and retrospective.[86]

I believe that the above nine successive stages of awareness may be further reduced to five phases: the nonframed (1), unframed (2, 3), framed (4–6), deframed (7), and reframed (8, 9). In these five phases one can recognize a characteristic pattern of ordinary narrative whereby action in a scene rises to a climax (4–6) and then falls off to a temporary resolution. Furthermore, I believe that in the full nine stages of suture, an additional pattern is manifest whereby feeling and belief alternate so that a spectator's 'experience' in one stage is followed in the next by his or her 'discovery' of some fact through the experience.[87] Overall, the spectator's feeling for time, which becomes doubly intangible (9), is matched by a gradual loss of spatial presence (4), which instead becomes infused with the presence of absence (5) — that is, of some thing intangible, lacking, or missing in what is seen. Thus, the purity and innocence of the photograph (1) and the film image (2), as well as the unbounded delight felt by the spectator in the film image (i.e., cinephilia; 3), are slowly but steadily eroded. The emerging 'presence of absence' becomes so "haunting" (i.e., another form of cinephilia; 7) that it calls forth a new shot (8), but one that is destined to alleviate only momentarily the anxious feelings connected with absence and loss.

Oudart's approach to the movement of a spectator's attention is not confined to a spectator's eye movements (2) nor based on a slow dawning of meanings (6). Rather, he draws on Lacanian theory to incorporate a spectator's unconscious in the overall process. For Lacan the unconscious is structured as a language and for Oudart that language interacts with the "signifying Sum" (6), which has been produced through the explicit language of cinema. For Oudart, hidden and repressed processes of the unconscious underlie what he calls the Absent One (5, 7, 8). Here is how Oudart defines the Absent One:

> [E]very filmic field traced by the camera and all objects revealed through depth of field — even in a static shot — are echoed by another field, the fourth side, and an absence emanating from it.[88]

> Every filmic field is echoed by an absent field, the place of a character who is put there by the viewer's imaginary, and which we shall call the Absent One.[89]

The Absent One seems to be conceived by Oudart as a diegetic *character* who is temporarily out of sight but who has been put into an unseen space by a spectator's imagination (unconscious?). Although the Absent One is revealed in the next shot, a new absence, or Absent One, arises from the spatial field that is excluded from the new shot. That is, even after an absence or gap has been sutured by the following shot, absence reappears because the new image, while closing one gap, opens a new one. Thus, for Oudart, a pervasive sense of *incompleteness* clings to the image. This leads Oudart to mourn the "tragic and unstable nature of the image" and the "tragic nature of [cinematic] language."[90] He laments that objects on the screen are destined to lose their "innocent" nature (in stage 4). The result is that film space for Oudart is marked by an essential "ambiguity."[91] Embodied in every image, there is no escape from ambiguity. Earlier sections of this chapter have analyzed the importance of ambiguity as a driving force within certain genres and film theories as well as within critical practice, language use, radial categories, and accounts of our fascination with film.

Disputes have emerged, however, over the exact nature of absence and of the Absent One. Daniel Dayan claims that what is absent, and still deferred in the following shot, is the sight of the camera itself and the apparatus of production. Dayan interprets this to mean that what is permanently masked through endless framing and reframing is the *ideology* that is speaking the fiction.[92] Dayan identifies this practice with classical Hollywood cinema, whereas Oudart believed that suture should be a *goal for all* films.[93] One reason, perhaps, that Dayan confines suture ("entrapment,"[94] an enforced forgetting) to classical Hollywood cinema is that he takes Oudart's starting point — which is a conception of the frame as the visible *composition* of a shot (cf. definition 5 of the frame with stages 1, 2, and 3 of suture) — and then extracts from a *sequence* of these shot compositions the rules of Hollywood continuity editing. This is done in spite of the fact that Oudart emphasizes that what is at stake in suture is not the "exchange" between two shots but the prior exchange in a *single* shot between what is visible in the image and what is recognized as a *lack* or *echo* in the same image from an imaginary field (i.e., the spectator's sensation of absence, an Absent One, *in* a single, visible image).[95] As Oudart sees it, there is always something missing (amiss?) in the immediate image.

For Kaja Silverman, "suture" names a set of semiotic processes that have deep psychological consequences, specifically, "the procedures by means of which cinematic texts confer subjectivity upon their viewers."[96] Suture is the set of active and hidden processes that, like the unconscious, work upon a passive and unsuspecting spectator/subject.

> Thus a [character's] gaze within the fiction [as in, for example, shot/reverse shot] serves to conceal the controlling gaze outside the fiction; a benign other steps in and obscures the presence of the coercive and castrating Other. In other words, the subject of the speech [a fictional character] passes itself off as the speaking subject [as an author].[97]

Silverman draws a line between the inside ("within") and the "outside" of a fiction. The inside of a fiction is an illusion or deception, just as what we believe to be true about our inner selves (conscious ego) is a misapprehension fostered by what lies outside conscious awareness — that is, the unconscious. Like a fictional character that we may identify with in a film, consciousness "passes itself off as the [true] speaking subject." Thus, Silverman sets up a series of 'containers,' each with a boundary: conscious/unconscious, self/Other, fiction film/real world, character/author, character/character, and shot/reverse shot. Suture functions to maintain the boundaries of each container, and create unity and "coherence," by concealing the 'cut.'

> Thus cinematic coherence and plenitude emerge through multiple cuts and negations. Each image is defined through its differences from those that surround it syntagmatically and those it paradigmatically implies ("this but not that"), as well as through its denial of any discourse but its own. Each positive cinematic assertion represents an imaginary conversion of a whole series of negative ones. This castrating coherence, this definition of a discursive position for the viewing subject which necessitates not only its loss of being, but the repudiation of alternative discourses, is one of the chief aims of the system of suture.[98]

Silverman deploys a further set of oppositions: syntagmatic/paradigmatic, presence/absence, positive/negative, and 'present' discourse versus one or more 'absent,' alternative discourses. These oppositions based on the linguistics of Ferdinand de Saussure mark the construction of *difference* itself, of a boundary line that is taken to be the founding gesture of all meaning. This dividing line may then be mapped onto *gender* difference, and onto male versus female. "Indeed," says Silverman, "the entire system of suture is inconceivable apart from sexual difference." Since Lacan characterizes the symbolic value of the female gender role in terms of castration (lack, loss, absence of the phallus, otherness to the male, repudiation), this means that suture in the end will function to the detriment of the female viewer.[99] "Coherence and plenitude" for the viewer are purchased at the price of what is 'absent'; in the case of sexual difference, the hidden 'coherence' of patriarchy — which underpins film generally — acts to disempower or neutralize the female.

William Rothman raises a new set of vexing issues about suture. His starting point is a notion of the frame as the view of a character — the prototypical instance being a point-of-view shot (definition 9 of the frame above). Instead of the unconscious, or Absent One, Rothman says that the spectator is reacting to visible cues on the screen, and to film conventions, in filling out a sequence and making it meaningful.[100] By contrast, in two important essays Stephen Heath carefully revises the nature of suture in order to shift it away from imagery and onto the very processes of *narrative discourse* (definition 13).[101] In this way Heath begins to move away from the two ideas that suture is anchored in a *shot* and that a shot functions to *conceal*.

The most recent theory of suture belongs to Slavoj Žižek, who blends Ernesto Laclau's concept of hegemony, Lacanian psycho-analysis, semiotics, and some of Rothman's ideas to describe both "standard suture" and a more "radical" form he calls "interface."[102] For Žižek the unit of film narration ("enunciation") is the shot. Žižek begins with a series of well-known types of misaligned and paradoxical objective/subjective shots, which are given a Lacanian explanation.[103] "Interface" arises when shot and reverse-shot are condensed within a single image (e.g., through a reflective surface in the mise-en-scène, superimposition, or split screen), evoking an uncanny, "*spectral* dimension."[104] Ordinary reality is seen to have another side in that "a part of drab reality all of a sudden starts to function as the 'door of perception,' the screen through which another, purely fantasmatic dimension becomes perceptible."[105] What has been "repressed" (e.g., alternative narrativizations, genre conventions, psychic trauma, ideology, historical circumstances) returns like an "apparition" (Absent One?) to upset ("short circuit") our comprehension of a shot: "the excluded externality always leaves its traces within."[106] The reason is that we cannot ever comprehend the "whole" of reality that we encounter: if we are to be able to endure our encounter with reality, some part of it has to be "derealised," experienced as a spectral apparition.[107]

Žižek concludes that both standard suture and its radical, compressed form, "interface," do not erase or conceal outside forces but, instead, provide the medium for their expression.[108]

The approaches discussed above may be summarized as follows. Oudart's starting point is a conception of the frame as the visible composition of a shot (definition 5), whereas Rothman begins inside the diegesis with a character's point-of-view shot (definition 9; that is, Rothman, unlike the others, assumes the existence of a fiction and does not attempt to analyze its nature or effects). Heath begins with the processes of narration (definition 13). For Dayan, the starting point is the frame as the real edge of whatever is recorded on the film emulsion by an actual camera (definition 1); these celluloid frames will accumulate and become a "shot" after the camera is turned off.[109] Silverman begins with the presence of an image (perceived as a whole; definition 3) that will be distinguished from other images (syntagmatically and paradigmatically) through differences established in the editing by, for example, orchestrating character glances; these shot differences, then, at a larger scale will be mapped onto semiotic processes and onto the subject by way of sexual difference, again through Gestalt-like principles (e.g., identification; definition 14) modeled on the 'good continuation' of individual shots (cf. definition 3), thus forcing all the parts to become whole and continuous once more. Žižek's radical form of suture, "interface," is an elaboration of how something may suddenly and strangely appear overlaid on the ordinary world, like a ghostly mirror reflection upon an invisible window (definition 8 [iii]). Žižek would seem to urge that we take the polysemy of the word "look" seriously: the world has a layered and ambiguous look, as do we when we look (with our hidden backgrounds). Ultimately, all versions of suture point toward unconscious states (definition 14; e.g., fetishism) that are said to underlie an emotion (*jouissance* for Oudart;[110] a feeling for a character through the conventions of film for Rothman), or a deceptive value ("unity" of subject position for Heath), an ideological belief (e.g., commodity fetishism; cf. Dayan), a gendered identity (Silverman), or the return of an "excluded externality" through an everyday object that is functioning as an adventitious "door of perception" (Žižek). The central problem addressed by suture is the relationship between a spectator's response to film and his or her hidden, inner self (i.e., drives and memories) because framing in film is assumed to replicate the split in a spectator between conscious and unconscious activities (cf. definitions 14 and 15). Other definitions and interpretations of framing are denied or ignored.

Before drawing some conclusions about suture, I would like to consider what I take to be nearly its opposite, a kind of 'antisuture.' Pascal Bonitzer defines an effect he calls "deframing" (*décadrage*). Hints of what is at stake may be found in Heath's notion of "disframing" and Metz's "deframing" (see definition 14). Bonitzer says deframing is not simply an oblique or paradoxical camera angle (i.e., what I referred to earlier as an 'eccentric' view) but, rather, an angle or camera position that is only partially, or not at all, motivated and that, further, interrupts the narrative by permanently concealing something of interest. Bonitzer speaks of shots from "strange" angles that show "bodies alluringly fragmented" or "limbs suggestively truncated," that are seen too close or held too long, that contain banal objects or reveal "inadequate reflections in clouded mirrors," or are empty. The result is that "a sense of mystery, of fear, of semi-nightmare, takes hold of the spectator," which is not dispelled by a subsequent reframe, pan, or countershot. Bonitzer's examples come from modern painters and such filmmakers as Dreyer, Bresson, Antonioni, Duras, Eustache, and Straub and Huillet.[111] This "scenography of lacunae" creates "a non-narrative suspense" — "a tension that persists from shot to shot and which the 'story' does not eliminate." As with suture, there is a psychoanalytic undertow:

> In Deleuzian terms it needs to be said that the art of deframing, the displaced angle, the radical off-centredness of a point of view that mutilates the body and expels it beyond the frame to

focus instead on dead, empty zones barren of decor, is ironically sadistic. . . . Ironic and sadistic inasmuch as its off-centre framing, as a rule frustrating for the spectator and disfiguring for the "models" (Bresson's term [for actors]), is the response of a cruel mastery, a cold and aggressive death-drive: the use of the frame as a cutting-edge, the living pushed out to the periphery, beyond the frame . . ., the focusing on the bleak or dead sections of the scene, the dubious celebration of trivial objects (such as the sexualization of washbasins and bathroom implements . . .), highlight the arbitrariness of this curious directorial gaze, one that perhaps delights in the sterility of its point of view.[112]

In a deframed image, something human has been lost or drained away, cruelly *dis*figured, but the spectator has arrived too late to witness how the frame/frame lines were *broken* and used "as a cutting-edge." Subsequent framings will not reveal the extent of the sadism that has taken place nor the remedy. The 'wound' to the film, as it were, will not be fully exposed or sutured, even temporarily. The deframed image, although still 'anthropomorphic' (though not necessarily 'anthropocentric'), has been mysteriously mutilated by "the sadistic irony of off-centre framing"[113] and what is human has been "pushed out . . . beyond the frame." A spectator infers that a violation has occurred within some human transaction but sees on the screen no cause, effect, or reaction. Something is permanently absent.

The theories of suture and deframing illustrate a general lesson about theories of framing. Every theory of framing is an attempt to describe in the broadest sense how the mind handles "discontinuity" — a perceived break, difference, or caesura. Narrative film, like natural language, is made up of an enormous number of discrete elements that are being variously integrated and juxtaposed on many levels. The crucial questions involve what should go together with what, on which level, and when. These questions cannot be answered in a mechanical way, because two elements that appear together may not belong together, while two elements that are separated may, in fact, belong together. In general, a theory of framing establishes a borderline and shows how it may be crossed, even if the crossing is blocked. Recall, for example, the bottom frame line of Oudart's illustration of suture in *The General* and the soldiers who suddenly and unexpectedly rise up through it, or the frame line we are not allowed to cross in Bonitzer's notion of deframing. In general, every theory of framing acts to place an initial diacritical mark that gives what is contained "inside" the frame the deictic quality "here" as opposed to something else "outside" the frame over "there" and "other." Framing elevates the notion of "difference" from a simple principle that distinguishes individuals to a constraint that distinguishes one class or group from another. But what, then, are the elements of film and narrative that are properly to be joined (grouped together) or separated (kept apart)? Which theory of framing will provide the proper diacritical and deictic marks? What will count as presence ("here") as opposed to absence ("there")?

Evidently, a theory about framing is no simple matter because it quickly leads into fundamental assumptions about the nature and workings of both film and narrative as well as the nature of comprehension, emotion, and how we discover value. Comprehending and reacting to a film is *not* a continuous act in the way that film runs through a projector or shots succeed each other. Comprehension moves in fits and starts on a tide of enigmas, hypotheses, feelings, partial answers, surprises, ambiguities, forking paths, mistakes, and — still lingering at the end — unrealized (but real) possibilities: what might have happened. For the spectator a basic problem is to understand how two elements in a film should be framed as being either contiguous or disjoint. Again, the difficulty is that two elements appearing together on the screen may be "separate," while an element appearing offscreen may actually be "contiguous" with something onscreen.

In watching a film, a spectator must determine relevant instances of "proximity" because judgments about proximity are essential to one of the most important methods of *causal* reasoning — that which locates "push-pull" causation. Where is it, exactly, that diacritic and deixis are affirmed or overcome? Stating the issue in this way, one can see that a theory of framing depends finally on the selection of a general theory of causation. Needless to say, there are many methods of causal reasoning and many kinds of causation and hence, many theories of framing.[114] A given theory of framing, as we have seen with suture and deframing, will usually string together several sorts of "frames" in accordance with its adopted principles of causation. (In deframing, for example, the spectator must see in subsequent "framings" that he or she will *not* see the cause or effect of the deframing.) As we will discuss in the next chapter, the problem of causation also concerns the limits of an "explanation." Thus, I believe, the concept of frame in its most general sense refers to the subtle, even intricate *restrictions placed upon the explanations* that are permissible for an occasion — the limits upon descriptions offered in answer to a question. When an explanation or description has been accepted and its details are well understood, causation is characterized as "linear" and a frame acquires a clear line.

With several sorts of frames operative, the word "frame" becomes *radial*. The main problem for any theory of interlaced "frames," such as suture and deframing, is to decide which assumptions and methods characteristic of a given frame (i.e., a frame under one of the 15 definitions) will be pulled along into the more comprehensive theory. Any single frame is probably inadequate as an explanation for the power of film, but a larger set of frames risks the confusion of becoming an arbitrary assemblage. I believe that one cannot strike a "balance" between a few and many frames in a purely logical or timeless way. Instead, one will need to consider embodied human abilities — basic cognitive and emotive responses — in relation to performance, that is, in relation to the actions, practices, and goals pursued in a particular environment.

ENVOI: THE INDEFINITE BOUNDARY

Finally, Wittgenstein reminds us that there are limits to thinking in a frame, and even to thinking in a sequence of frames. Meanings that are indefinite, blurred, or porous may have a use.

The sense of a sentence — one would like to say — may, of course, leave this or that open, but the sentence must nevertheless have *a* definite sense. An indefinite sense — that would really not be a sense *at all*. — This is like: An indefinite boundary is not really a boundary at all. Here one thinks perhaps: if I say "I have locked the man up fast in the room — there is only one door left open" — then I simply haven't locked him in at all; his being locked in is a sham. One would be inclined to say here: "You haven't done anything at all." An enclosure with a hole in it is as good as *none*. — But is that true?[115]

If we adopt for a moment "basic-level categories" for thinking about philosophical issues (as Wittgenstein frequently does), we can imagine some analogues to the situation of the man who has been locked in a room with only one door left open — analogues that may have powerful uses. For example, consider the plot of a classical film as it moves along a trajectory from one point through an open door to the next point (to a new room and scene) where each movement is subjected to partial and relative restrictions that act in relation to a path; or consider the tiny hole ("open door") in an hourglass through which sand drains away, measuring one kind of time found often in plots; or, finally, consider that there may be a point that is being communicated to the man in the room through the "sham" of being locked inside with an open door, just as narrative "fictions" (and fictions within fictions[116]) may well have a point and not be simply misleading or false.[117] If a few more doors and windows had been left open (but not *all* the doors and windows, producing a sieve), then one might have uncovered parallels with the methods of art cinema; indeed, "the man" in the room might not have been able to decide how to leave or if it was necessary to leave. In this analogy, the art cinema may be seen as approaching how we think generally in the cinema, neither entirely bottom-up nor top-down, neither entirely basic-level nor subordinate/superordinate, neither completely inside nor completely outside the film, but, rather, somewhere between the extremes of realism and relativism in an area where time runs in both directions. In this approach the images in a fiction film would be more like a rebus or horoscope than a telescope or microscope, and time would be a matter for interpretation, not a simple importation from the world.

We may now return to our initial question: Does the world dictate language or does language dictate a world? Or to put it differently, does language merely add a *tint* to the world we see? I believe this question cannot be answered using the container schema because the world does not entirely enclose, or determine, language nor does language entirely contain the world. No clear discontinuity between world and language will be found in order that a suture might be applied. Instead, we may imagine that language has only a fractional membership in the set "world" — that is, between 1 ("is a member of") and 0 ("is not"). I believe that the distinctions among subordinate, basic-level, and superordinate categories are meant to capture the sliding scale of inclusion/exclusion of language in relation to the world. The idea of a "degree of membership" in a set, however, is not as easy to visualize as is a container, such as a glass, that either holds a liquid or not, that either is tinted or not. This amounts to saying that the notion of a "fuzzy set" is not as clearly *embodied*, as is a "container," which has a definite surface and a depth. To invoke Wittgenstein's image of a man locked in a room with an open door: One may ask, with what degree of *certainty* can it be said that the man is in the room at a particular moment? That the man belongs and must stay within that room ('category') for all time?

Similarly difficult to visualize are the "in-between" notions of ecological conventions (Grodal), motivated conventions (Lakoff), moderate constructivism (Bordwell), and mild realism (Dennett). The notion of "radial meaning" (heterarchy) is yet another consequence of the partial inclusion/exclusion of language in relation to the world. It is no wonder that film theorists have had great difficulty in assessing whether *film* is to be thought of as being fixed in the world or in a language. Does the world dictate the framing of film or does the framing of film create a world? I have been arguing that the word "frame" by itself has no particular meaning other than its uses within various contexts, or language-games. Most film theories (including that of André Bazin) have been forced to create a tangle of meanings for "frame" and to suffer the attendant ambiguities. On the other hand, being "in-between," moving from one edge of a language-game to another, may be the best description we have of what a film theory is. The shifting and balancing of the many theories of suture and deframing illustrate generally how film theories form in order to reform. There is thus, I believe, a degree of ambiguity inherent in film theories. The effort to expunge all ambiguity is the desire to build a room for all occasions.

CODA: THE CAMERA

Now what shall we say about the entity that we call The Camera? Doesn't the camera *cause* a framing to be on the screen in each of the 15 senses of framing discussed above? More precisely, a camera may be said to cause a framing *after* one has specified in a suitable manner what it means to be "on the screen."

Perhaps we should turn the question around — let the tail wag the dog, for once. Because there are many ways of seeing the act of framing, perhaps there are many ways for the camera to be seen . . . or to be. Consider that the camera we see "moving" in animation is not identical to the physical camera on the animation stand (even if that camera were to move). Consider also that the camera we experience moving around Group Captain Mandrake, President Muffley, and Dr. Strangelove is *not* the same camera that moves around Peter Sellers. (Peter Sellers, but not the others, could be seen performing on a set in front of a camera in Stanley Kubrick's *Dr. Strangelove*, 1964.) Perhaps, then, there are many ways for the word "camera" to function in our discourse when we undertake to describe how we have experienced a film. That is, there may be many cameras (some incompatible, some indefinite) in our talk about cinema depending upon our goals.

I believe that the word "camera" is a radial concept that extends far beyond the properties of a (definite) physical apparatus able to record the real world and having a weight and serial number. I believe that the camera extends beyond — dare I say?

— photographicity, beyond pictured-ness, beyond even the visible and visual, and instead extends into the schematic and abstract wherein lies language and the language of film, where there is no genuine and exact description proper for all occasions,[118] where a camera is created to point out, and where getting the point means imagining a camera.

Chapter 5: **When Is a Camera?**

"SOCRATES: I should like, before proceeding further, to tell you how I feel about the [perfect or ideal political] state which we have described. I might compare myself to a person who, on beholding beautiful animals either created by the painter's art, or, better still, alive but at rest, is seized with a desire of seeing them in motion or engaged in some struggle or conflict to which their forms appear suited — this is my feeling about the [perfect or ideal political] state which we have been describing. There are conflicts which all cities undergo, and I should like to hear someone tell of our own city carrying on a struggle against her neighbors, and how she went out to war in a becoming manner, and when at war showed by the greatness of her actions and the magnanimity of her words in dealing with other cities a result worthy of her training and education. Now I, Critias and Hermocrates, am conscious that I myself should never be able to celebrate the city and her citizens in a befitting manner, and I am not surprised at my own incapacity; to me the wonder is rather that the poets present as well as past are no better — not that I mean to depreciate them, but everyone can see that they are a tribe of imitators, and will imitate best and most easily the life in which they have been brought up, while that which is beyond the range of a man's education he finds hard to carry out in action, and still harder adequately to represent in language."[1]

— Plato

"Our investigation is therefore a grammatical one. Such an investigation sheds light on our problem by clearing misunderstandings away. Misunderstandings concerning the use of words, caused, among other things, by certain analogies between the forms of expression in different regions of language."[2]

— Ludwig Wittgenstein

MOTION AND MOVEMENT

A living room appears on the screen. Soon there is motion: Space begins to slide toward the left, pushing objects on the left off the screen while new objects appear on the right. Objects that are near-by are moving more rapidly than those in the near background. Simultaneously, space that is seen through a window in the far background moves slowly in the opposite direction toward the right. Then the motion on the screen changes direction: Objects in the center of view suddenly begin to enlarge symmetrically at different speeds, moving faster and contracting lengthwise as they draw nearer but becoming increasingly distinct along diagonals emanating from a central point while, at the same time, objects away from the center of view enlarge in asymmetrical patterns, until each abruptly vanishes with a final blur and bending into the immateriality of extreme closeness at the edges of the screen. What is occurring?

In response to patterns on the screen, the human brain has computed a familiar set of differential speeds and trajectories for the objects, thereby recognizing that the objects are in motion, though not in movement, because it is the *viewpoint* on the objects that is changing: At first the viewpoint changes through the act of moving sideways *toward the right* (which we are able to visualize by using the cue of motion parallax), and then the viewpoint alters direction to move *forward* through a place (which we visualize by using the cues of texture gradient, foreshortening, linear convergence, and synthetic perspective). Other mathematically possible arrays, if they had been realized, would be seen only as noise or as mysterious abstract designs, not as movements of a viewpoint through a place. It does not matter how the various objects that possess differential speeds have themselves been produced on the screen: whether the objects have been, for example, drawn by hand, generated by a computer, or imprinted by photography; or, whether the speeds of the objects have been, for example, created by a rotating cylinder and drum of mirrors (Émile Reynaud's Praxinoscope), achieved by the flip-book principle (Herman Casler's Mutoscope), or radiated by mechanical or electronic projection. In the appropriate circumstances, the viewer will experience a directed *motion* that is localized to a screen — a change from one *condition* or state of the screen to a new *condition* or state.

If, in addition, we ask *what* moves or is moved — that is, if we wonder not just about the impression of motion, its speed and direction, but also about the nature of the *thing* possessing a viewpoint that is in physical or figurative *movement* from one *location* to a *new location,* creating the motion on the screen[3] — then we might risk proposing such substantives as a character (whose moving viewpoint is shown through a moving point-of-view shot), a narrator (who is presenting a story), an author (who corresponds with our sense of a developing narrative argument or commentary on the story),[4] an invisible, perhaps inquisitive, observer (if we ourselves at the time happen to be inquisitive), a cameraman, or simply a camera (or, a frame or a framing or a series of photographs) that happens to be in movement. If we were to choose the word "camera" as the nucleus for a description of the living room example, then we would say that the camera begins by moving to the right (making foreground objects move to the left as seen through the camera's viewfinder), followed by a change in direction in which the camera moves forward (making objects move toward the camera); or, still more briefly, we might say that the camera tracks right, then dollies forward.

But what sort of person, entity, or camera-thing have we thus imagined to have a viewpoint that changes? Whatever it is, it is not defined or governed strictly by the coordinates of the two-dimensional perceptual space of the screen or even by the properties of the three-dimensional space depicted on the screen (because a locale does not define a thing present in the locale) — nor does it matter whether the space is stationary or in motion — for the hypothetical entity exists in some other, very different conceptual domain. For example, a "person," such as an actor or author, is defined in a conceptual domain that includes notions of a discrete body, sentience, intentional states, personality, dispositions to act, and a social identity, and is not defined by his or her surrounding space, notwithstanding a person who is a "neighbor." A "fictional" person, or character, also possesses at least these

153

features. Thus, the first question I would like to consider arises: Which new contexts will be relevant in defining the entity that has a "viewpoint" that is being portrayed on the screen in terms of two-dimensional and three-dimensional visibilia? After addressing this question about entities-having-viewpoints that are defined in new contexts, we will be in a position to move to a second question: How do the *movements* of these entities help explain the motion and change that is seen to occur on the screen and within a depicted space, as well as help explain other important motions and changes that may be experienced in less tangible, less visible spaces when, for example, we follow an argument (moving from point to point), read, listen, narrativize, feel, remember, or entertain thoughts? These latter motions, both literal and figurative, are closely related to the problem of "meaning."As Wittgenstein observes, "Meaning some-thing is like going up to someone," like being "oneself in motion."[5] As we shall see, the ideas of "viewpoint" and "camera" are knotted up with processes of "meaning" and with multiple kinds of motion.

Figurative motions are part of everyday perception. We rou-tinely ascribe these motions to entities in figurative movement. Socrates provides an illustration when he offers several metaphors based on literal movement in order to aid the reader in following his argument (see epigraph). The reader is encouraged to make meaning by moving from point to point through the argument, as if he or she, as Wittgenstein says, "were in motion." In general, it is the reader who puts himself or herself 'into motion' because not every point that is to be 'followed' in an argument will be made explicit; that is, some points along the path must be presumed, filled out, interpreted, or identified only in a tentative way by the reader. The reader will sense himself or herself in motion and/or sense other things in motion: New thoughts may appear on the 'horizon' and draw closer, coming into greater clarity, while others will be abandoned. Needless to say, different readers, and the same reader on different occasions, will likely take different paths through a particular argument, or see different things in movement, even if the 'destination' remains the same. And it is the reader, too, who finally must make sense of the argument by 'applying' it, by 'going up to things,' by finding and recognizing specific objects and problems in his or her *present-day world* that will make the argument relevant (or irrelevant).

I wish to continue discussing figurative motions and reading because I believe we are engaged in the same activity when watching a film. Let's briefly examine the figurative motions offered by Socrates for the reader to experience. Socrates is entertaining an abstraction — the perfect political state. He does this by imagining figurative movements: the *actions* of a perfect state in relation to the *actions* of real states that he has known. Both of these sorts of actions are metaphorical (though not metaphorical in the same way), because a political state, whether ideal or real, does not act or move in the way that a person acts or moves when he or she is walking or grasping an object. One of the actions of real states that Socrates approves of as being like the actions of a perfect state is the "suitable war."[6] In a war, of course, the literal actions are undertaken by soldiers. In order to convey to the reader a sense of the *potentiality for perfection* in a real state, Socrates compares the perfect state to "beautiful animals" that are "alive but at rest." He says that his *feelings* about the perfect state are analogous to the feelings of a person who "is seized with a desire of seeing [the beautiful animals] in motion." Socrates implies that it is through action and movement (appropriate to the form of each animal) that the beautiful animals realize their being; that is, part of their beauty (or is it a *precondition* of their beauty?) is the ability to achieve the precise style of movement "to which their forms appear suited." For Socrates the beautiful animals are most alive when in movement. Socrates implies by analogy that the perfect state will be realized through appropriate action and movement (e.g., through the "suitable war").

Furthermore, Socrates says that the beautiful animals need not actually be real but may be "created by the painter's art." In this way Socrates brings the perfection of a state and the beauty of living animals into the realm of aesthetics. Note that Socrates is not saying that the painting he imagines will depict the animals as if they were in movement but, rather, that the painting will simply depict them at rest, *ready* to move. Socrates, in fact, does not approve of movement being represented in painting, whether incipient or 'actual' movement (for example, an animal about to begin to take a step or else in midstride), because he believes that painters are only capable of *imitating* the real, and thus what is achieved by painters is a thing that is still further removed from the perfection of the real than is the real itself. In this way of reasoning, the 'potential' movement of something is closer to 'perfection,' because both 'potential' and 'perfection' are less visible than 'incipient' or 'actual' movement. For Socrates it is a search for the perfection of the real that validates the aesthetic and not the reverse; that is, the aesthetic does not validate the real through pleasing form or by imitation. (In this passage Socrates merely hints at his distrust of artists; I will not here pursue the details of his arguments against painter-imitators.[7]) Nonetheless, Socrates does suggest that a person may "celebrate" the state "in a befitting manner" through the (poetic, aesthetic) use of spoken or written "language." Indeed, Socrates himself has used language to tell us about the perfect state and to tell us about himself and the situation in which he is speaking. ("Now I, Critias and Hermocrates, am conscious that I myself should never be able to . . ., and I am not surprised at my own incapacity; to me the wonder is . . . — not that I mean to depreciate them. . . .") In doing so, Socrates has employed a sequence of words in order to create movements of our emotions and in order to foster beliefs that are literal with respect to our state of mind but metaphorical with respect to various movements of our body (like walking or grasping) and metaphorical, as well, with respect to the movements of beautiful animals who are "alive."

To summarize: Socrates employs nine different kinds of figurative movements (actions) to propel his argument. They are as follows:

1. The *felt* action of being "seized with a desire" to see the perfect state (cf. Socrates' first words which also speak about desire: "I *should like* . . . to tell you how I *feel* . . ."; and, later, "to me the wonder is . . ."; and, "I am not *surprised* at . . . ")
2. The felt action of an *ideal* beholder of beautiful animals either painted or alive ("I might compare myself to a person who. . . .")

3. The potential actions of *painted* animals
4. The *potential* actions of living, beautiful animals
5. The actions of a *perfect* state (that would go "to war in a becoming manner")
6. The actions of a real *state* (though real, these actions are metaphorical because a state does not have legs and eyes, much less a mouth that would permit a listener to judge "the magnanimity of her words")
7. The *symbolic* actions that may be conveyed through the use of words in a narration ("I should like to hear someone tell. . . .")
8. The *ineptness* ("incapacity") of the actions of "poets present as well as past" (i.e., the actions of these poets are no real actions)
9. And finally, and most important for Socrates, the exercise of *skills* acquired from a proper "training" and "education" that will facilitate and guide a person's actions on different occasions, and grant to a real poet the ability to use language ("to represent in language")

The reader who follows Socrates' argument must interconnect at least nine different *frames* in which distinct kinds of "movements" may occur. Socrates' principal aim is to train and educate, to move the listener or reader. Without prior knowledge of the *forces* that govern the figurative movements, however, the student will fail to make the philosopher's argument come alive like a beautiful animal in motion. Similarly, I will argue that unless a film theorist or analyst fully understands which frames of figurative movement are being invoked by a particular use of the word "camera," he or she will fail to appreciate the argument being made and to appreciate what makes it possible for someone to make the argument.

In the sections that follow, I will continue to explore Wittgenstein's association of meaning with movement along a path. We will see how Wittgenstein's approach to language differs fundamentally from that of Socrates. For now it is enough to notice that Wittgenstein's connection of meaning to movement turns away from the idea that meaning is like a preexisting rule that is learned and memorized (a single, predetermined path or an equation). Nor does "real" meaning exploit some natural bond between person and thing, between a person and the perfection of a thing. "Meaning something" for Wittgenstein is not a rule or special mental state but, rather, seems to be part of a *behavioral act*: moving toward another person, being in action, doing or using something to accomplish a purpose, making time for something to happen (not merely "pointing to" or "imitating" some object). It seems that "meaning something" for Wittgenstein is living and moving and working toward a goal — that is, being in a concrete situation in which one makes decisions not within an a priori calculus or through universal resemblance or by causal law but in light of one's values, activities, and myriad interests. In "meaning something" we *choose* 'to go up to someone,' to act in a certain manner. Meaning is not 'delivered' or 'brought' to us, but made by us with a concrete aim in view. The symptom of meaning-making is that in using language one risks many *analogies* — that one is constantly trying to fit an analogy to a problem at hand. Meaning is relative to use and is not absolute — neither a perfection to be found nor something through which perfection is found.

Thus, Wittgenstein's approach to meaning allows one to see how Socrates is making meaning with reference to metaphors and models that move us from one region of language to another in an attempt to solve a problem (in this case, the problem of identifying the perfect state). Wittgenstein's approach is the one I will adopt in thinking about the word "camera." I believe that to understand what is meant by the word — that is, how we seek to move up to someone through using it — it will be necessary to evaluate how it acts within a complex of words and within one or more frames of figurative movement. I will also try to weigh the analogies that join these frames, because Wittgenstein warns that joining incompatible frames leads to "misunderstandings."

Using Wittgenstein's analogy, which connects meaning with motion, I will think of the object 'camera' (whether this object is taken to be literal or figurative) as 'meaning something' through the way that it is able 'to go up to persons and things and be itself in motion,' such as through an act of continuous reframing. As we shall see, however, motion (or its lack) *on the screen* is not a reliable indicator of the state of the camera's movement, nor is literal camera movement the only kind of camera movement.[8] Various technical issues become prominent here, such as the nature of the image appearing on the screen (i.e., its phenomenal nature) and the relationship of camera movement to film *editing* (i.e., to a change in the camera's position between successive shots even though we do not see it in motion, such as a series of shots moving closer to an object). There are also deeper issues involving the relationship of a movement to its *cause,* which will require us to search for greater clarity about the nature of causation as well as how the word "cause" functions in our talk about the world and the analogies we choose to build. That is, what sort of metaphors and frames do we typically use in thinking about "causation"? How do we use the concept of "causation" to move an argument forward? I will examine all of these questions in this chapter.

Although the problem of the perfect political state Socrates discussed is not an everyday topic, the nine kinds of abstract movements that he invoked in an attempt to solve the problem are quite familiar. That is, all of us are well aware of the action of a state, the potential movement of an object in front of us, the actions of animals depicted in paintings, the action of language, an action that is inadequate to a purpose, the changes brought about through education, and, especially, the feelings that emerge when one is "seized with a desire" or experiences "beauty." These and other figurative movements are enacted according to scenarios that are derived from scenes not unlike the one imagined at the beginning of this section in which motion in a living room appeared as the projection of the movement of a viewpoint. Indeed, "being in a living room" is a standard example of how the mind makes use of a frame-based, knowledge representation system in long-term semantic memory. Later I will consider the living-room scenario and related scenarios in more detail. To repeat: I believe that many types of abstract motions, movements, and projections[9] are based on ordinary activities, for example, arguing, reading, planning, remembering, entertaining thoughts, and projecting stories out of one's daily routine. When these everyday activities are implicated in our use of the word "camera," the notion of a camera will become more complex than its physicality. The question "What is a camera?" will give way to "When is a camera?" When — under which circumstances — does the description "camera" become apt?

The basic reason for this change from "what" to "when" is that watching a film is much more than watching the geometries onscreen created through the optics of the physical camera-machine. In watching a film, we employ all of our mental abilities in evaluating abstract motions, movements, and projections. Not least, we continue to be seized by many desires — only one of which is to see beautiful animals and other things come alive in splendid motion on the screen. Socrates might have condemned the camera as the ultimate tool of imitation, but only by forgetting its capacity for abstract movements. I believe that there are many legitimate cameras in different regions of our language. If so, then no one camera will be the natural one while the others are dim enigmas labeled unorthodox or incoherent, described through catachresis.

MOTION PICTURE

Let's return to the experience of motion on the screen, which we tend to take for granted. An examination of the details, however, will reveal unexpected intricacies in the sensory judgments we make and will suggest that even here cameras are being projected. The basic fact about watching a film is that we do not see each photograph separately but, rather, several photographs almost at once, producing what might be called the experience of a "hyper-photograph." The human visual system, unable to resolve the distinct photographs, interprets the small differences between successive photographs as a continuous *movement* from one dense array of elements to the next; that is, the intermittent photographs give rise to a sense of duration, an unbroken time. Changes in the differences between successive photographs account for the variety of speeds with which objects appear to move on the screen. (By contrast, film moves through a projector at a constant speed, while photographs flashed on the screen do not move at all.) The sense of duration created through hyper-photography is a necessary condition for objects to be seen to be in *continuous* movement, or else, like a tableau vivant, seen to possess at least the *possibility* of continuous movement though unmoving. Hyper-photography is also necessary for a given *viewpoint* to remain stable or, alternately, for the viewpoint to be seen to be in continuous movement. As indicated earlier, the viewpoint may be said to have its origin in any one of several entities, such as in a "camera" offscreen.

Hyper-photography, however, is not a sufficient condition for the perception of continuous movement on the screen, as shown by pixillation effects and the freeze frame, which may occur in a film that is projected normally. It should be remembered that the special kind of duration created through hyper-photography is *not itself* truly continuous, because the shutters of both a camera and a projector block out the light much of the time (typically about 389 milliseconds each second during projection — that is, the screen is black nearly 40 percent of the time); hence, many moments of a recorded event (including moments when the camera may be in movement) are *permanently* missing and can never appear on the screen, even when the screen happens not to be dark. Although the intervals between photographs are precisely measured, the intervals themselves are not displayed photographically; that is, only part of the recording process is ever made visible on the screen. Nevertheless, the spectator believes that he or she is, in principle, seeing "everything" that occurred in front of the camera — whether the camera was moving or not — because no gaps or breaks can be detected. The spectator may imagine that it is only a matter of "slowing down" the film in order to see a previously unseen moment.

The spectator's irresistible feeling of "continuity" through hyper-photography raises many complex perceptual issues.[10]

Hyper-photography can generate the appearance of an object in continuous movement, even when the object has not actually moved. In standard frame-by-frame, motion-control photography, for example, neither an object nor the camera is in movement during the exposure of a frame — they move only between exposures — yet one or both may be seen to be smoothly in movement when the film is projected. The same is true of a modern "multiple-camera" system, based on the work of Eadweard Muybridge in the 1870s, in which a large number of still cameras are fixed in a configuration and operated by a computer either simultaneously or in a sequence of exposures separated by less than a millionth of a second. In this system none of the cameras move, nor, surprisingly, is there always a camera for each image because morphing software may be used to create intermediate images. Nevertheless, on the screen it appears as if a single camera were smoothly following an action or else moving around an action that is mysteriously "frozen," slowed, or shown in time-lapse (as in Andy and Larry Wachowski's *The Matrix*, 1999). The speed of the apparent camera movement on the screen is determined by the spacing of the fixed cameras. In general, the converse is true as well: Actual movements of a camera or an object may not register on the screen because the movements were too fast or too slow with respect to exposure time, or else the movements of camera and object were exactly coordinated, canceling each other out, because movement of all material things is *relative*, not absolute.[11]

Jean Mitry notes that in a tracking shot, "the change in perspective caused by an *actual* change of position implies — and indeed includes — a real movement."[12] Thus, there may be cases in which a spectator *infers* real movement from a change in perspective because, say, the middle portion of a moving camera shot has been elided. But even when a camera does not move, the spectator may see another kind of hyper-photographic motion on the screen. This may occur when shots from different setups are *juxtaposed* in the editing of a scene. What is moving in this situation? Does a camera "jump" from one position to the next? Is it a physical camera that has this property?

Mitry describes a phenomenology of the spectator's feeling of movement when shots are edited:

> In everyday reality, we can only "totally" perceive static objects; we are dominated by movement. The fact that we can be in only one place at one time means that we are incapable of perceiving quickly moving objects; we catch only a fleeting glimpse of them. . . . Now, in the cinema the multiplicity of viewpoints restores to us not only the feeling of space but also its corollary: the feeling of movement. Editing allows us instantly to change our observation point, i.e., our position: *we move faster than the object in motion* and, for this reason, we dominate it.[13]

In many films the spectator is not supposed to notice the "jump" between shots; he or she is simply meant to experience a smooth, rapid movement that is faster than an object of interest. So-called "continuity" rules of editing have been developed by filmmakers to hide certain kinds of discontinuous motions. The editing device of "matching on action" illustrates some of the perceptual issues involved in portraying continuous change for a spectator even though the actual motion on the screen is not continuous (not continuous in several senses, as will be discussed). The match on action uses the movement of an object "across" two shots in order to suggest a single continuous action. A "node" of the action (a brief pause) is sometimes selected as the moment during which to cut to a new shot, or else a node may be created by interrupting the action with a frame line or an element of decor (for example, as a character walks toward screen right). The new shot typically involves a significant change in angle (at least 30 degrees) and/or a change in distance from the moving object, and is taken from the same side of the axis of action (the 180-degree rule). If the distance, for example, is closer to the action in the new shot, then the movement of the object (say, a character's arm raising a glass) is artificially slowed by the actor during the shooting of the second shot so that the *motion appearing on the screen* in the second shot will be a better match for the motion appearing on the screen in the more distant first shot. The reason is that a constant velocity will produce *different* speeds of motion on the screen, depending on the distance between the moving object and the camera. That is, when an object is close, its motion subtends a larger angle on the screen than when it is far away; hence, the speed of the motion *on the screen* will be greater the closer an object is to the camera. The aim is to match the speeds of the motions on the screen in the two shots so as to give the appearance of a single, continuous motion.

Furthermore, in a match on action, a small part of the movement of an object will often be left out ("elided") or else replayed ("overlapped") in order to make the match seem even smoother. The intricacy of these adjustments in the two shots is no doubt related to the very limited capacity (and limited time) of a spectator's short-term memory: Certain changes made evident in the second shot require immediate processing (e.g., a change in angle and scale requiring a mental adjustment in sizing to preserve the shape and, hence, identity of the object that is moving), leaving less memory resources for the overall context in which the changes occur. In the case of a match on action, part of the "context" for the changes in the new shot is the "motion" of an object that appears to be the same object and the same movement that was recognized in the first shot. That is, when motion in the new shot matches the *memory* of motion in the previous shot, no new processing seems to be necessary. The spectator then sees a continuous single movement of a single object. Because in fact the two shots have been made at different times and the action repeated (and slowed or speeded up or changed), there will be many combinations of motions and movements of an object, a camera, and a context that will be involved in producing a "motion" across two shots that will be noticed or not. One aspect of the art of editing consists of being able to manipulate variables in order to create various sorts of perceived continuities and discontinuities in the motion that is being pictured, no matter what the actual continuities and discontinuities were during filming.[14]

To further complicate matters, it is possible in certain kinds of cases, both on the screen and in the world, to perceive an object moving in the wrong direction or the wrong object to be in movement or to perceive motion when no object is moving, and in some of these cases, the motion is not being falsely attributed to some object — it is simply seen as a "pure" motion appearing on the screen or in the world (i.e., pure speed in a particular direction without the sense of a physical object being in motion). We may also see the movement of light even though no light is moving and we may experience paradoxical movement — that is, movement that is impossible for real objects, such as seeing a rotating spiral expand but not become larger. Moreover, by allowing certain "narrative" factors to intrude in our judgment, still larger, rather formidable concepts of mobility may be posited, such as Gilles Deleuze's "movement-image" and "time-image."[15]

These considerations raise an important point concerning the spectator. It is entirely normal for a spectator to fail to recognize that hyper-photography conceals the fact that something is permanently missing from the camera record, that light is not continuously present during projection, and that continuity rules of editing conceal or alter motions that are on the screen during shot changes (e.g., the match on action). Recall that something is permanently missing at every moment from one's normal vision of the world: We do not see that the blind spots in our retinas leave two black holes in the space in front of us (which our brain fills in by making guesses), nor do we see that the optical image on each retina is upside down and drastically curved. Moreover, the human perceptual system does not operate on the model of the cinema: In the brain there are no tiny moving pictures, no screen, no vantage point, no light, and no sound. Most times we see selectively what is present before us, but in other situations we are perfectly adept at not seeing that something is missing — and at not seeing what is present — as well as seeing what is not present because overall these sorts of processing and attention strategies offer major survival advantages (e.g., perceptual constancies that offer simplicity, speed, stability, and tolerance, without normally impairing accuracy). In some cases our perceptual system is incapable of seeing a mistake, even though we may know about the error in other ways (as in certain perceptual illusions). More important, these same

165

kinds of situations exist at higher cognitive levels where mental schemata operate to mask information that doesn't fit and to fill in gaps by making approximations and guesses where knowledge is absent.[16] Often we have no knowledge that what we see has been the result of an approximation or guess.

Later I will argue that the term "camera" should be understood against the backdrop of a diversity of bodily processes and judgments ranging from the perceptual to the cognitive, from the emotive to the motive. I believe that when a film critic speaks about a camera, he or she is tacitly invoking some theory of one or more human abilities that a camera is said to mimic, explore, refuse, transcend, and so on. The term "camera" becomes a shorthand way to make assertions about the meanings to be found in a film, *assuming* that a particular bodily process is the most prominent at that moment and operates in the assumed way. Thus, I will argue in general that it would be better to think of a "camera" less as an inert machine reprinting a strict visibility and more as a moderately open, rhetorical framework accommodating a diversity of what may be envisioned by different critics and spectators as they imagine specific perceptual and psychological effects. My present point, however, is limited to the claim that there is no absolute, perceptual definition of motion, movement, or immobility on a motion picture screen on which to build a self-evident notion of the camera.

CAMERA FICTION

What really is our idea of a "camera"? When we choose to speak, for example, of the *movement* of a camera as an explanation for a motion we sense on the screen, what is meant? Does a spectator, for example, think of the *specific* camera leased by a studio, having a certain weight and serial number that was in movement during the making of a shot? It seems unlikely that a spectator would even know which actual camera to think of. Perhaps, then, a spectator thinks of a very generalized camera with many possible weights and serial numbers — thus creating the image, as it were, of a *universal* camera. But this may still be too concrete. Instead, the spectator may be thinking of an *abstract* camera; that is, some sort of "box" with a lens, diaphragm, shutter, and film, accompanied by hazy thoughts of a cone of vision, light rays, refraction, chromatic aberration, mechanical parts, and laws of chemistry. Yet this abstraction may be too detailed: Perhaps simply a (silent) "box" would do — the camera reduced to an *ideal form*.[17] The problem, however, is that none of these notions of a camera seem to be pertinent, at least to the experience of a *fiction*. Knowing that some camera operated in the past to shoot the film, or knowing how a camera operates generally, is quite different from knowing how a camera functions in a film fictionally and narratively as well as quite different from one's experience of fictional, narrative, and discursive movements.

When we engage with a film, the viewpoint that we are given is swept into consciousness (working memory) along with the event that is being viewed, thus making both viewpoint and event equally sensate and available to the mental processes that are building meaning using the resources of long-term memory. We do not normally say, "Someone once set up a motion picture camera near a tree so that I could now look at a series of photographs that apparently show that there were some leaves moving on a tree." Instead, we say, "Leaves are moving." Once the spectator seizes on the (apparent) fact of the matter, he or she does not imagine that the tree and its moving leaves exist only as if seen through a particular, onetime peephole (or camera lens) such that the tree might really be only cardboard and the wind only an electric fan, but rather the spectator feels that the tree-leaves-wind exist as if they had been simultaneously seen through *many possible* angles. In seeing the tree, the spectator builds up a *generic* image of a tree (and its significance), rather than merely seeing something that was photographed from a specific angle. Seeing the tree "fictionally" merely builds further on this generic image of a tree. For example, the tree would become "fictional" if James Bond were seen standing under it, because "James Bond" is a generic abstraction (though a particular generic abstraction). Thus, what we see in a shot may have many invisible (abstract and mental) components. Nonetheless, we believe that these invisible components are *on* the

167

screen and, though not exactly *photographed*, have at least been "put there" or invoked by a camera.

Similarly, the question of how a prop (e.g., a tree) got into a film or was filmed, or who placed it in the film, is not the same as asking what it is doing in the film and what significance can be ascribed to the spectator's experience of seeing the prop fictionally with other fictional objects — that is, of seeing the prop as being something *else* in *another time and place* than the time and place in which it was filmed and of seeing it with *a new set of connections and affinities* to things than to the things present in the environment in which it was filmed. Hence, in a fiction film it makes no sense to ask whether a camera, or a prop, might have lied to us, or to ask what a camera might have concealed (or made explicit) in a shot, for a fiction is neither true nor false in the simple way that a physical camera either does or does not take a photograph of a thing. When interpreting a fiction, it will not help much to think of a physical camera that sees or overlooks or is blind. It is not the metaphor of camera *sight* that is at fault, but rather the mental image we have of "the thing that made the photograph." Once we form a mental picture of this sort of physical camera, we are locked into the implicit features that are pictured, and thus we forget that there may be other kinds of mental pictures for other occasions that depict a process of imagistic thinking based on very different causal processes (fictional and narrative), or that depict thinking not based on images at all (propositional and superordinate), hence pointing to other kinds of "cameras."

Here is an illustration of a camera that calls upon a "fictional" mindset: If one had been on the set during the filming of *Dr. No* (Terence Young, 1962), one would have seen Sean Connery and seen an actual camera and perhaps looked through it, but, even so, one would still not have seen James Bond or been able to converse with him. Even if we could magically talk with James Bond, what would we be able to talk to him about?[18] When Sean Connery moves across a set, we do not see James Bond in movement. We are merely seeing the creation of motion on photographs. To see James Bond in movement, we would need to see the film, and we would also need to watch with a certain attitude. Perceiving fictionally, I believe, cannot be equated with knowing the details or principles by which an artifact has been assembled in order to be perceived. The spectator's contact with a fiction is something in addition to, and quite other than, the facts of the artifact. That is to say, the physical camera is not identical to the camera through which we see fictionally.

The issues surrounding fictional viewpoints and fictional entities are so important that I would like to discuss a second example in greater detail. Let's consider a stage production of Bertolt Brecht's *The Threepenny Opera* in which a spotlight reveals the fictitious prostitute Low-Dive Jenny precisely by casting actual light on the actual actress who plays her, Lotte Lenya, perhaps.[19] To be complete, however, one should also include a description of the *fictional* light source that illuminates Jenny, perhaps the moon or lamplight or some source that may be unseen by the audience but that is presumed to exist in Jenny's world. If one were in the audience during a performance of the stage play, and *thinking like a lighting director*, one would see how an actual spotlight provides a certain quality of actual light around Lotte-as-Jenny, or, alternatively, if one were reading the script of *The Threepenny Opera* that included the stage direction, "General stage lights dim while spot comes up on Jenny," one would know how a lighting director might stage this action with whichever actress might be playing Jenny in whatever theater that might have been chosen to stage the drama.

On the other hand, if one were in the audience and *thinking fictionally* about Jenny and her world, one would see, for instance, only the moon, not a spotlight. (One might also be thinking fictionally about Lotte, but that would not be *The Threepenny Opera*.) This conclusion about being in the audience and seeing the moonlight would not be changed even if *The Threepenny Opera* became self-conscious at a particular moment and used Jenny to call attention to the spotlight in a direct address to the audience (for example, by making remarks about the cardboard moon and stagehands), because in that case, Jenny would no longer be quite the same character as before (she would become a narrator, though she might later return to being a prostitute in moonlight) and the "spotlight" that she would thereby reveal to us would no longer be quite the same as before — it would now have been made part of the *story* of *The Threepenny Opera* (for a story need not be limited to a diegesis). In short, through the agency of a self-conscious Jenny, the spotlight has become *a prop* incorporated into *The Threepenny Opera* and no longer light for the moon or a spotlight that is used generally to stage dramas other than *The Threepenny Opera*. One could also take the spotlight, as it were, in the opposite direction by employing its light metaphorically onstage — for instance, as light from heaven expressing the idea of grace — and, again, the general conclusion is not changed, for though a spotlight causes the light, the resultant illumination onstage is still not the light that is seen by the audience as coming from heaven bringing a state of grace. One cannot reduce light from heaven or the moon to a spotlight.

The relation between spotlight and moonlight is equivalent to the relation between Lotte and Jenny. But, one might protest, isn't one of Lotte's facial expressions (or way of walking) identical to Jenny's, whereas I have argued that spotlight and moonlight are not identical and not symmetric? The answer is that Lotte's facial expression is *not* identical to Jenny's because Lotte and Jenny are not in identical situations. It seems clear that Lotte (her past life, personality, present situation, wife of Brecht's collaborator Kurt Weill, antagonist in a James Bond film, *From Russia with Love*, 1963) cannot be identical in all particulars to Jenny, even if we imagine the facial expressions to be similar. (What *causes* a facial expression? Is the cause the same for both Lotte and Jenny? How many actresses may play Jenny?) I believe that we should say that there is something *less* of Lotte in Jenny or, alternatively, that there is something *more* to Jenny than Lotte. That is, for the audience, Jenny represents a surplus of meaning with respect to Lotte (emergent meaning, if you like). This surplus of meaning (i.e., the fiction) is what is lost when one collapses Jenny back into Lotte, moonlight back into a spotlight.

Part of the problem here is that the word "cause" is tacitly being used in two different senses when we think about the "cause" of the moonlight. For a lighting director, the spotlight causes the moonlight, because when the spotlight goes out, the moonlight ends. This is not true, however, for someone interpreting fictionally, for the reason that moonlight is not caused by a spotlight but by the sun; thus, if the spotlight goes out, the moonlight does not end but continues to be seen in mind as a fact of Jenny's world. Consider an analogous situation in which the script of *The Threepenny Opera* is being read (or heard) *as a story*. Here moonlight exists without either a literal, figurative, or imagined spotlight. For example, in "The 'No They Can't' Song" from *The Threepenny Opera*, a person will read about a special "moon over Soho" that exists "When you first fall in love and the moonbeams shine." The reader imagines the moon, and day and night, but not a spotlight illuminating the moon. In a larger context, however, the song is about the pretense and self-deception of young love and how a phrase like the preceding one about moonbeams, in fact, is merely, as the song says, a "line," an affected "bit." Only at this moment does the moon promptly vanish in irony — as subtly predicted by the 'negative' contained in the song's title and first line ("No, they can't . . ."). One might continue thinking about the lines in the script and argue that a more important cause of the need for *The Threepenny Opera* to shine a light on Lotte using a spotlight might be the eighteenth-century theatrical drama that it reworks and builds upon, John Gay's *The Beggar's Opera*. In this sense, another fiction is (apparently) the cause, the source, of the spotlight. That is to say, the spotlight lights *because/when* a script (Gay's, Brecht's) is taken to be an instance of the *kind* of thing that *can do* this, can illuminate by a rhetorical figure ('Now, I see what is meant by the song.'). The illumination achieved through figuration may be just as real as that achieved through a spotlight, even though that does not make them the same.[20]

Therefore, one should say that a spotlight and the moon both cause light on the stage, that both Lotte and Jenny send someone (Raúl Julia; Mac the Knife) to "prison." I believe that the same dark ambiguity about the "cause" of light onstage underlies the expression, "Lotte causes Jenny" (i.e., a "cause" in what situation?). Instead of seeking a single kind of causation for all occasions, it would be better to recognize sets of causes, and types of actions, that are arranged in layers or strata. (Many events besides light coming from a spotlight-moon would seem to possess "adjacent" causatives.[21] Plainly, we will need to examine the general nature of causation, though I will defer this inquiry until the section after next.) A "stratified" arrangement of causes might allow one to claim that moonlight "supervenes" on light from a spotlight or that Jenny's voice "supervenes" on Lotte's voice.[22] Moreover, it seems incorrect to assert that the spotlight occurs chronologically "before" the moonlight or that Lotte's voice occurs "before" Jenny's; each pair of events would seem to occur simultaneously, as if there were really only a single event in each case, but two distinct descriptions depending on the pertinent "cause" — that is, depending on what problem is being addressed in what situation.

Another possibility for separating moonlight from spotlight would be to employ the distinction between "mention" and "use." A word that is quoted is being mentioned rather than used, for example, if one were to write: "the word 'illuminate,' which may be used to indicate an action, has ten letters and does not rhyme with 'rhyme.'" The word "illuminate" as well as the second appearance of the word "rhyme" are being mentioned (quoted) but not, in the first instance, used. (In fact, the two mentioned words are also being mentioned in this book in an illustration about mention and use.) Note that whether the words "illuminate" and "rhyme" are being mentioned or used, causes are still at work in producing the utterance and its effect on a reader even though each word's *spelling* is unchanged; indeed, one could not mention a word unless it were, in fact, spelled the same as when it was being used. By analogy, one might say that light *from* a spotlight is being used to illuminate Lotte (a "use" of light) while at the same time light is being "mentioned" *with* a spotlight in the context of a moonlit night on stage, which produces a kind of "rhyme" between the mentioned "light" and the presumed moonlight illuminating Jenny (a "mention" of light).[23] When light is mentioned, some of its properties (but not all) are being highlighted — that is, exhibited so as to be noticed. Mentioning light does not amount to an assertion that the spotlight is the moon or is the light of the moon. This suggests to me, as with the notion of supervenience, that what is important in thinking about mention and use (and fiction and nonfiction) is not the nature of the material of an entity (whether made up of letters of the alphabet or light) but how and *when* that material is mobilized — that is, *when* it may be set in movement to create motion for some purpose in some situation. In attending to the mobility of something, it is a mistake to think that physical causation is the only true cause at work while other causes/interactions directed at other purposes are mere variants or imprecise ways of speaking.

Now suppose that a camera were to be set up to record a performance of *The Threepenny Opera*; that is, the purpose of the camera would be to record actual actors and their actual movements in actual light on the stage. It is certain that a spotlight onstage will cause the film in the camera to become exposed, but what light will be seen by a spectator when looking at the resulting photograph? Will a spectator see a spotlight or moonlight? In order to answer this question, one would need to know how someone is looking. What is the relevant action that someone is looking to find: the action of a spotlight in disclosing Lotte due to the prior action of a lighting director, or the action of Jenny lit up by the moon, or, indeed, some other action (e.g., the 'brilliance' of Bertolt Brecht)? Accordingly, one may ask whether the "camera" is really the same in each of these cases, that is, whether the rationale for the view and what is viewed is identical across all cases.

Perhaps enough has now been said about *The Threepenny Opera*. Let me summarize my argument by recalling a platitude about Edwin Porter's *The Great Train Robbery* (1903) that has wedged its way into every aspect of film history, theory, criticism, and aesthetics. It is often asserted that at the close of the film "a fictitious robber fires a fictitious gun at actual spectators by pointing the gun at the camera." When the gun is thus "pointed," is it still a fictional gun or has it become real? Or is it neither? What is "the camera" as a thing to be "pointed at"? How must a spectator be looking to be frightened? I believe that this claim is near nonsense despite its common sense because it confuses multiple frames of reference instead of discriminating between types of causation and ways of looking.

173

Though the sentence is grammatical, there is a deeper sense in which it is thoroughly ungrammatical, because, as Wittgenstein might say, its words have been drawn from different regions of language or, more precisely, drawn from different languages.

Let me state a conclusion based upon the above examples from *Dr. No*, *The Threepenny Opera*, and *The Great Train Robbery*: In order to avoid serious misunderstandings, one must be clear about what it is that language is being employed to do — about what specific work one wishes to accomplish with a form of expression, no matter whether the instrument of expression is a spotlight, moonlight, a camera, the skill of an actress, words spoken by a fictional character, a prop, or the words of a critic. One cannot discern the "use" of an expression or object in the abstract but, instead, must weigh a person's method of looking and listening and his or her abilities and goals in a particular situation. A "use" may rather be a "mention" within a context that is not immediately visible. The moonlight mentioned onstage, for example, is not as visible as the spotlight, because the light from the spotlight must be seen *as if* it were from the moon. A spotlight, when it illuminates, does not have a single use, or effect, for all occasions, and hence the causality associated with its "light" is not fixed for all occasions. Similarly, the "light" that is reflected to a "camera" is not absolute, but relative to a situation in which it is seen to function. The light that exposes an emulsion in a camera is not the light that functions fictionally on a stage. Or, as one might say, light on stage is being framed in two different ways by two "cameras."

RELEASING AND RECEIVING

Noël Carroll writes instructively about a fictional character's relationship to a spectator. I believe that his remarks may be expanded to suggest what kinds of roles a camera may play when a spectator is interpreting fictionally. Carroll says,

> [I]nsofar as we share the same culture as the protagonist [of a horror film], we can easily catch-on to why the character finds

the monster unnatural. However, once we've assimilated the situation from the character's point of view, we respond not simply to the monster, as the character does, but to a situation in which someone, who is horrified, is under attack.[24]

Although the spectator is able to understand the character's viewpoint and share in the character's disgust and fear, Carroll also emphasizes that the spectator is inevitably outside and external to that view: We respond not just to a concrete, apparent situation (a specific character resisting a malevolent, palpable creature) but also more broadly to "a situation in which someone . . ." That is, the spectator frames the situation quite differently from the character because the spectator has recourse to kinds of information that the character does not know at a particular time, may never know, can never know, or would have no interest in knowing. The audience may be truly concerned for the character, but the emotions felt by the audience will never be identical in all respects to, or as intense as, those of the character.[25]

A character has emotions because he or she acts on a belief, whereas an individual in an audience has emotions because he or she is entertaining a belief through construing a narrative pattern. (For some theories, a spectator's emotion is based on something less than a belief, such as an "evaluation," "judgment," "appraisal," "preference," or mere "thought.") Characters and their circumstances are, after all, fictional and represent only a prompt for the spectator, who must bring to bear on the fiction his or her own memories, desires, anxieties, curiosity, cultural knowledge, wonderment, dread, self-deception, values, ambivalence, and so forth. An individual spectator will amplify and make salient (fill in, fill out, reorder, revise) that which exists on the screen as merely a series of *unfinished, hollow, and indefinite* referents (*a* situation, *some*one, *an* action, *some*time), perhaps not unlike seeing some thing in a Rorschach inkblot.

An individual has emotions at the movies not because he or she mistakenly believes the fiction true but, rather, because he or she is expending energy in reacting to something that is familiar.

175

The individual makes it familiar (generic) by reworking what is partially indeterminate on the screen. A thought is frightening to a spectator only because he or she imagines how the thought may connect to a fearful situation, or type of fearful situation, outside the movie theater. Implicit in watching a film are questions about why a story is being told: What values and real situations are implicated in the story? Why are these fictional events worthy of attention? Whose interests are being served through the telling of the story? Again, a spectator is engaged in a different activity from a character, even if the result may be that an emotion felt by the spectator is similar to one felt by the character.

Although a spectator may well imagine that he or she is "inside" a fiction (or "inside" a character), he or she is in a different place within the fiction from the view that appears on the screen. This is demonstrated by the fact that although a person normally cannot recall the exact shots or their sequence in a scene, he or she can easily describe the locale, remember the action, pinpoint doors and furniture, fill in details, overlook certain "mistakes" in continuity, visualize moving about within the scene to assume new angles, and draw pictures of the scene from angles that were not shown (for example, from an ideal overhead view).[26] These abilities show that our essential comprehension of a scene is much deeper than what happens to have been shown, or is being shown, in the fragments of space provided by a relatively few shots. The reason is that when we look at a shot, it is embedded within everything that we have previously learned, inferred, and assumed about the significance of ongoing events as well as embedded in expectations about the future of these events. Most important, our comprehension does not escape our values and life experiences, our place in a nonfictional world. Thus, what we are constructing when we see a shot on the screen is decidedly nonlocal and nonvisual in nature — namely, patterns and connections that give underlying form to an event. We are not memorizing lists of shots, angles of view, or miscellanies of visibilia, but using long-term memory to assemble a mental matrix that permits us to freely visualize and feel in ways that have been projected through the fiction from ordinary belief.[27]

No image appears simply in a "present-time" removed from thought, memory, and expectation, at least in narrative discourse. Therefore, one should not speak of *the* camera at all, but of many separate superimposed cameras corresponding to multiple (even incompatible) interpretations that are simultaneously operating during a shot. In *Dr. No*, for example, do we see both Sean Connery and James Bond in the same image, or separately in two kinds of overlapping images? In a point-of-view shot, do we see only a character's private view, or — in another way of looking — do we see an image that is being presented by a higher-level, implicit narration in order to reveal information and advance the plot? But, when we look again, don't we see that this higher-level narration is itself being presented (as a device, convenience, conceit, mask, or frame) by a still more powerful narration in order to delay and *hide* developments in the story so that the plot will not just halt, but will continue, and in due course will have a proper *end*? [28] How do characters who have a point-of-view (whether or not seen in the film at a given moment) come to exist? (I am referring here to characters, because a spectator does not believe that a point-of-view shot represents the actor's view, such as Sean Connery's view.) I believe that the spectator creates and appropriates a character's view as needed to aid comprehension during the unfolding of a narrative pattern that has a "point." Thus, it is misleading to visualize a film image in a story as being singular merely because it has come from a single photograph or a single shot.

When we watch a film, we are not painstakingly reconstructing the view of the/a physical camera, step by step — or identifying with it, or becoming equivalent to it — but, rather, we are crisscrossing through time: remembering, imagining, feeling, filling out, and applying one or several *developing models or schemata* that make possible our conscious acts of perception. Our visual knowledge of a scene is neither identical to, nor determined exclusively by, the visible and audible features of a shot or a sequence of shots. Instead, a camera in a fiction film is a global construct that is at least partly projected by the viewer's mental state and, hence, like the notions of "character" and "diegesis," is more than the

177

sum of what is literally heard and appears on the screen during a shot or a sequence of shots. In this way of thinking, a "camera" comes to function almost as the spectator's *mini-theory* of film comprehension — that is, as an emblem for his or her beliefs about the creation, watching, and interpreting of a film.

Christian Metz offers a graceful and apposite remark:

> When I say that "I see" the film, I mean thereby a unique mixture of two contrary currents: the film is what I receive, and it is also what I release, since it does not pre-exist my entering the auditorium and I only need close my eyes to suppress it. Releasing it, I am the projector, receiving it, I am the screen; in both these figures together, I am the camera, which points and yet which records.[29]

SUSTAINING AND OTHER CAUSES

> "[T]here came a morning when something rather peculiar happened to him. And this thing, which as I say was only *rather* peculiar, soon caused a second thing to happen which was *very* peculiar. And then the *very* peculiar thing, in its own turn, caused a really *fantastically* peculiar thing to occur."
>
> — Roald Dahl, *James and the Giant Peach*
> (Chapter 2, original emphases)

I have been arguing that our comprehension of film is not restricted to the limited views offered by shots and a physical camera. What we come to know and contribute to the film as we construct its fictional world exceeds what the screen shows. This casts doubt on the claims of some writers who take photography to be the essence of film and the preeminent cause that stimulates and authorizes our responses.[30] The emphasis on photography presumes that the crucial fact about film is that something has thrown a part of itself — its outline, texture, or movement — onto the screen. Film is seen as an art of "moving shadows." Even if an object happens not to be in movement, it is said to endure on the screen, and this abstract movement of the object (in the flow of time rather than across space) is said to be directly recorded on film — a shadow seized and held firmly in place. This causal approach, often identified with the theories of André Bazin and Siegfried Kracauer, insists that the movements and persistence of an object are captured photographically by film despite the annoying mechanical and perceptual "technicalities," metaphors, fictions, and figurative projections that surround pictorial motion and movement (discussed in the preceding sections).

Our fascination and respect for photography come in part from a seemingly insurmountable asymmetry: We feel that a blurred or dim picture is a picture of something that has sharp or bright lines, while we feel that a picture with distinct lines cannot be an approximation of something that is blurry. The same may be said of motion on the screen: Though it may be blurred or partial, it must be of a movement that is from *one precise point* to another. The belief is that no matter how distorted a photograph, certain basic facts of the world — some of them at least — will make their *presence felt* in the photographicity of film.[31] Thus, an indistinct area in a photograph will be assumed to be a function of the medium (e.g., focus, exposure, resolution, or registration), much like a window that has been streaked with rain. What is not specific to the medium is inessential and contingent, an obstacle to perfect functioning and perfect vision. In this approach, seeing by a spectator depends on overcoming physical obstructions and imperfections in the medium. The argument proceeds as follows: *But for* the limitations of the instrument, we would be able to see, not just a few points in space, but each point in space, and each point of a color, clearly and distinctly, because real space and real color, even if toned, supposedly have the property of being composed of clear and distinct, minute bits packed tightly along continuous and dense lines. Something seen to be blurry or tinted is simply imperfect because it is seen to have too many or too few lines, or more than one proper color.

The folk theory of looking at the world as if through a "window" — where some things are imagined to be sharp (i.e., real) and others blurry (i.e., imperfect or subjective) — may underlie the idea in some branches of philosophy and jurisprudence that a strict test or rule (which draws sharp lines) is fundamentally *more accurate* than a vague, open rule (which makes lines fuzzy; cf. the rules of law stated in the Bill of Rights).[32] Sometimes we forget that when we look at the world, some movements actually are "indistinct" (for example, in peripheral vision or at dusk) and that some movements alter the appearance of an object and make lines "indistinct." Hyper-photography itself is a "blurring" of the distinction between individual photographic frames. This raises the question: Under which conditions should we say that an object actually is?

To summarize: The asymmetry involving sharpness and blurriness in a photograph reaffirms the conventional "window" image we have for looking at the world. The photographic asymmetry, like the fundamental one between cause and effect, is taken to be the mark of a unique and irreversible photographic or microscopic process whose unidirectional nature situates us firmly as being located *at one end* of its working upon the world (like a periscope that locks us in place). Moreover, our memory, too, may be conceived as being (imperfectly) photographic.[33] It is not surprising, then, that the power of the *photographic* in a picture may be extended even further in order to model the whole of cinema: its history, ideology, aesthetics, and realism, as well as explaining the reactions of its spectators.[34]

Causal theories of representation look backward in time, searching for an origin that can explain how the past has been sharply focused into a present participle (overcoming "noise" in the system). A branch of physics or engineering usually provides the covering laws that are taken to define cinema as a photographic medium — for example, laws that describe how the chemical activity of a film emulsion makes past and present contiguous. One aim of invoking such physical laws is to locate the camera within an intricately linked chain of events passing through the medium or else to detect the camera as an instantaneous spot *sustained* on a dense "tapestry" (the world) by a meshwork of hidden causal fibers.

But this focus seems to be too narrow. An element may be necessary or sufficient for an outcome but still not be the most "important," or the most "prominent," in a causal sequence with respect to its benefit *for*, or its impact *on*, us. For instance, having a match to strike seems to be more important in the usual circumstances than that there be oxygen in the air or that the Earth be in a stable orbit around the sun (both of which are taken for granted); having a script for a film would seem more important than the presence of silver halides in the film emulsion or the presence somewhere of phosphor dots that are capable of flickering on a television screen. In addition, we do not find it helpful to reduce ordinary actions and events to the operation of the four fundamental physical forces — the strong nuclear, weak nuclear, electromagnetic, and gravitational forces. The reason is that there are innumerable types of daily interactions on a human scale that are better described in an ordinary language which plainly marks the relevant motivation for motive push and pull.[35] When we speak of "past" and "present," we are most often referring to a sense of time measured on a human scale and to a kind of time that is *made significant for our memories and interests*, for our problems and projects. This is not the same kind of *history* as that of photons that have, or have not, alighted upon silver halides. A different history requires a different language.

The types of causation that are proposed by photographic theories of film representation are both too local and too strong.[36] These theories are reminiscent of the reduction of moonlight to a spotlight in *The Threepenny Opera* on the assumption that talking about the moon onstage is inexact and inaccurate ("blurry"), whereas filaments and electricity provide the real truth about light, like a photograph in sharp focus. On this basis theorists of "new media" conclude that the essential qualities of film cannot be photographic because new technologies make it impossible to tell the difference between a photograph and a computer-generated picture. Such arguments miss the point, because they are premised on the need for a perceiver to attain *certainty* in his or her judgments based on acts of perceiving. (Descartes sought just this measure of certainty but was forced to give up on sensory data and rely instead on a kind of introspection.) When looking at an image, what is it that one is supposed to be certain of? A connection to the world, if it is to be true?[37] I have been arguing that the physical connection of photography to the world is not the issue. A connection to the world may be causal (and thus truly representative, even "typical") in many ways *other* than "physical." And these other ways cannot be reduced to the physical.

I believe that instead of searching for a single sort of causation at the root of everything, one should begin by searching for causes of different sizes and strengths arranged in layers or strata. This would be an acknowledgment that causes in one layer are relatively autonomous from other layers and that analysis should proceed in a horizontal manner along a layer, rather than seeking to penetrate through layers to reach the base. I believe that the most important and prominent causes for understanding how a spectator thinks about a "camera" will be causes from a "middle level" that correspond to the world that we normally inhabit, a world of middle dimensions (i.e., neither the small-scale world of quantum fluctuation nor the large-scale world of galaxy movement). In fact, it would be more accurate to speak of a still-smaller world of concern, a middle world of levels within the middle world, which would include ordinary language and folk theories.

I will return in later sections of this chapter to a discussion of various "mid-mid-sized" causes, but first we must examine the general notion of causation and how theorists deploy it in an effort to fashion an *explanation*. This will help solve misunderstandings that arise when a set of causal terms is selected to explain what a camera *can do* in order to define what sort of object it is. I will attempt to show that the notion of "causation" is more complex than might appear. Not all types of causation are physical in the same way. Moreover, because causation is tied to "explanation," it has an intimate tie to how we use language.

I will begin with the example of a table in a room. I would like to illustrate the innumerable types of causation that surround the table. In fact, it may be instructive to think of the room as a sort of "medium" acting between the table and its users. How should one isolate those causes that are deemed "important"? Here are some causes:

> In the room, the floor and the legs of the table act as "sustaining" causes that keep the top of the table in *position* to sustain a different substance, a shadow of the table, that *appears* on the floor (and whose size is responsive to — is caused by — the *fact* of the size of the family that uses the table) at the same time that the floor and table legs keep (sustain) the top of the table level as (generally) *envisaged* by a carpenter who caused the legs to be attached (decorating them according to the *fashion* of the time) as well as by the *resolve* of a person who later (specifically) caused the table to be *carried* into the room (where the presence in the room of air to breathe was *necessary*) and who, by continuing to *not act*[38] to upset the table, causes it to stand at the ready — in all *probability* — remaining in a fit condition to support (sustain) the dishes for tomorrow's meal (during which a cup will sustain a liquid) that will be brought to the table *because* it is a standard social *practice* and *because* it stands reflecting light causing an *impression* on a person who *can see* where to bring the dishes (though walking into the room does not cause the walls to change color or the room to change shape), incidentally causing the person who brings the dishes to *infer* that the table had been legally purchased (i.e., acquired through a socially regulated *exchange*) and is nice to look at (as judged *aesthetically*), which inferences cause a change in the person's overall *beliefs* that sustains a new conviction, eliciting also a pleasant *memory* of an unrelated passage in a favorite book (the effect of a college education that was *expected* of members of the family) with the unintended consequence of remembering the need to *plan how* to buy brushes and paint for the walls *conducive to* a result whereby *someone* will undertake to do the "necessary" painting . . . and so on. (By the way, what causes an "example" to appear in a book and what sustains it?)

My example is meant to hint at the large number of causes at work in a prosaic situation, indeed a number almost uncountably large. I also mean the example to emphasize the enormous range of *types* of causes with varying strengths, tendencies, possibilities, and the myriad interrelationships that are working to bring together quite disparate things, including materials, physical forces, conditions, percepts, partial ideas, general ideas, inferences, intentions, inclinations, forbearance, feelings, expectations, plans, abilities, procedures, behavior, fashion, social rules, facts, catalysts, probabilities, and other things. Despite these many complications, however, we ordinarily reduce causation to something simple that fits with an immediate interest, and the mechanism for doing so lies in language.

The concept of "causation" refers to change. But which of many changes are of interest? There are two kinds of change: either an overt change — a coming into existence or an important change in state — or else an inertia or resistance to change — a persistence. The latter is called a *sustaining* cause.[39] Is there a sharp line between these two kinds of change, and, if so, from what point of view must we look to see the line? Ordinarily we think of a cause not in terms of inertia or constraint but as some active force or energy, a power or agency that compels or produces evident change. Obviously, motion and movement, and how we see and talk about them as instances of change, involve such "positive" causation. But, of course, there may be causation at work where there is no motion and/or no movement; this is the less familiar causality of *un*changing states due to the presence of sustaining causes. Note that a sustaining cause actively *works* to produce no change; it is not something that *potentially* may occur in the future nor something that a person has omitted or *not* done (notwithstanding the fact that a failure to act may cause something to happen which, in turn, may lead to legal liability). Think of table legs working to sustain a tabletop and the tabletop holding the legs upright, or stones sustaining each other in an archway, or a lens in a spotlight sustaining our view of the gestures of an actor onstage while, at the same time, sustaining attached and cast shadows elsewhere onstage that obscure our view. I will continue to probe the nature of sustaining causes in what follows because this peculiar notion of "unchange" or "inaction" seems to be deeply embedded in our decisions about what constitutes a positive "action" bearing upon an object. That is, the notion of sustaining causation would seem to lie behind (sustain?) our talk about the prototypical form of causation that features a striking change brought about by what I will term a "positive" or "mobile" causation.

I wish to propose the following analogy: Positive or mobile causation is to sustaining causation as a property is to a substance. This formulation brings out the close connection between causality and ontology. Just as a property may occur and undergo change in many different particular things, but requires a substance in order to appear, so positive causation may appear and make changes, but only against (i.e., only when sustained by) a background of causative immobility. What moves or changes moves only *relative to* a chosen frame of causal reference. Thus, to take as an example the adage "the more things change, the more they stay the same," one may inquire, in each specific case of putative "change," which particular frames of reference will make the adage true and which frames will make it false. It would seem that sometimes we think of a camera's relationship to film in the same way — namely, as that of a positive or mobile cause to a sustaining cause, like a property to a substance. The key question about the camera will involve which frame of reference (which sustaining cause, which "substance") is to be chosen when a particular causal problem is to be solved about film.

When we consider less tangible, less literal forms of mobility, we draw closer to the problem of causation in general, to *its* causality. I believe that when we talk about causation, we are disclosing what is relevant to our interests in the context of practical interactions with a world, that is, disclosing our immersion in a "form of life" (Wittgenstein) or a "way of worldmaking" (Goodman). In talking about causes, we frame a world by creating categories that make similarities — "things like 'c'" are regularly followed by "things like 'e,'" forming the larger category "things like 'c-e.'" (If the category is fuzzy, then the causation may be fuzzy, probabilistic.) We create categories, differences, and hierarchies in order to divide and parse the world into significant types of pieces with respect to our interests. These pieces then become part of a "language" within which modes of change and interaction may be described. The aim is to indicate how relevant temporal "parts" work to make up a *whole*, how a "duration" is formed.[40] For example, in the epigraph above from Roald Dahl, three events are said to be causally linked — all are alike in being "peculiar," though each remains distinct by being called "only rather," "very," and "really fantastically" peculiar. Once a thing or part is "peculiar," it is perhaps inevitable that it become more so, and also less so.

Wittgenstein emphasizes the connection between causation and language in the following way:

> Whenever we say that something *must* be the case we are using a norm of expression. Hertz said that wherever something did not obey his laws there must be invisible masses to account for it. [For example, one might explain a planet's observed eccentric behavior by saying that there must be some other planet attracting it.] This statement is not right or wrong, but may be practical or impractical. Hypotheses such as "invisible masses," "unconscious mental events" are norms of expression. They enter into language to enable us to say there *must* be causes. . . . We believe we are dealing with a natural law *a priori*, whereas we are dealing with a norm of expression that we ourselves have fixed. Whenever we say that something must be the case we have given an indication of a rule for the regulation of our expression, as if one were to say "Everybody is really going to Paris. True, some don't get there, but all their movements are preliminary." . . . The statement that there must be a cause shows that we have got a rule of language. . . . We ought not say that there are no causes in nature, but only that we have a system in which there are no causes. Determinism and indeterminism are properties of a system which are fixed arbitrarily.[41]

Wittgenstein argues that choosing a set of categories and a proper segmentation (a grammar) has important consequences.

Two of Zeno's paradoxes, for instance, render movement impossible; that is, movement is impossible within the terms Zeno uses to describe the world. (His terms divide "distance" and "time" into a series of precise mathematical points designed to create a clear and sharp picture of the world. Recall the discussion at the beginning of this section.) Think also of the causal ramifications of making a distinction between mind and body — one of the preoccupations of Western philosophy — or of the causal fallout from the distinctions posed by John Searle in his Chinese Room argument about artificial intelligence.[42] A segmentation is designed to specify which "parts" will belong to an "object," thus setting into motion the appropriate *sustaining* causes. A part, however, may also be an object with its own parts, and an object may be merely a part connected to something else; moreover, something that previously went unnoticed, may suddenly become relevant as a part or an object. Stipulating parts and objects is vital for framing and describing a "causation" that will properly fit the pieces. Just as two parts exist because a distinction has been drawn between them, so the "causal" part of an interaction between two things is distinguished from the "effectual" part of the interaction. Simply marking the passage of time, however, is not sufficient to define causation, even though marking time is necessary for causal reasoning. A chronology is necessary for causal reasoning, because a cause cannot precede its effect and an effect cannot work backward in time to create a cause. A chronology, however, is not sufficient for distinguishing cause from effect, because real time is a continuum, while dividing cause from effect requires a sharp discontinuity, a disjunction of some sort. This disjunction is supplied by the segmentation — the language — that has been adopted for prescribing parts and defining objects according to our immersion in a situation or problem.

As an illustration, consider the act of writing with a pencil as opposed to scratching a blackboard with a fingernail. In both cases the same motive force (muscles, arm) in the same temporal sequence of linked events is applied to a similar end (making a mark); yet in the former we focus on the pencil as an effect (of how the arm moves), while in the latter we focus on the blackboard (or the annoying sound) as the effect. We do not say that the arm compels the movement of the fingernail in the same way that the arm compels the movement of the pencil. The reason is that our attention is usually drawn to the actions of certain *independent midsized objects*, not drawn to what we deem to be simply sustaining causes or background causes that are tied up with *mere parts* that constitute an object. We take the pencil to be an independent object, while the fingernail is a mere part. The following are all things we assume to be "mere parts" when we distinguish writing with a pencil from scratching with a fingernail: the fingernail, the fingers gripping the pencil, the wood holding the pencil lead in place, oxygen in the blood, nerve impulses, calories from ingested food, molecules in the blackboard, screws securing the blackboard to the wall, a wooden frame holding the blackboard in place so that it might be scratched, a medium of air for the transmission of changes in kinetic molecular energy originating in a scratch on a blackboard, and a psychical mechanism alert to a particular sound. Now suppose that the pencil were taken away but the hand continued to move, perhaps absentmindedly: Is its movement now a *cause* of some figures being drawn in the air? Is it instead an *effect* of something? Is it neither cause nor effect? Don't we need to *interpret* this situation in order to assign cause and effect? Think also of a pencil bouncing down a hillside: Is the pencil writing? Do we say that the movements of one end of the pencil are *both* the cause and the effect of the movements of the other end? (We cannot: Instead we must invoke causes that sustain each other.)

The problem of segmenting into a series of "parts" that are relative to one another — that is, breaking up the temporal continuum to find the exemplary description for our purpose, to designate a relevant "cause" and "effect" — can be extended backward from the arm-with-pencil to the problem of disengaging mental events such as "willing" the arm to move the pencil. In this situation, however, it may be a mistake to think that a single vocabulary in a universal language of causation can account for every set of segmentations (partitions) that we may wish to make and that we may find useful for forming a causal expression. As

Wittgenstein observes, "Let us not forget this: when 'I raise my arm,' my arm goes up. And the problem arises: what is left over if I subtract the fact that my arm goes up from the fact that I raise my arm?"[43] The answer, I believe, is not to say that "nothing" remains, which would lead to the result that behavioral facts simply coincide with mental facts; rather, the answer is that what remains is a boundary between *two different regions of language* across which obvious analogies may be wrong. To put it differently, causation exists in layers or strata that are fit to different scales and problems. For this reason I believe that one should be wary of assimilating an expression such as "I took a photograph" to the expression "Light reached the film emulsion." (Cf. a theory that explains film in terms of its "photographicity.") Such a correlation produces the following analogy: "*Arriving* at a decision to take a photograph is like *pushing* a button on a camera." The "mental" (first-person) and "physical" (third-person) cameras in these expressions may not be sufficiently alike to function in analogous ways as "parts" of a single causal sequence that can be encompassed by a single form of expression. Aren't we being misled by the physical presence of a camera into thinking that "arriving at a decision" can be fused to "pushing a button," and that both events are as physical as the camera? Perhaps both events are indeed physical, but then shouldn't we say that they involve different physics?

I believe that this line of reasoning supports the distinction that I have previously urged between the expressions "I see James Bond" and "I see *that* Sean Connery is acting in the role of James Bond." I am trying to suggest that the general notion of causation needs to be broadened and deepened from the sort of physical causation tied up with film theories built upon physics and photographicity — theories that celebrate "moving shadows," as it were. I believe that when causation itself is viewed in relation to language, it will be seen to have different uses in different situations. A camera, too, should be seen relative to the specific language that we have chosen in framing problems of concern to us. It is not that causation doesn't exist in nature (for we have important projects that concern nature) but, rather, that causes are

189

everywhere — positive and sustaining — and they do not decide an issue apart from the discourse that states the issue.

In answering causal questions, much depends on how we choose to look and for what purpose. Where attention is focused, causation becomes mobile, or positive, while the rest is at rest, or, rather, the remainder is causation that sustains. In choosing to focus our attention, we place a frame around something. When a given frame is thus in place, it *sustains* the elements that are the focus of our interest. If we focus on the presence of a shot onscreen, for example, we might say that the four sides of the shot act as "sustaining" causes of the image and its content, much as the four legs of a table keep the top and its objects (its content) in place. (Indeed, the word "tableau" comes from "table" and from "tablet." In this mental picture, the frame appears in a tangible form, distinct from its "content," and so easily leads to the thought of a *tabula rasa*.) I have been arguing, however, that although the physical causation of photography may sustain a film image onscreen, it will not, in general, sustain the "meaning" of the image, because the causal background for "meaning" is not physical causation but the interests and problems of humans. For this reason, commentary offered by a critic on the meaning of a shot is relevant to fashioning and refashioning a theory of film. To paraphrase Wittgenstein, 'what the thing film is is the class of things it does.'[44] A theory of film is not simply an objective statement about physical causes and, as such, is not permanent but subject to change.

In the previous chapter we found many kinds of frames at work in film theories. This makes it unlikely that an absolute frame exists that will determine the nature of film or its parts for all cases; rather, an object such as film would seem to become appropriate to a frame because the frame is relative to a problem, process, goal, or some type of behavior. In short, I believe that an object is relative to a situation in which certain kinds of things can happen in a kind of 'action-game' specified by a "language-game." My present concern is with a camera-object that 'appears' on the screen only because it *sustains* a viewpoint, or meaning, through the framing of a shot. We come to know this camera-object through what we experience, feel, and come to believe when assessing and reassessing the meanings of a film. These meanings are not limited to the moment-by-moment meanings of what is on the screen during projector time. Instead, a camera emerges from a wider set of discursive practices, from its fit within a variety of language-games.

The ultimate question concerns *how and when* causality is to appear *in our language* as a frame with which to explain a "game" being played (or a "grammar" being followed) when we make meaning.[45] The interests that shape these forms of expression must not be assumed to be uniform or transparent across our language. As Wittgenstein suggests in the epigraph, language is divided into regions of various sizes and strengths. Making analogies between these regions based on similar ways of speaking, he says, may cause (!) misunderstandings.[46] Thus, more than a formal analysis of language into uniform rules will be required in order to deal with the many uses that we may make of the vocabulary of causation. How, then, should language be analyzed in a nonreductive way?

WITTGENSTEIN

"Philosophers like to follow Aristotle in saying that philosophy begins in wonder. My impression is that philosophers nowadays tend to associate the experience of wonder with the explanations of science rather than, as in Wittgenstein and Austin, with the recognition of our relation to things as they are, the perception of the extraordinariness of what we find ordinary (for example, beauty), and the ordinariness of what we find extraordinary (for example, violence)."[47]

— Stanley Cavell

"I want to say: it is characteristic of our language that the foundation on which it grows consists in steady ways of living, regular ways of acting."[48]

— Ludwig Wittgenstein

Wittgenstein argues that language should be grasped in terms of the vast diversity of uses and applications of words in *accomplishing* purposes with the things around us. He argues that language should not be analyzed by focusing on the homogeneity and limited range of sonic and written forms or by seeking uniform formulas. (Here are some uniform formulas about language: 'every word signifies something,' 'every word and its parts are signs,' 'the word "negation" has a single meaning and essence,' 'language is communication.') For Wittgenstein language is not made of bits and pieces that are to be carefully assembled to form a picture of the world. Instead, Wittgenstein draws an analogy with instruments in a toolbox that, I believe, bears also on the nature of causality and its intimate connection to language:

> Imagine someone's saying: "*All* tools serve to modify something. Thus the hammer modifies the position of the nail, the saw the shape of the board, and so on." — And what is modified by the rule, the glue-pot, the nails? — "Our knowledge of a thing's length, the temperature of the glue, and the solidity of the box." — Would anything be gained by this assimilation of expressions? —

To me this suggests that when language is understood to be inextricably intertwined with *particular* acts and actions — a "form of life" as opposed to 'rules' or the naming of 'definite' objects — it grows to encompass relevant forms of causality as well, or, rather, that causality should not be understood in a narrow, technical way that assimilates actions into one or a few formulas (e.g., 'every tool modifies something — either itself, an object, or our knowledge,' 'every tool is capable of mobilizing physical force,' 'causation is physical force,' 'causation modifies something'). Instead, causality should be opened up to the differentiation of numberless specific contexts in which actions are used and applied to accomplish very different goals in differing ways, in which human 'action-games' are woven into "language-games."[49] That is, rather than splitting language into larger and smaller parts vertically, as it were — into syntactical phrases, words, morphemes, phonemes, letters, and so forth — Wittgenstein divides it horizontally into (overlapping) regions that map into kinds of projects and uses. Wittgenstein stresses that understanding and interpreting involve a skilled performance that is fit to the plan of a game, not to feelings or conscious states of mind.[50] He asks, for example, what it could be like to know the alphabet "all the time." Is it in consciousness? When we are speaking or reading, do we recite the alphabet silently to ourselves?[51] Is this how we come to know meanings?

In the toolbox example, the "nails" are the potential 'sustaining' causes that help maintain a shape or, as Wittgenstein says, maintain the "solidity" of the box. Presumably, then, to talk about causes as 'sustaining,' absent a practical context (e.g., when someone says that nails simply "modify" a thing's solidity), is exactly the sort of overgeneralized classification that Wittgenstein warns against because it is independent of a pragmatic situation in which our aims and interests are able to define the useful objects, their parts, and (in)actions. In this sense, what is taken to be 'sustaining' is simply the effect of how we have chosen to segment and speak about our actions and, thus, how we speak about that which binds and holds a variety of acts together in a given setting. Here language, like nails, is being properly used to give shape to a project, and, in turn, language can be judged against that project. Absent a situation, however, what 'sustains' is no more informative than what 'causes' or what 'is.' It is our choice of an expression, or rather an interlocking set of expressions, that creates a focus, that sets in motion a form of causality and defines what will be taken as not changing.

Wittgenstein warns against creating formulas such as 'every word signifies something' that give language a false sense of uniformity. I submit that the causal formulas concerning film in the accompanying figure 5.1 are misleading in exactly this way. These propositions are nearly vacuous. They are based on selecting some *fact* about film, positing a causality for the 'fact,' overgeneralizing the causality, and finally elaborating the result into an ontology, epistemology, and aesthetics of film where the favored causal principle is scaled to fit assumed

FIGURE 5.1   Nearly Vacuous Causal Formulas about Film

---

1. Film is made out of photographs (i.e., film is caused by a camera).

2. Film is sustained by photography (i.e., sustained by still frames on celluloid being held motionless one at a time at a fixed distance from a lens in a projector and focused on a screen).

3. Film form is defined (bounded, framed) by photography.

4. Film images are produced and exhibited by light (i.e., images are brought into being by the action of ambient light and reanimated through projection).

5. Film brings meaning to light (and brings to light meaning).

6. Film light is defined (bounded, framed) by its absence (shadowiness).

7. What film presents on the screen is only significant in terms of what is hidden from us and, therefore, the value of what we see is continually threatened.[52]

8. Film presents absence (i.e., absence is presented as what is not properly exposed, what is not photographed, what is only a photograph, what is elsewhere, what is not visible, what is not visual, and/or the *possibility* at any moment of any of these); more dramatically, film is ghostly — an interstitial, unrealized (derealized, irrealized) real.

9. Film is an interaction — a dialectic or tension or suture — between presence and absence, light and shadow (moreover, when film is held to be a photographic medium, sound will be measured by *its* visibility, i.e., whether the source of a sound is present onscreen or absent offscreen).

10. Film is continually changing through intermittent movements of presence and absence, light and shadow, seen and unseen, sound and silence, imagined and unimagined, unimagined and unimaginable.

11. Film movements are caused (have a direction, are directed).

12. Film presents the present — an ever-new present experience of change — by leaving the former present behind (for example, by leaving behind the time of a spectator in a theater [the time of film projection]; or by leaving behind the time of a character who is in movement and constantly changing his or her physical viewpoint and "point of view"; or by leaving behind the time of an event by narrating a new event).

13. Film is an experience of time.

14. Film is an experience.

15. Film guides us through an experience.

---

modes of film experience. Film then becomes a 'tool' that serves to 'modify something.' The antidote to such overgeneralization is not, however, an empiricism, as we shall see, but a greater sensitivity to the empirical — that is, to certain practices of cinema and ways of talking in particular circumstances.

Propositions 1–15 of figure 5.1 push one toward a deceptive assimilation between camera and experience, as when one protests: "But the word 'camera' must surely name a particular *thing* that *guides us* to a particular experience of a photograph or image! The camera surely causes us to have a particular experience of a photograph through a related experience of form, lighting, space, time, movement, causation, meaning, feeling, belief, and/or self-awareness, among other experiences that we have in watching a film." The answer is: When you say this, you are *thinking of* a particular experience of being guided in a film, which forces an expression on you that makes it seem as if there were something *common* to all forms of guiding, that there is a guide, and that the camera is it. You are thinking of your experience not only through the medium of film but also through the medium of the concepts "because," "influence," "cause," "connection," and even "through," which seem to share a definitive, core meaning (as in looking *through* a window that sustains a view).[53] The concept of *guiding*, for example, would seem to presuppose a continuous act along a continuous path revealing a continuous set of experiences for a witness who is within some setting. But, one may ask, how many forms of "continuous" experience may be said to exist? How does one decide *when* certain changes of impression, but not others, belong together as the effects of being guided and that, by virtue of these impressions, become parts of a setting? What sort of large-scale mental "picture" or "scene" must be constructed from these diverse parts to contain the relevant actions of guiding and the effects of being guided?

A more cautious approach would be to assume that there are many and incompatible ways of being a guide (and of being a cause) and that, rather than just one, there are many cameras operating in different regions of our language activity as we consider the various places and 'action-games' that concern (relate to, affect, are affected by) cinema. In order to speak of a camera as a guide, one must *feel the effects of being guided*, of having been presented points of interest for consideration; that is, one's course — one's movement in a fiction and in a narrative — must be altered, and one must perform under this influence in some way — and probably in several ways — by, for example, having feelings, remembering, expecting, being surprised, narrativizing, fantasizing, learning, behaving, and speaking in response to being guided. Being guided has many parts and different parts on different occasions. If our guide is to be a camera, it will be different things on different occasions, and it will be relative to *our performance* (i.e., relative to our behavior while being guided and our explanations to ourselves and others about having been guided) and not just relative to the physicality of a photograph or to the physical objects seen in a photograph. Are there not many kinds of experiences that viewers may have with a film that will support feelings of having been guided? Although we may do many things with, and to, a camera and, for that matter, a computer, neither of these objects can itself be guided because neither is sentient, except metaphorically.

Might a camera be a sort of abstract guide — either in the sense of a "universal" guide that is a composite of several possible guides or else a "theoretical" guide made up only of essential and idealized parts? (This question is analogous to an earlier question in the section, "Camera Fiction," about whether a spectator thinks of a camera as being either a "universal" camera or a "theoretical" camera.) As Wittgenstein argues, to be a guide is not reducible to a material thing, to a subset of possible materials, or to a metaphysical thing, but must include the responses of the person being guided as he or she experiments by fitting new perceptions back onto circumstances, thereby finding a relevant sense of "being guided" by a guide. Trying to define a "guide" in the abstract is like trying to define a "cause" or a "tool" in the abstract. To imagine a camera as being a guide, it would not do to remember a film (for then one would be guided by a single experience) nor to imagine an imaginary film (for then again one would be guided by a single experience); instead, one would need, perhaps, to think of a camera as functioning like a guide word at the top of a dictionary page or a key word in a database, both of which are something different, and are employed in a different context, from a word with the same spelling that appears in the main part of the dictionary or database.

Perhaps another way to imagine a camera as a guide would be to think of a camera as functioning like a photograph on the cover of a book that contrasts with the same photograph inside the book. In this way, being guided by the cover photograph will appear in conjunction with emerging ideas as one reads with the cover in mind — that is, with an evolving set of questions one wishes to answer. Being a guide depends not on the existence of a word or a photograph or an object but on the way in which a person creates new patterns by continuously modeling *changes* in his or her perception against a point of departure and an imagined destination. Thus, the photograph on the cover functions in a different way from the same one inside the book. As suggested by these analogies with a dictionary, database, and book, I believe that a camera is characterized less by its physicality than by its relationship to a structure of information — more exactly, its relationship to an individual who is making information useful. A 'camera' emerges as a way of thinking about the course of one's thinking. In watching a film, our thoughts *adjust*, moment by moment: The point against which we measure these adjustments (departure, destination) is a 'camera.'

Let's bring Wittgenstein's ideas to bear on the analogy of a 'camera' with the cover of a book. A photograph on a cover is usually taken to be a 'sample,' or 'picture,' of the contents of the book. For Wittgenstein, both a "picture" and something offered as a "sample" may become a guide for a person through his or her act of "regarding" it. (The etymology of the word "guide" includes "to look after," "to know.") This directly raises the issue of perceiving: How might an object cause a reaction that may then *alter or guide* what the object is seen to be doing to us when we look at (regard) it, thus becoming something different before our very

197

eyes and acquiring a new meaning? I am claiming that a camera we imagine as a guide is not identical in all respects to the camera that manufactured the photograph, just as a photograph on the cover of a book is not identical in all respects to the 'same' one inside the book. What a thing 'is' depends on *which relations* are being selected as the most important when one is looking at or thinking about the thing.

The analogy of a 'camera' with the cover of a book may be extended to looking at (regarding) a film. Just as the sudden realization that a photograph in a book is like the one on the cover will cause a change in the nature of the photograph inside the book, so a shot in a film that is recognized in retrospect to have been a point-of-view shot will change the nature of what was first seen. The same dawning of awareness also happens with a shot in a film showing a particular character that leads a viewer to see the character as being *typical* of a type of character (that perhaps he or she has known in daily life), or a shot that initially depicts something specific but then is seen to conform to a kind of plot or standard iconography or else to summarize a scene or embody the title of the film or of another film. In all these instances, after the shot has been 're-recognized,' it changes into something different, though it may change back or change again. A camera, too, is not always 'the same,' but is subject to being 'reframed.'

One way that Wittgenstein approaches this problem of 're-recognition' is through the notion of what he calls the "dawning" ("flashing" or "changing") of an "aspect" of a picture or a sample. An "aspect" for Wittgenstein is experienced directly (i.e., effortlessly, rapidly) and extends far beyond his well-known examples of ambiguous pictures such as the duck-rabbit and Necker cube with their twin aspects and other enigmatic representations such as puzzle-pictures. An "aspect" for Wittgenstein also includes, for example, seeing a feature as being particular or general (e.g., seeing a sample leaf as being typical of a particular kind of oak tree or *else* seeing it generally as being from a typical tree); noticing a family resemblance when looking at someone's face; detecting emotions such as hesitancy, timidity, and sadness; seeing fictionally (e.g., seeing moonlight in a spotlight in *The Threepenny Opera*); and experiencing certain aesthetic effects.[54] Although the duck-rabbit has become a popular symbol for Wittgenstein's ideas, it is misleading to the extent that it implies that an aspect dawns only like the gestalt of a form. Wittgenstein's many examples show that, in general, an aspect depends on a sense of *familiarity* that, in turn, is a function of memory and learning. The dawning of an aspect might be focused on a physical object, of course, the perception of which turns on familiarity, but it may equally be focused on a situation or representation in which our 'preferences' are being recognized. Preferences and aesthetic values are familiar in a far more complex, and intense, way than the mere perception of gestalt form, because they depend on the manner in which we *wish* to look and talk as well as on the way we normally think and act. Thus, for Wittgenstein, aspects and their dawning arise in a range of cognitive and emotive situations. The camera, too, if it is to be a guide, must be part of a process of recognition and reconfiguration.

Wittgenstein stresses that after an aspect has dawned (flashed, changed), we see the object or event as something new, or see something new in it, even though the physical characteristics of the object or event have remained unchanged. What sorts of 'causes' are responsible for a change when the object or event itself (e.g., a photograph) has remained physically the same? The range of Wittgenstein's examples shows that aspects may dawn through many operations of mind. For example, aspects may arise from illusory patterns of stimuli (i.e., bottom-up), or from a task one is performing (i.e., top-down), or from cross-modal or lateral processing (as in synesthesia; or, as in 'lateral' continuity rules in film, e.g., the convention of sound perspective which matches audibility and visibility), or from 'perceptual metaphors' (e.g., visualizing a knight's move in a chess game in terms of a distinctive 'shape'), or from effects of memory. Moreover, Wittgenstein's use of pictures to illustrate the process of dawning raises the question of whether all pictures, including the 'pictures' on our retinas, pose puzzles of seeing aspects or of seeing things under alternative cognitive descriptions.

That is, in looking at a picture and trying to 'recognize' it, we may be searching for various kinds of resemblance that put the picture into one or numerous 'families.' It would seem reasonable, as well, to conclude from Wittgenstein's arguments that words may have nonconscious 'aspects' that may dawn.[55]

One might say generally that aspect-perception is a form of *framing*, or of reframing, an object by seeing it in a new context. On the other hand, perhaps 'framing' cannot be suitably defined in a general way: the preceding chapter presented framing as a radial concept dependent on a dispersed series of descriptions/situations with *no essence*, i.e., there was no set of necessary and sufficient conditions that defined all and only the forms of framing without utilizing a specious overgeneralization. Instead, the preceding chapter argues that a theorist selects one type of framing or aspect-perception as *prototypical*, in order to *sustain* the resemblances that he or she believes to be relevant.

Where might the 'camera' fit in Wittgenstein's scheme? Is the camera a cause or an effect of aspects? Would the 'camera' be *prior to* each of the "aspects" of an image that may dawn (and, if so, in what sense would it be prior: chronologically? logically? causally? practically? grammatically?)? Another possibility is that the 'camera' occurs to us as an afterthought where it merely *sustains* aspects or simply *belongs to* aspects (as a physical shape, and the shape of a certain move, belong to a chess piece[56]). Perhaps the camera appears to us *during* the recognition of aspects as a sum of all the "aspects" of an image. (Note that a sound may cause an aspect to dawn in an image, or a sound may produce an image in the mind of a spectator, and, by guiding us in these ways, the sound may function as a 'camera.') I have posed this array of questions in order to indicate some of the epistemological problems that arise when traditional causal analyses based on photographicity collide with linguistic and imagistic analyses based on the production of mental "aspects" that dawn or flash from memory to guide a spectator. Are we guided by a photograph on screen or by tacit prototypes of objects and events?

MENTAL CAMERA

> "I wanted to say that it is odd that those who ascribe reality only
> to things and not to our mental images move so self-confidently
> in the world of imagination and never long to escape from it."[57]

> — Ludwig Wittgenstein

I have been arguing that "the camera" is a composite entity whose
"unity" and "conspicuousness" from shot to shot are always
a matter of ongoing judgments that are being made relative to
(a tacit theory about) being guided through things of interest. We
do not so much "see through" or "with" the camera's eye (eyes?)
as we employ the term "camera" to name and mark a place in our
stream of thought. A camera does not rule over our thought about
how a text is seen; it is merely an occasion, one of many, during
which we consult, negotiate, and confabulate about a text.[58] A
camera represents a phase of our thought, much as point of attack,
in medias res, backstory, turning point, climax, and epilogue
represent phases of our comprehension of narrative causality. Of
course, one may freely stipulate that the term "camera" will be
used exclusively to refer to a physical object. I would submit,
however, that for a critic — though not, of course, for a historian
of film technology — this obvious meaning is banal and that *no
critic uses the term "camera" to refer to a piece of equipment.*
Rather, a critic speaks of the camera in the ways most helpful
to his or her interpretive and evaluative projects.[59] The camera,
absorbed into these projects of responding to films, acquires a
flexible, metaphorical identity, better adapted to the causality of
ever-new and emerging contexts that are being summoned from a
spectator's memory. The pertinent question then becomes: How is
a particular critic using the word "camera" to do something — to
say something about how one watches?

Consider a critic who speaks of "Hitchcock's camera."
In this connection one doesn't hear about the cameraman,

cinematographer, or art director, even though these individuals were persons who actually looked through a camera and were directly concerned with the look of a shot. It remains "Hitchcock's" camera because the critic is not really designating an object but, rather, alluding to *how the object was manipulated* as an instrument of Hitchcock's predilections, willpower, and *aesthetic* persona (no matter how contradictory, incomplete, ambiguous, accidental, failed, forced, or unconscious such authorial intentions may have been — indeed, a certain amount of obscurity in Hitchcock's motives is convenient, for it allows the critic his or her own place in the fashioning of the artifact's effect and, specifically, in the telling of a story about the use of a "camera"). Ordinarily, the expression "Hitchcock's camera" is invoked when the critic is dealing with a particular film, such as *Vertigo* (1958) or Brian De Palma's *Obsession* (1976), and making an argument not about a physical camera but about a distinctive kind of story, its characteristic modes of telling and tone, and notable (and quite disparate) elements of film style and technique.

Here is an experiment: Recall a shot from Hitchcock's *Vertigo* and try to imagine the camera that made the shot in a way that is completely separate from *Vertigo* or "Hitchcock." What would such a camera be like? Is this the camera that critics discuss when analyzing the film? Far from narrowing the definition of a "camera," critics routinely enlarge the notion of "camera" to include many other elements of style and theme. For example, a critic may conceive of the editing in *Vertigo* as a sequence of camera setups (a critic may say, "the camera cuts to a close-up. . . ."); mise-en-scène in *Vertigo* as shaped by camera position, lens focal length, and film exposure; character movement in *Vertigo* as determined by blocking for the camera; narration as movements of the camera "between" shots; sound in relation to what is visible onscreen; theme as a matter of what the camera shows. For a critic, Hitchcock's camera is mental rather than physical and is tied to the density of a film's total experience. Hitchcock's camera resides in a discerning eye that is able to search for it even in films by other directors (e.g., *Obsession*), rather than being confined to a thing that had bulk and was moved on a set. For these critics, it is only after the camera *came to be Hitchcock's* that it came into *true being*.

There are many difficulties to express when one moves beyond the "physical" camera and tries to summarize how the term "camera" will be employed while watching a film. Sometimes becoming entangled in one's own prose is evidence of underlying complications in attempting to define a term. For example, John Kreidl applies ten analytical concepts to each of nine early Jean-Luc Godard films in an effort to understand the interpretive process. Two of his concepts are "camera ontology" and "spectation by the camera." He defines "camera ontology" as follows:

> By camera ontology, I mean the camera's creation for the viewer of *a* world mediated by the camera itself, the sense of space-time the viewer is given by the shots in the film that we see as well as by the off-screen space the projected film suggests. What we see in film that produces in us a sense of being is seen only through the camera's eye. This "symbol," in Sartre's words, of the images in motion, moderated by the camera, is what we ontologize to give us our sense of being while we watch the film. *Breathless* [Godard, 1960] features a vital, ontological use of the camera as composer of experience: the jump cut. The way Godard uses jump cuts at certain points to *affect the meaning of the film* is much more important than that he uses it to "pace the film quickly" or to "avoid using establishing shots to save money." They (the jump cuts), as used by Godard, are *not editing devices* to speed up the pacing, thought up by an editor, but cuts conceived by the direc-tor to make us ever aware that the world of this film is limited to the discontinuous images presented to us. In *Breathless*, there is no off-screen space, no "world elsewhere," something that may account for its popularity with young Americans in 1960, sub-merged in the immediate and the fads of the moment, which they found the film expressed back to them.[60]

Although some writers may reject the camera of an auteur like Hitchcock or Godard, their search for the camera still concludes by endowing it with an animated, metaphorical status. Consider an argument by Jean-Louis Baudry:

> And if the eye [of the spectator] which moves is no longer fettered by a body, by the laws of matter and time, if there are no more assignable limits to its displacement — conditions fulfilled by the possibilities of shooting and of film — the world will be constituted not only by this eye but for it. The mobility of the camera seems to fulfill the most favorable conditions for the manifestation of the "transcendental subject." There is a phantasmatization of objective reality (images, sounds, colors). . . .

Baudry draws on the words of Jean Mitry for support: "In the cinema I am simultaneously in this action and *outside* it, in this space and out of this space. Having the power of ubiquity, I am everywhere and nowhere."[61]

Hugo Münsterberg expresses similar beliefs:

> [Film] can act as our imagination acts. It has the mobility of our ideas which are not controlled by the physical necessity of outer events but by the psychological laws for the association of ideas. In our mind past and future become intertwined with the present. [Film] obeys the laws of the mind rather than those of the outer world.[62]

Thus, although Baudry, Mitry, and Münsterberg develop different theories of film, they nevertheless would seem to agree that the movement of a physical camera is neither necessary nor sufficient for the movement of a spectator's eye/idea/mind. Because spectators do not literally move from their seats, and a camera is in some way the 'source' of every shot in a film, it is difficult to see how the claims of these three writers about the "mobility" of film could be true unless their conceptions of the camera go beyond that of a physical piece of equipment.

The vital movements of film, however, may not be exclusively psychological but may draw upon a preexisting, *natural* affinity that a perceiver has with the movements of the world. According to Jean Epstein:

The cinema is a particular form of knowing, in that it represents the world in its continuous mobility, as well as a general form of knowing because, once it addresses all of the senses, each will be able to surpass its physiological limitations. . . . [W]e can already measure the significance of the change that the cinema — in its expression of the external and internal movement of all beings — has brought to bear on our thinking.[63]

For Epstein, "art" in film is composed only of the "photogenic," which he defines in terms of an essential mobility that exists in the world:

A moment ago I described as photogenic any aspect whose moral character is enhanced [amplified] by filmic reproduction. I now specify: only mobile aspects of the world, of things and souls, may see their moral value increased by filmic reproduction. . . . Photogenic mobility is a mobility in [the] space-time system, a mobility in both space and time. We can therefore say that the photogenic aspect of an object is a consequence of its variations in space-time.[64]

Epstein firmly believes, as do the later theorists Siegfried Kracauer and Walter Benjamin, that the camera is not a leaden mechanism but something that has the power to reveal the mobile world by transforming and surpassing the merely visible.[65] Movement of the camera in Epstein's theory becomes a privileged technique, because it may point to, coincide or correlate with, fundamental forms of positive mobility linked to changes in the world and changes in thought:

[Cinematography] discovers movement where our eye sees nothing but stasis. . . . All those authors who are currently multiplying the moving camera shots in their films do so not out of some affectation of style. They are instinctively obeying a primary law of their art. . . .[66]

For Gilles Deleuze, the camera of the "time-image" connects directly to movements of the mind.

[T]he fixity of the camera does not represent the only alternative to movement. Even when it is mobile, the camera is no longer content sometimes to follow the characters' movement, sometimes itself to undertake movements of which they are merely the object, but in every case it subordinates description of a space to the functions of thought. This is not the simple distinction between the subjective and the objective, the real and the imaginary, it is on the contrary their indiscernibility which will endow the camera with a rich array of functions, and entail a new conception of the frame and reframings. Hitchcock's premonition will come true: a camera-consciousness which would no longer be defined by the movements it is able to follow or make, but by the mental connections it is able to enter into. And it becomes questioning, responding, objecting, provoking, theorematizing [sic], hypothesizing, experimenting, in accordance with the open list of logical conjunctions ("or," "therefore," "if," "because," "actually," "although . . ."), or in accordance with the functions of thought in a *cinema-vérité*, which, as Rouch says, means rather truth of cinema [*vérité du cinéma*].[67]

In sum, for these five theorists, the mobility and causation associated with the camera have an irreducible mental aspect — an "aspect" that arises, or "dawns," Wittgenstein would say, because all of our mental abilities are applied when we look, not just our ability to see basic shapes, color, depth, and motion on the screen. Wittgenstein argues that we have an intimate bond with the world through our language-games and descriptions, because they project our interests and further our goals. It is thus a misleading simplification, I believe, to define the camera as a piece of equipment and assume that the definition will serve as a basis for any question one may ask about a camera. Similarly, a definition of the "frame" as a straight line on the screen will not advance all questions about a frame (see chapter 4).

I would like to present a detailed illustration of one of the typical ways that a critic may talk about a shot in a film. It is an insightful discussion because the critic, Gerald Mast, has enmeshed both the "camera" and the "frame" within our practical interests. As spectators, we entertain a fiction for the ways in which our practical knowledge and emotions may be summoned and remodeled through depictions of narrative causality and psychological agency. For a critic, a camera's *effect* on a spectator normally becomes part of what it is to be a camera, to be the camera of that shot and framing. The critic describes the sense of what he or she has seen in a film by picturing the effect on his or her own seeing. The appropriate contexts for these effects, though often cued in some manner, are *not* determined by the film, because the causes of an interpretation are much more complex than bottom-up stimulus and response or mere chains of association discovered on the screen. The screen is both a cause and a *focus* for our attention.

My illustration of these ideas is drawn from a discussion by Gerald Mast of the framing of a shot from Charles Chaplin's *Easy Street* (1917). Mast's description attempts to portray how the film is working on us through various narrative, performative, stylistic, and psychological frames. Even though the shot is not directly "subjective," we come to picture the inner vision of the character being portrayed by Chaplin because the multiple top-down frames that are invoked by Mast blur the lines among motion, moving, motive, and emotion with the result that the camera is more mental than physical:

> The three areas of the shot, right, center, and left, have been translated into three areas of thought: consideration, action, reconsideration. If we were to chart the *mental action* of the shot [which concerns the decision whether or not to apply for a job as a policeman], rather than its physical pattern of movement, we would come up with something like this: Charlie [Chaplin] considers a possibility [right] but rejects the idea [as he moves center to left]; reconsiders it [left then back to right] and rejects it again [center to left]; reconsiders it [left then back to right] and resolves to take the action [right] but is frightened away [center to left]; then reconsiders his hesitancy [left], decides to take the action [left to center], but is frightened away again [center to right]; then reconsiders his hesitancy once again [right] and finally summons sufficient energy and resolution to perform the action successfully [right to center]. The pattern of *thought*, of *motion*, and of *position* in the frame is *identical*. If Charlie ever

evacuated this frame, if he ever crossed beyond the frame's left boundary, the shot (and this *plot* motif) would end, and Charlie would never become the policeman this film requires him to be. (Of course, Chaplin could play the little trick of leaving the frame but prolonging the shot on the 'empty' space until Charlie reentered the frame to reconsider his decision. This alternative would in no way diminish the power of this frame, this space, as an area for thought. Chaplin simply does not like to trick the frame line in this way; he wants to establish it as a concrete boundary to thought.) It is significant that this shot is itself a complete *little story*, with a beginning, middle, and end [corresponding to right, center, and left]. It is also a perfect circle of both action and movement (it begins and ends with Chaplin moving from the right edge of the frame). The structure and symmetry of the shot could only be destroyed by a cut. Chaplin is far more aware of what a frame is — both in terms of psychologizing space inside the frame and defining the boundary between on-frame and off — than those critics who wish he would cut more often."[68]

WHEN

"[H]e said that the actual word 'beautiful' is hardly ever used in aesthetic controversies: that we are more apt to use 'right,' as, e.g. in 'That doesn't look quite right yet'. . . . The question of Aesthetics, he said, was not 'Do you like this?' but '*Why* do you like it?' . . . What Aesthetics tries to do, he said, is to give *reasons*, e.g. for having this word rather than that in a particular place in a poem. . . . *Reasons*, he said, in Aesthetics, are 'of the nature of further descriptions'. . . ."[69]

— G. E. Moore's account of a lecture by Wittgenstein

I have argued that causation is arrayed in *strata* that relate to different ways of mobilizing terms, of being embodied and disembodied in worlds made. Each stratum provides a new frame for the basic terms used to analyze a film, such as "camera." I would like to clarify the motivation for this enlargement of the meaning of "camera" by considering our experience of *motion and change*, not on the screen (where still images alternate with blackness and nothing literally is moving anyway), but in more abstract realms, such as when one detects the ebb and flow of a conversation or lecture, reads a novel, looks into a painting, personifies a thing, narrativizes a few weeks of one's life, plans ahead, or searches for words to express a problem. After all, if a camera is to exist in abstract realms and is to act as a guide for us, then so, too, will such attributes of the physical camera as "moves toward" or "moves alongside." My purpose, then, in considering abstract forms of "moving" (as with the earlier example from Socrates) is to show that such abstractions do not exist in a vacuum but are connected in a radial fashion to a variety of ordinary ways of perceiving, employing rhetoric, and living in a world and, hence, are not easily reduced to an all-purpose, general definition.

Abstract motions are frequently projected from our model of everyday life. In this model we visualize ourselves in a place with midsized, composite objects that move by being "pushed and pulled." Think, for example, of a living room with a table, picture window, picture hanging on a wall, parquet floor, and furnishings. Objects differ from each other and from their parts, and differ in their possibilities for movement (e.g., the wooden table is different from the wooden floor, and the table moves differently than does the inlay of the floor). These objects of everyday life are conceived as solid and compact, not diffuse like a vapor, a grid of fine wires, grain in wood, or dishes scattered on a table. These objects are middle-sized, unlike electricity or the weather, and are stable, not transitory like a sound or ice cube, or intangible like a feeling or words on a grocery list.[70] The objects exist on the same scale as our bodies and are salient for us (are "of consequence") precisely because they can be "pushed and pulled" in familiar kinds of ways to accomplish familiar tasks. I believe that this model of our concrete world becomes, in effect, a *medium for thought* that sustains a distinctive rhetoric of action.

The living room I have described is no doubt familiar because I have used "basic-level" categories in describing it.[71] What is the significance of this basic level? Lakoff and Johnson argue that such categories match up with evolution and natural selection:

> In the natural world, basic-level categories of organisms are genera. That means that they are for the most part determined by their overall part-whole structure. The part-whole structure of a class of organisms is, significantly, what determines whether it will survive and function well in a given environment. Thus, part-whole structure determines the natural categories [i.e., the basic-level categories] of existing genera. And it is what our perceptual and motor systems have evolved to recognize [through gestalt perception] at the basic level. That is why we have tended over our evolutionary history to function optimally in our basic-level interactions.[72]

Other models (causal strata) may be built upon the concrete ("living room") model of our world. That is, new "containers" or "frames" holding new sorts of abstract, moving objects may be envisioned in order to explain events of interest. In particular, a camera may be conceived as a special kind of "container" that moves among objects, removing them to its interior.[73] Here are a few additional examples of ordinary but *abstract* movements and changes occurring in models that are extensions of a concrete model of the world: I have moved *away* from a previous life; I have moved *closer* to winning the chess game; my car *falls* in value each month while my son *grows to resemble* his parents who *rise* to the occasion when he *raises* his voice; I *plan* someday to move the blue and brown books from the shelf to the desk; looking into the distance, I judge the *length of time* that it will take to run to the landmark; I will reach the landmark *inside of* five minutes (i.e., with*in* a "container" of time of a definite size); I *visited* the film-philosophy website; words on my computer screen are *sent* and ideas are *exchanged*; now I *grasp* what is meant by the title of the painting.

In these examples "movements" by certain hypothetical objects — entities and concepts that are theoretical, quasi-theoretical, folk-psychological, analytical, critical, heuristic, hermeneutic, nonconscious, and so on — are working to model our feelings of motion and change when we watch, listen, read, narrativize, think, and remember, that is, when we seek to explain our awareness of an impending change by fitting it back into a basic-level pattern of change. The abstract movements illustrated above draw upon such ordinary (top-down) competencies as the following: contrasting present time with the past; knowing the strategy of a game; knowing the economics of car ownership; implementing folk biology and folk psychology (i.e., folk causality); scheduling one's future activities (so as to puzzle over a problem in philosophy); imagining present or future duration as a space or container; and creating a handy analogy for the process of *communication* based on, for example, thinking how one might carry a piece of paper across a living room to the window where the light is brighter (to where "I can now see clearly . . ."). Still other important kinds of abstract thought are built upon a basic-level model of the world. For example, objects and persons may be imagined in a *narrative frame* by using a source-path-goal schema in which an initiating force is seen to have begun the movement of objects and persons along a *trajectory* (sustained by the path, but encountering obstacles) toward a decisive end.[74] Psychological changes of a person (his or her "life story") may also be modeled in the same fashion, for instance, when one ponders the "arc" of a character in a story.

Many superordinate and subordinate models are routinely built upon the "living room" model of our world in order to extend our reasoning abilities and to invoke a new stratum of causation. These models (as illustrated above) work to solve problems in a wide range of new situations by *preserving the inferential structure* of the basic-level. Everyday human reasoning, including the comprehension of fiction films, is not based on formal categories of logic or on probabilistic logic but, instead, is derived from basic-level categories, prototypes, radial concepts, metaphors, frames, schemata, imagery, and heuristics.[75] In this manner powerful inferences are generated that shape everyday percepts, beliefs, emotions, and actions.

If there is a top-down component to our experience of abstract sorts of motion, then it suggests that many concepts not specific to film (cultural, economic, historical, political, hermeneutic) — including concepts not yet invented — will be relevant to thinking about and comprehending film. Therefore, one of the tasks of theorists and critics is to formulate concepts that make *new forms of causality* relevant to our interests. In particular, it seems to me that abstract movements of each of the eight cameras analyzed in chapter 3 have helped to bring to light a variety of aesthetic devices, social values, and historiographical principles, thus making a contribution toward revealing the worlds we have inferred and desired.

When top-down components become relevant to our experience of film, no definitive catalogue of all possible types of motion and change can be drawn up because no definitive catalogue of all possible types of top-down perception can be drawn up. For a "camera," the six variables of pan, tilt, rotate, track, dolly, and crane exhaust only a single domain of possible motions created by movements of a physical thing *with respect to* the three spatial dimensions. But, one may wonder, is the camera limited to moving only in a model of the world based on a living room, and not also within other, abstract spaces?[76] Adding zooms, rack focus, optical printer effects, and special effects expands the inventory of motions but leaves the original domain little changed. The reason is that within the concrete, "living room" model of the world, the *viewpoint* of such a camera is tied to what a person might see who moves about the room. By contrast, if the living room were to be viewed from within a fireplace atop burning logs or from under a parquet floor that had suddenly become transparent in certain spots, then the normal viewpoint would be seen to be subjected to the perspective of another, more abstract model of action in the world (e.g., seeing the living room framed by a counterfactual of what *could* be seen *if . . .*, or framed through a hypothetical *wish*, or offered as a *symbol* for something else). Needless to say, there are many possibilities for abstract "viewpoints" involving both sight and insight and, hence, many cameras that move in ways other than the physical, just as moonlight on a stage illuminating Jenny moves differently than a spotlight illuminating Lotte.[77]

Abstract models of the world may lie *beneath*, as well as above, the "living room" model of the world. A model that lies beneath will attempt to dissect concrete, midsized objects into a fine web of formal, stylistic, physical, or mathematical relations. One such model (liable to the paradoxes of Zeno) analyzes locomotion as a specific mechanical displacement against a three-dimensional geometrical field of *zero-dimensional points*. These points are the minimal units or "parts" of space that are used to define a movement by a physical object. In this "mathematical" model of space, a given movement must be continuous from one point to the next — it must occupy each point in turn without skipping a point — and no two objects can occupy the same point at the same time. Such a definition of movement will produce the six variables of camera movement mentioned above as well as descriptions of the internal movements of a camera when it, too, is seen to be composed of many, still smaller parts in space that occupy points (lens, gate, shuttle claw). If one begins with the mathematical model of zero-dimensional points, then it seems as if camera movement can be exhaustively analyzed and defined for real space because nothing seems to be smaller than an infinitesimal point. If this is accepted, the reduction, as in Zeno's paradoxes, is complete. From the standpoint of such a scheme, higher-level abstractions are taken to be approximations or fictions (i.e., not real and ultimately dependent on something occupying points) and one is left with the notion of a camera that moves only from one point to its neighbor without skipping points or being in two places at once.

Nonetheless, in describing "camera movement" critics do not rely exclusively on the mathematical model but, rather, most often entwine *three* descriptions springing from mechanical/mathematical, concrete, and cognitive/emotive frames. For example, a critic may assert that a certain *panning shot* (mechanical) reveals that a *stagecoach traveling across a landscape* (concrete) is *vulnerable* (cognitive/emotive). Note that each of the three descriptions refers to a different type of "movement" in a different frame of reference because, strictly speaking, the panning camera is not part of the reality of a moving stagecoach and, further, it is not the moving stagecoach

213

that is "vulnerable" but its occupants for reasons unrelated to a panning camera or the horses pulling the stagecoach. This is to say that the attributive word "vulnerable" is not a concrete description of the "stagecoach" but, rather, that the word is hinting that *the spectator should be afraid* for what may happen to the occupants of the stagecoach. (An occupant of the stagecoach, of course, may, or may not, feel "vulnerable.") Accordingly, the word "vulnerable" draws on an unstated, abstract model of human emotions and how emotions may be elicited in spectators by a set of circumstances. The precise configuration of this model of the emotions, and whether it lies above or below our concrete model of the world (or else is roughly congruent with our concrete model of the world, as in behaviorism), depends on the details of the theory that is chosen to model or display — put on view — the emotions.[78]

Vivian Sobchack, thinking of a scene from John Ford's *Stagecoach* (1939), elaborates on the three descriptions (mechanical, concrete, and cognitive/emotive) that typically make up a critic's 'description of camera movement':

> Such descriptions [of camera movement] proceed to point to the cognitive and affective functions of *mechanical* locomotion and then, in a vaguely causal manner, link these functions to *human* meaning. Thus, a *pan* is described as a particular rotation of the camera on its vertical axis from a stationary point that functions, for example, to establish the contiguity of screen space, and leads the viewer to understand and feel from this expression the "sweep" and "scope" of a Monument Valley landscape and the fragile vulnerability of the stagecoach crossing it. How this transformation of the originally mechanical into the secondarily human, of determinate locomotion into responsive and meaningful movement occurs, or how it can be argued and justified, is hardly touched upon. Thus, there is something unsatisfying and inappropriate about such descriptions of camera movement in the discipline's basic works. . . . [These descriptions] seem to have nothing to do with our *experience* of camera movement on the screen as meaningful. . . . We understand the "sweep" and "scope"

of a landscape or the "fragile vulnerability" of a particular object not because mechanical locomotion has somehow been transformed into cognitive and emotional [semiotic] codes. Rather, we understand the movement precisely because we never regarded it as mechanical in the first place. The theoretical transformation of camera movement into mere motor locomotion, into discrete and determinate movements in geometric space, is *secondary* — an objectification of an original experience that is *then* seen as problematic in regard to the human meaning it conveys. Camera movement as experienced, however, is *not* a problem. We understand it and its projects in lived space as we understand ourselves in spontaneous motion and responsive activity in the world.[79]

Sobchack asserts that we experience camera movement and its purpose in "lived space" in the same way that we understand ourselves and our activities when we are thinking about ourselves as embodied in, and living in, a concrete model of the world: "[C]amera movement echoes the essential motility of our own consciousness as it is embodied in the world and able to *accomplish* and express the tasks and projects of living. . . . As Maurice Merleau-Ponty tells us: 'Consciousness is in the first place not a matter of "I think that" but of "I can."'"[80] Perhaps we might add that the usual tripartite description of the camera is a mini-narrative, a story about a camera movement, in which the "mechanical" part of the mini-narrative defines the narrator's position *outside* the "concrete" story events, while the "cognitive/emotive" part is meant to solicit the interest and participation of the viewer: 'I can, I might.'

Are we, then, to give up our tripartite descriptions of the camera (mechanical/mathematical, concrete, and organic/emotive)? It would seem that a mechanical description of the camera would be useful during the production phase of a film. But equally during production, a filmmaker may be entertaining abstract descriptions by imaginatively projecting *possible* experiences that a viewer may have when a scene of one sort might be filmed as opposed to another sort. For a critic the relevance of a given description of camera movement must be judged against the goal in offering the description.

Thus, it seems futile to search for a single type of "pure" description for what the camera can do, either a mathematical formula that is always true (*a priori*) or a clever metaphor that will fit all occasions and can be stretched to cover all facets of the mind. Even general metaphors that link the camera to an attentive eye, window, picture frame, mirror, scientific observation, communication, expression, magic lantern, moving shadow, illusion, dream, machine, or commodity seem to fail in being exhaustive (cf. the eight cameras in chapter 3 and the radial meanings of "framing" in chapter 4).

What is surprising is that we continue to think that, in spite of everything, there must exist a reliable, immutable definition for a camera, a fundamental fact of camera-ness that needs only to be finally uncovered. We insist on tying the camera to human concerns and to drama — a drama of creation by an artist, a drama of characters, a drama connected to our lives and desires — rather than identifying the camera with a mathematics/mechanics, yet we are still amazed that the human drama cannot be reduced to a single situation or framed by a single model for all humans. We continue to think that there must be a definite, *right description* or reason — neutral and exact — that fits a camera and fits all our experiences of being guided by a camera. We believe that a description of a thing is ultimately traceable to the essence of the thing — the core set of necessary and sufficient conditions that govern its existence. In order to resolve these puzzles and avoid misunderstandings, we will need to look more closely at what constitutes a "description."

UNDER DESCRIPTION

"It was marvelous, I said to myself that day on the subway, that I could have forgotten so easily. In the official version of my life [my] nickname does not appear. People have asked me, now and then, whether I have ever had a nickname and I have always replied, No, it is funny but I do not seem to be the type that gets one. I have even wondered about it a little myself, asking, Why is it that I have always been Mary, world without end, Amen, feeling a faint pinch of regret and privation, as though a cake had been cut and no favor, not even the old maid's thimble or the miser's penny, been found in my piece. How political indeed is the personality, I thought."

— Mary McCarthy, "C.Y.E."

I would like to suggest that the question about how to employ the term "camera" when looking at a film needs to be rephrased as follows: We must inquire through *what set of judgments*, based on which beliefs and desires, is a "camera" *seen to have* certain properties, that is, *when* does a camera come to exist *under descriptions that we offer* of the functioning of the text, under labels that we apply to the text in order to *picture* (to model) a series of photographs (or film) as having been seen picturing (modeling) motion and change.[81] If one objects to this formulation by saying that the "camera" must either exist or not — that it cannot exist at some times but not at others in a film — then one's thought is being dominated by the concept of a "physical" camera and the associated causality of imagery rather than thinking of the causality of a perceiver's interaction with imagery, how a film is made to mean by a perceiver, and how a perceiver feels *guided* by a "camera" in certain ways at some times but not at others. Thinking of a physical camera is not the same as engaging with the symbolic functioning of a film — that is, with the ways in which a film solicits labels and perceivers apply descriptions. The question of *when* also involves the time of looking — that is, the social setting, the historical circumstances — which frames our interest in looking. An examination of historical circumstances is relevant because it assists in determining what it is possible to say at a given time, what judgments can be made, and what (when) descriptions become persuasive.[82] Judgments, like one's personality, have a political edge.

There is no absolute object with an essential set of properties but only objects and properties seen under diverse descriptions
within contexts that are acceptable to various people in various
degrees at different times. As Richard Rorty declares:

> The essentialist philosopher, the one who wants to hold on to the
> notion of "intrinsic, context-independent, property," says that the
> "it" which inquiry puts in context *has* to be something precon-
> textual. The antiessentialist rejoins by insisting that it is contexts
> all the way down. She does so by saying that we can only inquire
> after things under a description, that describing something is a
> matter of relating it to other things, and that "grasping the thing
> itself" is not something that precedes contextualization, but is at
> best a *focus imaginarius*.[83]

Rorty is not alone in believing that a thing materializes only
"under a description." He elaborates:

> The way in which a blank takes on the form of the die which
> stamps it has no analogy to the relation between the truth of a
> sentence and the event which the sentence is about. When the die
> hits the blank something causal happens, but as many *facts* are
> brought into the world as there are languages for describing that
> causal transaction. As Donald Davidson says, causation is not
> under a description, but explanation is. Facts are hybrid entities;
> that is, the causes of the assertibility of sentences include both
> physical stimuli and our antecedent choice of response to such
> stimuli. To say that we must have respect for facts is just to say
> that we must, if we are to play a certain language game, play
> by the rules. To say that we must have respect for unmediated
> causal forces is pointless. It is like saying that the blank must
> have respect for the impressed die. The blank has no choice, nor
> do we.[84]

The idea that 'causation is not under a description, but an
explanation of facts is' sums up a major portion of my argument
in this chapter about the relativity of the terms "movement" and

"camera." What is at stake with the term "camera" in critical discourse is not (usually) the camera's physicality and its ground for causal forces (i.e., the camera as a blank, the world as a die), but its status as an *explanation* for what is seen in a film. This is one reason why I argue that "photographicity" (i.e., the causality of photographs) cannot be extended into an ontology, epistemology, and aesthetics of cinema, indeed why *objective* (context-independent) facts cannot found a general theory, or explanation, of cinema. The many approaches to textural analysis in chapter 2 illustrate that facts about movements onscreen appear under broad categories (e.g., motivation, anthropomorphism, and point of view). The many theories of a camera in chapter 3 illustrate that facts appear under descriptions (and ultimately come from more extended descriptions, or theories, of cinema). The many theories of a frame in chapter 4 illustrate that radial meaning is a consequence of facts having been placed under descriptions. In parallel fashion it seems to me that one of the recurrent problems in analyzing and watching documentary film is that the various types of causation that make the film *be* a "document" are too often combined in misleading ways with the "explanation" appearing in a given descriptive language of what is *being* documented, even if the explanation is left to the spectator or critic to produce (as in "direct cinema").

The existence of radial meaning suggests the inadequacy of the idea that language is *directed at*, or takes its meaning from, something *fitting* in the world — something in the world that fits it. The search for such a fit seeks to close or eliminate the middle ground between language and world, making both objective. In this futile search the relationship of "fitting" is taken as being external to language; it is a purported relation between the physicality of a word and the thing in the physical world that is said to fit it (now or at some future time). But this leaves out the cognitive processes intermediate between language and world that define what it is to be — what counts *as being* — a "fit." It leaves out *the uses* of language through which our thought and our body *project* signs onto the world according to rules (a "grammar") adopted to facilitate certain purposes in the world.

219

A film theory is an example of how rules may be legislated and laid down to govern the way we may act and speak — that is, to govern the 'moves' we may make according to the rules of a 'game,'[85] for example, the way in which we may project a notion of a 'camera' for a film. To take Wittgenstein's example and turn it into a question: is it true that there is a "piston" in the world that fits a "cylinder" of language — language as a 'hollow' form?[86] Suppose that there is no "piston" to fit a "cylinder" of language, or that different sorts of "pistons" fit it or "pistons" fit it metaphorically, or that the *descriptions* of "piston" and "cylinder" are radial. In these situations, one needs to look toward language *use* to discover meaning and to give up the idea that a film theory can be discovered that fits film perfectly objectively. There is no film theory that is purely objective in its description of film because there are no objective descriptions. There are only moves within a grammar or language-game.

A larger point can be made here about the nature of truth. As one moves away from isolating and manipulating the "name" of an event or thing toward weighing facts about an event or thing that emerge from "under a description," the standard for judging truth shifts from an inquiry into the name's *correspondence* to the world toward an inquiry into the *rightness*, or adequacy, of rendering a given description of the world, of creating a version. A central tenet in the philosophy of Nelson Goodman is the assertion that "rightness" provides a norm distinct from "truth" that judges how we use words:

> [R]ightness is a matter of fitting and working. Since rightness is not confined to those symbols that state or describe or depict, the fitting here is not a fitting *onto* — not a correspondence or matching or mirroring of independent Reality — but a fitting *into* a context or discourse or standing complex of other symbols.[87]

> For a concept with greater reach than truth, consider *rightness*. "Right" and "wrong" apply to symbols of all kinds, verbal and nonverbal. Not only statements but demands and queries, words,

categories, pictures, diagrams, samples, designs, musical passages and performances, and symbols of any other sort may be right or wrong. Moreover, rightness pertains to all the ways that symbols function. A symbol may be right or wrong in what it says, denotes, exemplifies, expresses, or refers to via a homogeneous or heterogeneous chain of referential steps; rightness, unlike truth, is multidimensional. . . .Rightness is plainly more complicated than truth and also more volatile, varying with circumstances that in no way affect truth.[88]

Every critical method will authorize certain kinds of descriptions that are implicitly historicized, as against others, of how a film is working upon us or 'guiding' us, as Wittgenstein would say. An appropriate subset of a given set of descriptions (a "schedule" of descriptions[89]) will be collectively taken to define (in the manner of a sustaining cause) the working of a "camera," that is, to define the rationale, the reason, for our having seen the significance of something. A "camera" is thus connected to our assessment of *rightness*, rather than *truth*. To speak of the truth of a camera or photograph is often a misleading simplification. In the end, the proof of a camera's existence will be displayed in images and sounds on the screen where a camera is no longer out of sight, out of mind, but seeing it — through the insight of descriptions — becomes believing, just as seeing a table in a living room (in the way we live our lives) invites us to believe in the rightness of a mode of ready-made conduct appropriate to the room and to invest our hopes generally in familiar objects and projects.

LANGUAGE

"SOCRATES: Excellent. And do you accept my description of the process of thinking?

THEAETETUS: How do you describe it?

SOCRATES: As a discourse that the mind carries on with itself about any subject it is considering. . . . I have a notion that, when the mind is thinking, it is simply talking to itself, asking questions and answering them, and saying yes or no. When it reaches a decision — which may come slowly or in a sudden rush — when doubt is over and the *two* voices affirm the same thing, then we call that its 'judgment.' [Cf. the two voices of Socrates and Theaetetus.] So I should describe thinking as discourse, and judgment as a statement pronounced, not aloud to someone else, but silently to oneself.

THEAETETUS: I agree."[90]

— Plato

The preceding section makes evident that of the eight cameras discussed in chapter 3, I prefer the final one: the camera as a descriptive, "semantic label" or "reading hypothesis." I prefer this notion of the camera because it readily opens onto a set of film theories that are firmly grounded in our language and verbal abilities. Language is our preeminent modeling system. We use it to find our imagined place among the many worlds of objects and events. Consciousness itself is unthinkable apart from the restless and unremitting phonological stream that echoes in short-term memory (the mind talking to itself, according to Socrates). Consciousness is a driving force and a primary form of motility with a definite direction. Consciousness is always *directed at* something, is always *of* something, not unlike a Socratic "dialogue" or kinesthesia or projection. Recall Wittgenstein's belief that "meaning something is like going up to someone," like being "oneself in motion."[91]

One cannot avoid thinking and living in words; nor can words avoid having been crafted by humans who are using them to solve problems of living in worlds. Indeed, the very *existence* of consciousness, as Daniel Dennett argues, "is too recent an innovation to be hard-wired into the innate machinery" and "is largely a product of *cultural* evolution that gets imparted to brains in early training."[92] (Consciousness, as we know it, and language, culture, and "art" are only about 50,000 years old; modern humans, Homo sapiens, about 100,000 years old; the first known human, Homo habilis, more than 2 million years old; the mammalian order of primates, 55 million years old.) I have asserted that a critic's camera inevitably acquires a metaphorical dimension as an instrument of thought. Therefore, I will propose the following figure for the camera as a "semantic label": Like an in-drawn breath, the camera acts in a transitional area between propensity and saying, between discourse and judgment, between problem and description, thus being more aural than visual.

Film is greater than what meets the eye because it must be taken up by consciousness, which imposes (often verbal) descriptions onto an object of interest and onto other objects in relation to objects of interest. Such a description, or "aspect" (in Wittgenstein's sense), is not an expansion of a set of neutral facts about an object — nor is it simply arbitrary, for we are always situated in a world that requires that we *act* — but, rather, the description is a hypothesis or viewpoint or powerfully condensed folk theory about the nature and significance of an object as being this or that kind of thing for a range of possible interactions. As Tzvetan Todorov says, "One cannot verbalize with impunity; to name things is to change them."[93] Can we not equally say, 'One cannot visualize with impunity; to see things is to see them under one or several aspects and hence to change them'? We are never really finished with a description — a 'seeing as (if),' a 'seeing in,' or, perhaps better, a 'seeing with' — for a description is always under adjustment in the ongoing process of conceiving and naming new segments of a world, segments newly seen as kinds and parts of things, in accordance with our present interests. A description of something is fluid because it includes *tacit* relationships to other objects that are *not* present and to memories of objects and descriptions; that is, a description already includes potential roles for us to play when the game expands and descriptions proliferate. Schematically: we see a as-is and present, and also a as-if b (or "about" b—where b is blank and not present, i.e., b remains to be filled-in and filled-out by a beholder), when circumstances are c under description d_1, which intersects radial descriptions d_2, d_3, d_4 .... One must still decide how to apply these (and other) terms; for example, how should the term "as if" be interpreted? One must choose a theoretical language-game in which to make moves. Or, perhaps, the initial question should be, which films are important to us?

What, then, is the object camera? Like film interpretation, a conception of the camera is less a discovery of the *factual what*, an absolute, than already a kind of functional description, or an *occasion when*, because a nominal camera will exceed what has been produced on the screen as soon as a spectator responds and performs as if guided by an unseen and mysterious cause. A camera cannot escape the occasion when a spectator imposes grammatical form on what he or she notices — when a camera-whatsit is given some expression in a region of language tied to a plan, activity, or game. A camera is outlined and filled in as a person applies thought within some frame — when a person acts to solve a problem by adjusting a metaphor. The word "camera," then, may be taken to be a gesture toward a meshwork of habits and actions and reasons that motivate our favored descriptions — descriptions that, in turn, lead to movements, both figurative and literal.

Notes

PREFACE

1. Gilles Deleuze, *Cinema 2: The Time-Image*, trans. by Hugh Tomlinson and Robert Galeta (Minneapolis: University of Minnesota Press, 1989), p. 280.

2. Stanley Cavell, *Cities of Words: Pedagogical Letters on a Register of the Moral Life* (Cambridge, Mass.: Harvard University Press, 2004), pp. 4–5. The quotation spans two paragraphs.

3. G.E. Moore, "Wittgenstein's Lectures in 1930–33," in *Philosophical Occasions*, 1912–1951, ed. by James C. Klagge and Alfred Nordmann (Indianapolis: Hackett, 1993), p. 114 (original emphasis). See, e.g., Ludwig Wittgenstein, *Philosophical Investigations*, trans. by G.E.M. Anscombe (Oxford: Blackwell, 3rd ed. 1967), §§ 106–133.

4. I will discuss in chapter 1 two ways of conducting an analysis, one of which, 'vertical dissection,' concerns 'building' and '(de)constructing,' and is shunned by Wittgenstein. On Wittgenstein's preferred approach to doing philosophy ("seeing connexions"), which I will associate with a method of 'horizontal intersection,' see, e.g., *Philosophical Investigations*, §§ 122–132, 435–436, and Hans-Johann Glock's *A Wittgenstein Dictionary* (Oxford: Blackwell, 1996), "philosophy," pp. 292–298. Notice that analyses marked by 'vertical dissection' share a language with the building trades: foundations and materials; larger and smaller rooms (cf. categories and "areas" of inquiry; compartments and departments); hallways, conduits, and movements from point to point; doorways, openings, frames, thresholds, together with a carpenter's associated "reveal" (!); the opposition between inside and outside; and, regularity and rationality (blueprints, design). Notice, too, the "independence" of the builder/analyst from what is built. For more on the idea that a theory or an argument may be likened to a building, see George Lakoff and Mark Johnson, *Metaphors We Live By* (Chicago: University of Chicago Press, 1980), chap. 17, "Complex Coherences across Metaphors," pp. 97–105; and p. 46.

5. George Lakoff and Mark Johnson, *Philosophy in the Flesh: The Embodied Mind and Its Challenge to Western Thought* (New York: Basic Books, 1999), chap. 24, "How Philosophical Theories Work," pp. 541–542, from part III, "The Cognitive Science of Philosophy," pp. 335–548.

225

6. After providing the reader with 20 epigraphs, Cavell begins his book with these two sentences:

> The first of the epigraphs I have placed as guardians or guides at the entrance to this book — 'I know that the world I converse with in the cities and in the farms, is not the world I think' — opens the concluding paragraph of Emerson's 'Experience.' It captures one of Kant's summary images of his colossal Critiques, epitomized in the Groundwork of the Metaphysics of Morals, namely that of the human being as regarding his existence from two standpoints, from one of which he counts himself as belonging to the world of sense (the province of the knowledge of objects and their causal laws, presided over by the human understanding), and from the other of which he counts himself as belonging to the intelligible world (the province of freedom and of the moral law, presided over by reason, transcending the human powers of knowing).

Incidentally, Cavell's use of the metaphor "entrance" in the first phrase of the first sentence suggests an 'open door' that 'frames' a 'path.' Such metaphors are not without consequence. See chapter 4 below, definition 8 of the word "frame."

7. I will argue that it does make sense to speak of a 'language' of sense-impressions. Wittgenstein will be a strong presence in the chapters to follow, so let's get started with his view on this question:

> The fluctuation in grammar between criteria and symptoms makes it look as if there were nothing at all but symptoms. We say, for example: 'Experience teaches that there is rain when the barometer falls, but it also teaches that there is rain when we have certain sensations of wet and cold, or such-and-such visual impressions.' In defence of this one says that these sense-impressions can deceive us. But here one fails to reflect that the fact that the false appearance is precisely one of rain is founded on a definition.

> The point here is not that our sense-impressions can lie, but that we understand their language. (And this language like any other is founded on convention.) *Philosophical Investigations*, §§ 354–355; cf. § 392.

Here I believe Wittgenstein is pointing toward an integration of language and body. He is not suggesting that philosophy or language be 'reduced' to the everyday. What is important are 'basic-level categories' derived from sense-impressions that set in place "criteria" that, in turn, make embodied existence sensible and whole through the use of language. For Wittgenstein, philosophy is not a device for transcending ordinary and 'imprecise' language nor is language used to transcend or merely gloss sensation. Furthermore, I believe that film theory as a species of philosophy has taken too little note of its own use of language and its relationship to a human mind that is embodied (sense-impressions, symptoms). See chapters 4 and 5 below.

8. I discuss the connection of language and film at the end of chapters 1, 3, and 5.

9. See, e.g., Wittgenstein, "Cause and Effect: Intuitive Awareness," in *Philosophical Occasions*, pp. 368–426; Lakoff and Johnson, *Philosophy in the Flesh*, chap. 11, "Events and Causes," pp. 170–234.

CHAPTER 1: THE LIFE OF A CAMERA

1. Nelson Goodman, "Foreword," in *Ways of Worldmaking* (Indianapolis: Hackett Publishing Co., 1978), x.

2. Béla Balázs, "The Face of Man," in *Theory of the Film: Character and Growth of a New Art*, trans. Edith Bone (1945; repr., New York: Dover, 1970), 60; cf. 91, 92.

3. Christian Metz, "Problems of Denotation in the Fiction Film," in *Film Language: A Semiotics of the Cinema*, trans. Michael Taylor (New York: Oxford University Press, 1974), "Conclusion," 145 (original emphases); cf. sect. 10, 142–43.

4. Roland Barthes, "The Death of the Author" [orig. 1968], in *Image, Music, Text*, trans. Stephen Heath (New York: Hill and Wang, 1977), 143, 146.

5. Ludwig Wittgenstein, *Philosophical Investigations*, trans. G.E.M. Anscombe (1953; repr., Oxford: Blackwell, 3rd ed. 1967), §§ 371, 373 (original emphasis); cf. § 383.

6. Barthes, "The Death of the Author," 147 (my emphasis).

7. Barthes, "The Death of the Author," 148; and see the Barthes epigraph. Barthes also says:

> [W]riting is the destruction of every voice, of every point of origin. Writing is that neutral, composite, oblique space where our subject slips away, the negative where all identity is lost, starting with the very identity of the body writing. (142)

The "death" of the author may be theorized in many ways, for example, through works by M. M. Bakhtin, Julia Kristeva, Tzvetan Todorov, Michel Foucault, and Monroe Beardsley. The displacement of the author has its roots in nineteenth-century hermeneutics (e.g., with F.D.E. Schleiermacher). For an account that, like Barthes, rejects theology and metaphysics in favor of a measure of historicism and nominalism, see Richard Rorty, *Contingency, Irony, and Solidarity* (Cambridge, U.K.: Cambridge University Press, 1989),

"Introduction" and Part I, "Contingency," xiii–69 (on the contingencies of language, selfhood, and community). On Wittgenstein's notion of the contingency of language (i.e., its dependence on certain needs, interests, and activities), see Hans-Johann Glock's indispensable *A Wittgenstein Dictionary* (Oxford, U.K.: Blackwell, 1996), "autonomy of language, or arbitrariness of grammar," 45–50. A sketch of Wittgenstein's main ideas is provided by A. C. Grayling, *Wittgenstein: A Very Short Introduction* (New York: Oxford University Press, 2001).

8. Barthes, "The Death of the Author," 148 (original emphasis). I am led to think of the doomed character, the "officer," in Kafka's "In the Penal Colony" as being a prototypical *reader* when Barthes says, "The reader is the space on which all the quotations that make up a writing are inscribed without any of them being lost. . . . " (148) Cf. also Peter Greenaway's *The Pillow Book* (1996).

9. See the Barthes and Kruesi epigraphs.

10. See the Barthes epigraph and "The Death of the Author," 147.

11. Here is how Jean-Louis Comolli expresses the shift from an Author or Camera as interpretive standard toward a 'set of readings':

> For our third proposition is as follows: the less the reading of a film can be attributed to its écriture [writing], and connected to its signifying system in a relation of production, the more the reading 'passes through' the film, thereby demonstrating its lack of density, and the more the film's 'reality,' *its maximum weight of condensation, lies in the weight and reality of its readings, so that what we need to read is no longer the 'film' but rather that which constitutes it: its readings.*

"Film/Politics (2): *L'Aveu:* 15 Propositions" in *Cahiers du Cinéma 1969–1972: The Politics of Representation*, ed. Nick Browne (Cambridge, Mass.: Harvard University Press, 1990), 164 (original emphases).

12. The "impersonal" mode of address may be compared to an implicit extra-fictional narration, i.e., narration by the so-called "implied author"; see Edward Branigan, *Narrative Comprehension and Film* (New York and London: Routledge, 1992), pp. 90–95 (Metz: film itself as a "potential linguistic focus"). See also Christian Metz, "The Impersonal Enunciation, or the Site of Film (In the margin of recent works on enunciation in cinema)," *New Literary History* 22, 3 (Summer 1991), 747–72, reprinted in *The Film Spectator: From Sign to Mind*, ed. by Warren Buckland (Amsterdam: Amsterdam University Press, 1995), 140–63; and Metz, *L'Énonciation impersonnelle, ou le site du film* (Paris: Méridiens Klincksieck, 1991).

My discussion of the impersonal mode of address in the present chapter makes use of the ideas of transparency, opaqueness, and surface. I will examine these ideas in greater detail in chapter 4 and will offer an alternate way (based on radial meaning) to think about how language "loses focus" and becomes "decentered" and dispersed.

13. John M. Ellis, *Language, Thought, and Logic* (Evanston, Ill.: Northwestern University Press, 1993), 5–6; see also 24–25, 34–40. Ellis concludes that certain features of Wittgenstein's notion of "language-games" should be understood in relation to evaluative and ethical uses of language; see, e.g., 79–80, 95.

14. See the Wittgenstein epigraph as well as Glock, *A Wittgenstein Dictionary*, "grammar," 153; see also "explanation," 111–14, "form of life," 124–29, "language-game," 193–98, "understanding," 372–76, and "use," 376–81.

15. For Wittgenstein, neither "language" nor "game" can be defined by necessary and sufficient conditions and thus both are radial in meaning. It may also be the case that the compound, "language-game," is radial and, further, that one game may be embedded in another. Wittgenstein, perhaps, seeks to put a halt to the interplay of games by saying that language-games are ultimately embedded in a "form of life." Nevertheless, it would seem that "form of life" is relative to some degree. Chapters 4 and 5 will introduce embodiment (i.e., effects connected to the human body and its interactions with the physical environment) as a limiting factor in certain conceptual schemes and in a realizable "form of life." Barthes's literary theory also incorporates the human body; see, e.g., *The Pleasure of the Text*, trans. Richard Miller (1973; repr., New York: Hill and Wang, 1975).

16. Ludwig Wittgenstein, *Philosophical Occasions*, 1912–1951, ed. by James C. Klagge and Alfred Nordmann (Indianapolis: Hackett, 1993), Appendix A, "Immediately Aware of the Cause" [notes taken by Rush Rhees, 1938], 408 (original emphases and ellipsis points); cf. 407, 195.

17. P. F. Strawson, *Analysis and Metaphysics: An Introduction to Philosophy* (Oxford: Oxford University Press, 1992), chap. 2, "Reduction or Connection? Basic Concepts," 17–28. I believe that Socrates' advice to Phaedrus is a classic statement of the 'reduction' method: "First, you must know the truth concerning everything you are speaking or writing about; you must learn how to define each thing in itself; and, having defined it, you must know how to divide it into kinds until you reach something indivisible." (Plato's *Phaedrus* 277b5-8; cf. 247c3-e5)

Broadly speaking, Wittgenstein's early work emphasized "reduction" and his later work "connection." On "connection," see, e.g., Wittgenstein, *Philosophical Investigations*, § 122; cf. §§ 91–92, 126; and *Wittgenstein's Lectures, Cambridge, 1932–1935: From the Notes of Alice Ambrose and Margaret Macdonald*, ed. by Alice Ambrose (Amherst, New York: Prometheus Books, 2001), Part I, § 10; Part II (The Yellow Book), §§ 1, 3. Cf. Richard Rorty, "Wittgenstein, Heidegger, and the Reification of Language," from *Essays on Heidegger and Others: Philosophical Papers, Vol. 2* (Cambridge, U.K.: Cambridge University Press, 1991), 50–65.

18. Charles L. Stevenson, "On the 'Analysis' of a Work of Art," in *Contemporary Studies in Aesthetics*, ed. Francis J. Coleman (New York: McGraw-Hill, 1968), 69–84. For an analysis of one type of dissective analysis, see, e.g., Tom Gunning's review article, "The Work of Film Analysis: Systems, Fragments, Alternation," on Raymond Bellour's book, *The Analysis of Film* [Bloomington: Indiana University Press, 2000], in *Semiotica* 144, 1/4 (2003), 343–57. A variety of analyses may be found in *Close Viewings: An Anthology of New Film Criticism*, ed. Peter Lehman (Tallahassee: Florida State University Press, 1990). On assorted genres and techniques of analysis, see esp., David Bordwell, *Making Meaning: Inference and Rhetoric in the Interpretation of Cinema* (Cambridge, Mass.: Harvard University Press, 1989).

19. Doing analysis by tracing "connections" may also be like wandering in a garden. See James Elkins, *Our Beautiful, Dry, and Distant Texts: Art History as Writing* (New York: Routledge, 2000), esp. such chaps. as 3, 7, and 10, "On the Impossibility of Close Reading" [i.e., on the impossibility of reductive analysis], "The History and Theory of Meandering," and "Writing as Reverie" [i.e., writing in relation to literal and figurative wandering in gardens].

20. Strawson, *Analysis and Metaphysics*, 19–20; cf. 24, 46, 64.

21. Gilberto Perez, *The Material Ghost: Films and Their Medium* (Baltimore: Johns Hopkins University Press, 1998), 91. Although in this passage Perez connects each of the cameras to a personal auteur (or perhaps auteur-narrator), such a connection is not necessary and may be thought of as only a shorthand way of describing a particular kind of experience by a spectator. For further discussion, see chapter 5 below, the section on "Mental Camera."

22. See the Barthes epigraph. More generally, Wittgenstein argues that "questions as to the *essence* of language, of propositions, of thought" are wrongly posed: "For [these questions] see in the essence, not something that already lies open to view and that becomes surveyable by a rearrangement, but something that lies *beneath* the surface. Something that lies within, which we see when we look *into* the thing, and which an analysis digs out." *Philosophical Investigations*, § 92 (original emphases); cf. §§ 90, 91.

23. According to Barthes, "Once the Author is removed, the claim to decipher a text becomes quite futile. To give a text an Author is to impose a limit on that text, to furnish it with a final signified, to close the writing. . . . In the [true] multiplicity of writing, everything is to be *disentangled*, nothing *deciphered*; the structure can be followed, 'run' (like the thread of a stocking) at every point and at every level, but there is nothing beneath: the space of writing is to be ranged over, not pierced; writing ceaselessly posits meaning ceaselessly to evaporate it, carrying out a systematic exemption of meaning [perpetual release of new meanings]. In precisely this way literature (it would be better from now on to say *writing*), by refusing to assign a 'secret,' an ultimate

meaning, to the text (and to the world as text), liberates what may be called an anti-theological activity, an activity that is truly revolutionary since to refuse to fix meaning is, in the end, to refuse God and his hypostases — reason, science, law." "The Death of the Author," 147 (original emphases).

24. On "piecemeal theorizing," see Noël Carroll, "Prospects for Film Theory: A Personal Assessment" in *Post-Theory: Reconstructing Film Studies*, ed. David Bordwell and Noël Carroll (Madison, Wis.: University of Wisconsin Press, 1996), 38–41, 57–58. For Carroll, the "pieces" of a theory should be the result of an attitude of openness about *disciplinary* boundaries — a sort of practical pluralism that values methodological experimentation. Although the theoretical questions and answers that are specifically addressed by the "pieces" have a historical dimension, they are still meant to be powerful generalizations and to be objective. Also, for Carroll, some hybrid methodologies are better than others. Note especially that Carroll's "piecemeal theorizing" is not the same as David Bordwell's call for "middle-level research" and a "historical poetics." Bordwell's approach sets aside certain abstractions and generalizations about film in order to concentrate on historicizing the *data* found by academic scholarship. See Bordwell, "Contemporary Film Studies and the Vicissitudes of Grand Theory" in *Post-Theory: Reconstructing Film Studies*, sect. "Middle-Level Research," 26–30; and Bordwell, *Making Meaning*, chap. 11, "Why Not to Read a Film," sect. "Prospects for a Poetics," 263–74.

25. See note 22 above.

26. On an "impure" film theory, cf. André Bazin's argument for "impure" film, "In Defense of Mixed Cinema" [orig. 1951], in *What Is Cinema?*, [vol. I], trans. Hugh Gray (Berkeley and Los Angeles: University of California Press, 1967), 53–75. Consider Bazin's rejection of ontology and hidden (entrenched) values in favor of connecting film to the relativity of culture and history:

> [W]e must say of the cinema that its existence precedes its essence; even in his most adventurous extrapolations, it is this existence from which the critic must take his point of departure. As in history, and with approximately the same reservations, the verification of a change goes beyond reality and already postulates a value judgment. Those who damned the sound film at its birth were unwilling to admit precisely this, even when the sound film held the incomparable advantage over the silent film that it was replacing it. (71)

27. Jan Simons, "'Enunciation': From Code to Interpretation," in *The Film Spectator: From Sign to Mind*, ed. Warren Buckland (Amsterdam: Amsterdam University Press, 1995), 203 (my emphasis). See also the epigraph from Christian Metz

(above) and Simons, *Film, Language, and Conceptual Structures: Thinking Film in the Age of Cognitivism* (University of Amsterdam: Ph.D. diss., 1995). Brian O'Leary makes a similar point: "[T]here are only a limited number of ways the mind can work, and these can appear across multiple sense modalities. Linguistics, which is an area that has been subjected to intense experimentation, theorization, and introspection over many decades, can perhaps serve as a heuristic for understanding other forms of cognition." O'Leary, "Hollywood Camera Movements and the Films of Howard Hawks: A Functional Semiotic Approach," *New Review of Film and Television Studies* 1, 1 (November 2003), 10. See generally Warren Buckland, *The Cognitive Semiotics of Film* (Cambridge: Cambridge University Press, 2000); and Buckland, "Film Semiotics," in *A Companion to Film Theory*, ed. Toby Miller and Robert Stam (Oxford, U.K.: Blackwell, 1999), 84–104.

28. See the Balázs epigraph.

CHAPTER 2: A CAMERA-IN-THE-TEXT

1. *Jean Cocteau: The Art of Cinema*, ed. André Bernard and Claude Gauteur, trans. Robin Buss (New York: Marion Boyars, 1992), chap. 3, "Poésie de Cinéma," sect., "*Orphée*," 160.

2. According to V.F. Perkins:

> Many of Ray's camera movements appear to be incomplete. Any simple guide to movie-making will tell you that a travelling shot must have a beginning, middle and end. Often Ray uses only the middle: the camera is already moving at the beginning of the shot, and the movement is unfinished when the next shot appears; or if the movement does end, it falls somewhere short of its apparent goal. Whole sequences are often built up from these "incomplete" shots so that the montage becomes a pattern of interruptions in which each image seems to force its way on to the screen at the expense of its predecessor (e.g. the introduction of Scott Brady's gang in *Johnny Guitar* [1954]). Ray is one of the most "subjective" of all directors. The world he creates on the screen is the world seen by his characters. His dislocated editing style reflects the dislocated lives which many of his characters lead.

Notice that Perkins treats the "incomplete" camera movements as an *editing* strategy involving "interruptions" and 'displacements' where "each image seems to force its way on to the screen" (not unlike, perhaps, a kind of 'jump cut'). The "beginning, middle and end" of standard camera movements, mentioned by Perkins, suggests a close tie to narrative structure, which is commonly said to have a beginning, middle and end. Indeed, Perkins argues that the incompleteness of Ray's camera movements is narratively motivated since it ought to be seen in terms of character 'subjectivity' ("dislocated lives"). Revealing character subjectivity is often the narrative motivation of last resort for a critic (see number 7 on my list of motivations involving "time" in the text above and number 13 on my list of "some kinds of movements"). Perkins, "The Cinema of Nicholas Ray," in *Movie Reader*, ed. Ian Cameron (New York: Praeger, 1972), 66 (original emphasis).

3. Several quite different aesthetic uses of unmotivated camera movements are analyzed by David Bordwell in *The Films of Carl-Theodor Dreyer* (Berkeley and Los Angeles: University of California Press, 1981), 153–64 (especially *Ordet*, 1954, and *Vampyr*, 1932); and Brian Henderson in "Toward a Non-Bourgeois Camera Style (Part-Whole Relations in Godard's Late Films)," in *A Critique of Film Theory* (New York: E.P. Dutton, 1980), 62–81.

4. Jean Mitry, *The Aesthetics and Psychology of the Cinema*, trans. Christopher King (Bloomington: Indiana University Press, 1997), 185 (original emphases); see also p. 186 on "purposeless movement." Mitry says, "The art lies in making these [camera] movements seem natural but at the same time necessary." (185)

5. V. F. Perkins, *Film as Film: Understanding and Judging Movies* (Baltimore, Md.: Penguin, 1972), 129.

6. This list of the basic elements of narrative, together with some additions and refinements, is taken from Edward Branigan, *Narrative Comprehension and Film* (New York and London: Routledge, 1992), chap. 1, "Narrative Schema," 18. See also Kristin Thompson, *Storytelling in the New Hollywood: Understanding Classical Narrative Technique* (Cambridge, Mass.: Harvard University Press, 1999); and David Bordwell, *Narration in the Fiction Film* (Madison: University of Wisconsin Press, 1985). Note that my characterization of narrative in the text is basically a "vertical," dissective analysis; see the third section of chapter 1 above, "How Should Analysis Proceed?"

7. *The Missouri Breaks* (Arthur Penn, 1976) opens with a scene that is seen in *retrospect* to have been in medias res.

8. Ben Brewster argues that the early history of cinema may be divided into three periods according to how props and film devices (e.g., camera movements and point-of-view shots) are narrativized, including time itself, which may be narrativized through an appointment or deadline for a character or through the circulation of an object from person to person. See Brewster, "A Bunch of Violets" (unpub. ms. 1995).

9. See, e.g., Jerome Bruner, *Making Stories: Law, Literature, Life* (New York: Farrar, Straus and Giroux, 2002); and Bruner, "Self-Making and World-Making," *The Journal of Aesthetic Education* 25, 1 (Spring 1991), 67–78.

10. André Bazin, *The Cinema of Cruelty: From Buñuel to Hitchcock*, ed. François Truffaut, trans. by Sabine d'Estrée (New York: Seaver, 1982), "Pan Shot of Hitchcock," 114–15 [orig. 1950]. Karel Reisz and Gavin Millar go further than Bazin by criticizing the implicit editing in the long takes of *Rope* for not being classical enough. Kristin Thompson criticizes Reisz and Millar for having an inadequate view of the function of "narrative" in *Rope* and in films generally. See Reisz and Millar, *The Technique of Film Editing* (New York: Hastings House, 2nd ed., 1968), 233–36; Thompson, *Eisenstein's Ivan the Terrible: A Neoformalist Analysis* (Princeton, N.J.: Princeton University Press, 1981), 266–67.

On the narrativization of shot scale, see generally Jacques Aumont, Alain Bergala, Michel Marie, and Marc Vernet, *Aesthetics of Film*, trans. and rev. by Richard Neupert (Austin: University of Texas Press, 1992), 225–30. Narrativizing shot scale means that the scale of a shot is being used to direct a spectator's attention to relevant action. Changes in scale will indicate the significance of events and will lead the spectator toward an appreciation of a character's emotions and motivation with respect to events.

A major theme in film theory has involved the study of the nature and effects of the so-called "long take," often accompanied by a lengthy camera movement. One variety of the long take is the plan-séquence, also known as "interior montage" and "latent montage." Here are a few works on the topic: David Bordwell, *On the History of Film Style* (Cambridge, Mass.: Harvard University Press, 1997); Vladimir Nizhny, "Mise-en-Shot," from *Lessons with Eisenstein*, trans. by Jay Leyda (New York: Hill and Wang, 1962), 93–139; Brian Henderson, "The Long Take," from *A Critique of Film Theory* (New York: E.P. Dutton, 1980), 48–61; David MacDougall, "When Less Is Less: The Long Take in Documentary," in *Film Quarterly: Forty Years — A Selection*, ed. by Brian Henderson and Ann Martin with Lee Amazonas (Berkeley and Los Angeles: University of California Press, 1999), 290–306; Jean-Pierre Geuens, "Visuality and Power: The Work of the Steadicam," *Film Quarterly* 47, 2 (Winter 1993–94), 8–17; Lutz Bacher, *The Mobile Mise en Scene: A Critical Analysis of the Theory and Practice of Long-Take Camera Movement in the Narrative Film* (New York: Arno Press, 1978); Daniel Arijon, "Twenty Basic Rules for Camera Movement" and "Punctuation by Camera Motion," in *Grammar of the Film Language* (New York: Hastings House, 1976), 380–84, 604–11. Noël Burch remarks that the "unbearably prolonged," long-held shot may have important aesthetic uses. See *Theory of Film Practice*, trans. Helen R. Lane (New York: Praeger, 1973), 53, 68 n. 2, 118, 127, 152; reprinted by Princeton University Press, Princeton, N.J., 1981.

11. I am here using terms proposed by David Bordwell for analyzing the flow of narration in a film. See figure 2.4 later in this chapter.

12. Herb A. Lightman, "The Fluid Camera," *American Cinematographer* 27, 3 (March 1946), 82; see also p. 103.

13. Cf. Lightman, "The Fluid Camera," 82, with V.I. Pudovkin, in *Film Technique and Film Acting*, trans. Ivor Montagu (New York: Grove Press, revised and enlarged ed., 1970), *Film Technique*, chap. I, part II [orig. 1926], five sections on "editing," 66–78.

14. I will examine embodied reasoning and related cognitive processes in chapter 4. Stronger claims for embodiment may be based on, for example, expressive, communicative, or psychoanalytic theories (see chapters 3 and 4), or on the phenomenological theory of Vivian Sobchack (see chapters 4 and 5). On the general problem of anthropomorphism and narration, see Branigan, *Narrative Comprehension and Film*, 109–10.

15. Vivian Sobchack, "Toward Inhabited Space: The Semiotic Structure of Camera Movement in the Cinema," *Semiotica* 41, 1/4 (1982), 318. In this formulation Sobchack is drawing on the work of Maurice Merleau-Ponty and Joseph Kockelmans. See generally James Peterson's notion of the "phenomenological schema" in *Dreams of Chaos, Visions of Order: Understanding the American Avant-Garde Cinema* (Detroit: Wayne State University Press, 1994), 77–80, and "holistic theories of narrative" in Branigan, *Narrative Comprehension and Film*, 156–57.

16. Sobchack, "Toward Inhabited Space," 324, 327.

17. Raymond Durgnat, "The Restless Camera," *Films and Filming* 15, 3 (Dec. 1968), 15 (my emphases). The two films are René Clair's *Under the Roofs of Paris* (1930) and *July 14th* (1933).

18. Forrest Williams, "The Mastery of Movement: An Appreciation of Max Ophuls," *Film Comment* 5, 4 (Winter 1969), 73.

19. Béla Balázs, *Theory of the Film: Character and Growth of a New Art*, trans. Edith Bone (1945; repr., New York: Dover, 1970), chap. 6, "The Creative Camera," 48.

20. Much has been written about the nature of literary point of view. Gerald Prince provides a schematic overview in *A Dictionary of Narratology* (Lincoln: University of Nebraska Press, 1987). Two dense but rewarding treatments of the topic are Boris Uspensky, *A Poetics of Composition: The Structure of the Artistic Text and Typology of a Compositional Form*, trans. by Valentina Zavarin and Susan Wittig (Berkeley and Los Angeles: University of California Press, 1973); and Gary Saul Morson, *Narrative and Freedom: The Shadows of Time* (New Haven: Yale University Press, 1994). A fine recent book is *New Perspectives on Narrative Perspective*, ed. by Willie van Peer and Seymour Chatman (Albany: State University of New York Press, 2001).

21. Norman Friedman, "Point of View in Fiction: The Development of a Critical Concept," *PMLA* 70, 5 (Dec. 1955), 1160–84.

22. Wayne C. Booth, "Distance and Point-of-View: An Essay in Classification," *Essays in Criticism* 11, 1 (Jan. 1961), 60–79; and Booth, *The Rhetoric of Fiction* (Chicago: University of Chicago Press, 2nd ed. 1983).

23. The explicit or implicit violation of the boundary between two narrative levels is one of the most important issues for a theory of point of view. For a discussion of some varieties of Genette's "metalepsis," and for terms from other theories addressed to the same issue, see Branigan, *Narrative Comprehension and Film*, 250–51 n. 32.

24. Gérard Genette's scheme for analyzing literary point of view has been notably influential. Figure 2.3 is based on his *Narrative Discourse: An Essay in Method*, trans. Jane E. Lewin (Ithaca, N.Y.: Cornell University Press, 1980; orig. 1966, 1969, 1972). Genette defends his system and offers some revisions in *Narrative Discourse Revisited*, trans. Jane E. Lewin (1983; repr., Ithaca, N.Y.: Cornell University Press, 1988). Three essays that seek to apply Genette's scheme to film are the following: Brian Henderson, "Tense, Mood, and Voice in Film (Notes After Genette)," *Film Quarterly* 36, 4 (Summer 1983), 4–17; Marsha Kinder, "The Subversive Potential of the Pseudo-Iterative," *Film Quarterly* 43, 2 (Winter 1989–90), 3–16; and David Alan Black, "Genette and Film: Narrative Level in the Fiction Cinema," *Wide Angle* 8, 3/4 (1986), 19–26. In this latter journal issue, see also Jeffrey S. Rush, "'Lyric Oneness': The Free Syntactical Indirect and the Boundary Between Narrative and Narration": 27–33; and Frank P. Tomasulo, "Narrate *and* Describe? Point of View and Narrative Voice in *Citizen Kane*'s Thatcher Sequence": 45–52. For more on levels of narration and free indirect discourse, see Charles Forceville, "The Conspiracy in the Comfort of Strangers: Narration in the Novel and the Film," *Language and Literature* 11, 2 (2002), 119–135. See generally Bordwell's *Narration in the Fiction Film* for commentary on Genette's scheme and proposed changes. See also Mieke Bal, *Narratology: Introduction to the Theory of Narrative* (Toronto: University of Toronto Press, 2nd ed. 1997).

25. Bordwell, *Narration in the Fiction Film*, 57–61.

26. Seymour Chatman, "Characters and Narrators: Filter, Center, Slant, and Interest-Focus," *Poetics Today* 7 (1986), 189–204; *Coming to Terms: The Rhetoric of Narrative in Fiction and Film* (Ithaca, N.Y.: Cornell University Press, 1990), chap. 9, "A New Point of View on 'Point of View,'" 139–60; and *Reading Narrative Fiction* (New York: Macmillan, 1993). See generally Shlomith Rimmon-Kenan, *Narrative Fiction: Contemporary Poetics* (London: Methuen, 1983).

27. George M. Wilson, *Narration in Light: Studies in Cinematic Point of View* (Baltimore: Johns Hopkins University Press, 1986), 4–5.

28. Jacques Aumont, "The Point of View," *Quarterly Review of Film and Video* 11, 2 (1989), 2–3.

29. Francesco Casetti, *Inside the Gaze: The Fiction Film and Its Spectator*, trans. Nell Andrew with Charles O'Brien (1990; repr., Bloomington: Indiana University Press, 1998), chap. 3, "The Place of the Spectator," 45–83, and "Glossary of Terms," 135–41. See also Casetti, "The Communicative Pact," in *Towards a Pragmatics of the Audiovisual: Theory and History*, Vol. 1, ed. by Jürgen E. Müller (Münster: Nodus Publikationen, 1994), 21–31. For an in-depth survey of various semiotic and enunciation theories, see Robert Stam, Robert Burgoyne, and Sandy Flitterman-Lewis, *New Vocabularies in Film Semiotics: Structuralism, Post-Structuralism and Beyond* (New York: Routledge, 1992), Part III, "Film-Narratology," 69–122, and Part IV, "Psychoanalysis," sect. "Enunciation," 159–162. See also André Gaudreault and François Jost, "Enunciation and Narration," in *A Companion to Film Theory*, ed. Toby Miller and Robert Stam (Oxford: Blackwell, 1999), 45–63; and Robert Stam, *Film Theory: An Introduction* (Oxford: Blackwell, 2000).

30. Douglas Pye, "Movies and Point of View," *Movie* 36 (2000), 2–34.

31. The first scheme in figure 2.10 for analyzing point of view is based on the principles of a case grammar and may be found in Edward Branigan, *Point of View in the Cinema: A Theory of Narration and Subjectivity in Classical Film* (Berlin and New York: Mouton, 1984). The scheme is refined in "'Here is a Picture of No Revolver!': The Negation of Images and Methods for Analyzing the Structure of Pictorial Statements," *Wide Angle* 8, nos. 3–4 (1986), 8–17. The six general elements in this approach may also be considered as more or less salient *cues* for hypothesis building; see Bordwell, *Narration in the Fiction Film*, p. 126. In *Point of View in the Cinema* I summarize the major categories of Friedman, Booth, and Kawin (from which figures 2.1, 2.2, and 2.11 in the text above are derived) as well as summarize the point of view theories of Hugo Münsterberg, André Bazin, and Jean Mitry; see Appendix, "Orthodox Theories of Narration," 190–221.

The second scheme in figure 2.10 for analyzing point of view may be found in my *Narrative Comprehension and Film*, chap. 4, "Levels of Narration," 86–124. This scheme is derived from Susan Sniader Lanser, *The Narrative Act: Point of View in Prose Fiction* (Princeton, N.J.: Princeton University Press, 1981). For applications of my approach, see Thomas Elsaesser and Warren Buckland, *Studying Contemporary American Film: A Guide to Movie Analysis* (London: Arnold, 2002), chap. 6, "Cognitive Theories of Narration (*Lost Highway*)," 168–94; and Warren Buckland, "Narration and Focalisation in *Wings of Desire*," *CineAction* 56 (Sept. 2001), 26–33.

One may conceive of a "level of narration" as a *bracketing* of knowledge in order to indicate the particular *scope* of the relevant quantifiers, connectives, predicates, and variables of (narrative) propositions. Overall, a "level of narration" is part of a *procedure* or process of knowing. But then, one may ask, who is it that acquires (has acquired) this "information" or knowledge? When we choose to imagine that the information is possessed by a fictional or hypothetical "narrator" in a text, "narration" will be seen as the *method* by which the narrator presents his or her (or its) knowledge to us; on the other hand, when we imagine what it is like for ourselves to possess information from a text, "narration" will be the *method* we use to talk about, explain, and expand upon the knowledge we have acquired (including our own explanations to ourselves). The connection, if any, between these two kinds of "narration" is neither direct nor causal, but is merely "partially motivated" through a "motivated convention," "ecological convention," "moderate constructivism," or "mild realism" (see discussion in chapter 4 below).

Both of my schemes for analyzing point of view reject communication models of narration in which, for example, an Author transmits (narrates) a message that is decoded by a perceiver who is then able to retransmit (narrate) what has been sent. Jan Simons skillfully connects my two schemes and places them within the broad context of a generative and cognitive semantics where a spectator's inferential activity replaces a process of "decoding." Many aspects of mind, including the emotions, are involved in making "inferences." This means that the information of a text is not simply contained *within* the text. See "'Enunciation': From Code to Interpretation," in *The Film Spectator: From Sign to Mind*, ed. Warren Buckland (Amsterdam: Amsterdam University Press, 1995), 192–206.

32. Theorists often overlook problems associated with evaluating the degree to which a perceived level of narration is *identifiable* or definite. Here are some *in*definite expressions in language: "a," "some," "somewhat," "somehow," "something else," "it," "this and that," "whatnot," "blah-blah," "now and again," "occasionally," "one day," "someplace," "somebody," "other." What follows is an illustration of indefiniteness at work in the imagery of a film. The opening titles of Jean-Luc Godard's *Pierrot le fou* (1965) conclude with the letters disappearing from the title "Pierrot le fou," leaving only the first "o" on the screen (revealing a movement from a definite name to something indefinite). Cut to the sight of a tennis ball being hit by a woman who is practicing on a bright day (does this shot already possess one or more oblique [indefinite] associations with the preceding "o"?); cut to a reverse angle through a fine wire fence showing a *diffused* view from behind the woman as she is seen volleying with another woman on a tennis court near a large statue of a decorated object that seems to be some sort of giant vase or cup; next, there appears a daytime shot of a man carrying some books while looking at other books by spinning two circular display racks outside a bookstore; and, finally, there appears a shot of distant

city lights, indistinct buildings, and trees reflected in two blurred, shimmering white streaks on the dark waves of a wide river with the last deep, red gleam of a sunset in a hazy blue sky. This shot would appear to represent a typical or occasional sunset that might be seen from a number of possible (indefinite) places looking toward a city. Over the final title card of the opening credits, and continuing over the four shots just described, a man says:

> After the age of fifty, Velasquez stopped painting definite things. He drifted around objects, like the air and twilight, catching within his shadows and airy backgrounds, the palpitations of color, which he transformed into the invisible core of his silent symphony. Henceforth, he captured only those mysterious interpenetrations of shape and tone that form a constant, secret movement, neither betrayed nor interrupted by any jolt or cataclysm. Space reigned supreme. It was as if an aerial wave, gliding over the surfaces, soaked up their visible emanations, defined and modeled them, then spread them about like a perfume, an echo of themselves, a scattering of impalpable dust.

Of course, not just shapes and colors (blues, reds, and neutrals in these shots) may be made indefinite and diffuse ("mysterious interpenetrations of shape," "palpitations of color") but also such narrative elements as action, event, causation, character (identification, personality, agency identity), motive, setting, argument, and theme. The opening shots of *Pierrot le fou* are relevant to the story, and to its ending, but not in a concrete way and perhaps not immediately, even though the shot after the river shows the man from the bookstore in a bathtub reading aloud about Velasquez and the film ends at the ocean. Only *certain* dispersed but potent details from these shots (which cannot be predicted) will be relevant coupled with a *method* of looking and narrating that might be characterized as itself drifting around objects in the manner of Velasquez, searching for mysterious interpenetrations and movements.

One might deny the existence of "indefiniteness" in film by saying that a shot is too "concrete" and shows only a time that is definite (a present time, or maybe a past time). However, the question would then arise, what sort of "camera" — what conception of a camera — allows one to speak in this way?

For a formal treatment of narrational definiteness and indefiniteness, see Branigan, *Narrative Comprehension and Film*, chap. 6, "Objectivity and Uncertainty," 161–91. The same issue of definiteness and indefiniteness arises with a photograph; see text accompanying note 3 in chapter 3 above and note 31 in chapter 5 above. See also George M. Wilson's argument that film narration at its most basic is understood by a spectator to be "indeterminate"; "*Le Grand Imagier* Steps Out: The Primitive Basis of Film

Narration," *Philosophical Topics* 25, 1 (Spring 1997), 295–318. Consider also the indefiniteness of the "bracket syntagma" and the "episodic sequence" in Christian Metz's eight-part "grande syntagmatique." Metz's category of the "autonomous shot" (e.g., the plan-séquence) hints that the syntagmatique need not be fixed to the existence of shot 'divisions' or the splicing of shots. Hence, for example, the 'indefiniteness' of the bracket syntagma (which offers typical samples of something or typifies a recurring event) need *not* be the result of the existence of multiple shots as if it were simply the 'abstractions' of editing that were responsible for creating a sense of indefiniteness out of the 'concreteness' of separate shots. See, e.g., Branigan, *Narrative Comprehension and Film*, 45, 140–42, 284–85 n. 32, and Metz, "Problems of Denotation in the Fiction Film," from *Film Language: A Semiotics of the Cinema*, trans. Michael Taylor (New York: Oxford University Press, 1974), 108–46.

33. Bruce F. Kawin, *Mindscreen: Bergman, Godard, and First-Person Film* (Princeton, N.J.: Princeton University Press, 1978), 18–19, 19 n.7, 21–22, 55–56, 112–116, 190; and Kawin, "An Outline of Film Voices," *Film Quarterly* 38, 2 (Winter 1984–85), 38–46.

34. Slavoj Žižek, "The Hitchcockian Blot," in *Alfred Hitchcock: Centenary Essays*, ed. Richard Allen and S. Ishii-Gonzalès (London: British Film Institute, 1999), 124 (original emphasis). More on the blot may be found in Žižek's essay, "'In His Bold Gaze My Ruin Is Writ Large,'" in *Everything You Always Wanted to Know about Lacan (But Were Afraid to Ask Hitchcock)*, ed. Slavoj Žižek (New York: Verso, 1992), 210–72. Several other essays in the book also address the blot or the "perverse object," the "Thing," or the "stain" that induces the gaze. The notion of a blot might be compared to James Elkins's approach to "the unrepresentable, unpicturable, inconceivable, and unseeable," in *On Pictures and the Words That Fail Them* (Cambridge: Cambridge University Press, 1998), chap. 8, 241–66; esp. 259–61.

35. Žižek, "The Hitchcockian Blot," 123–24, 129.

36. Žižek, "The Hitchcockian Blot," 124–125, 128. Žižek relies here on the theories of Lacan.

37. Žižek, "The Hitchcockian Blot," pp. 123, 125.

38. Žižek, "The Hitchcockian Blot," p. 128. Žižek relies here on Jacques-Alain Miller's commentary on Lacan.

39. Žižek, "The Hitchcockian Blot," 123, 126 (emphasis omitted), 137 n. 1, 138 n. 3.

40. The phallic candles atop the wooden chest in *Rope* are a reminder of the dead homosexual entombed below. Ironically, one of the candles (introduced by an unmotivated camera movement) is initially leaning sideways and is straightened by one of the murderers. This candle may function as a double blot because it both resurrects/re-erects the victim *and* is the requiescat that

lays him finally to rest as a dead 'stiff.' Recall that after the candles have been placed on the wooden chest above the corpse, one of the murderers will again check the 'sturdiness' of the candle that he had previously fixed.

We might continue to think about *Rope* in the spirit of Žižek by imagining a 'de-blot' that will unknot the plot. Later in the film, the maid removes the candles from the top of the wooden chest and attempts to open it, but she is prevented from doing so by the killers, resulting in a premature dénouement preempted. Nevertheless, at the end of the film the *rope/chest/candles/party* blots will finally be exposed (the curtains thrown open, the window opened) when professor-detective Rupert (James Stewart) provides the final lesson to all (after a lecture) by de-familiarizing what had seemed merely familiar and ordinary, thus revealing (finally) the concealed 'not' within the plot knot (i.e., thou shalt not kill) as well as the repressed 'not' of the film's story which is tied up with aspects of Hitchcock's life (bullying in the English private school system, experimenting with style, and philobatism). But what is it that is forbidden and denied perhaps too strongly by the plot? Is there a sexual 'not' that seems not completely a not? What sort of sexual 'practical joke' has been played on the victim's fiancée by the murderers *and* by the victim *and* by Hitchcock? On the aspects of Hitchcock's life mentioned above, see Peter Wollen, "*Rope*: Three Hypotheses" in *Alfred Hitchcock: Centenary Essays*, 74–85.

41. Žižek, "The Hitchcockian Blot," 129–30.
42. Žižek, "The Hitchcockian Blot," 127, 128, 129.
43. Žižek, "The Hitchcockian Blot," p. 129; see also p. 125.
44. In chapter 5, I will readdress from another perspective the problem of the various kinds of movements that produce motion on the screen. The result will be a new understanding of the nature of a "camera."
45. A strong statement by André Bazin about the importance of deep focus and the movement of a spectator's eye may be found in "The Evolution of the Language of Cinema," in *What Is Cinema?* [vol. I], trans. by Hugh Gray (Berkeley and Los Angeles: University of California Press, 1967), 23–40.
46. On the perceptual distinction between a zoom and a dolly (numbers 4 and 6 in the text), see, e.g., Joseph D. Anderson, "Moving Through the Diegetic World of the Motion Picture," in *Film Style and Story: A Tribute to Torben Grodal*, ed. Lennard Højbjerg and Peter Schepelern (Copenhagen: Museum Tusculanum Press, University of Copenhagen, 2003), 11–21.
47. For more on the "kinetic depth effect" that is produced by a camera in movement, see chapter 3.
48. The "follow shot" may be contrasted with what might be called an "avoidance," "evasive," or "runaway" shot, which is quite rare in films. For example, a camera might move left as the center of interest moves right. If the split

Projecting a Camera

between the camera's framing and the center of interest becomes pervasive, then one will reach a device like Bonitzer's "deframing" (see chapter 4). Still more extreme would be to dissolve the center of interest.

49. What distinguishes an active follow shot (e.g., when the camera is tracking with a character) from a passive follow shot (e.g., when the camera and character are riding in a car) is that the means of conveyance is narratively *un*motivated in the former (a camera mounted on a dolly moving on rails beside the character) but motivated in the latter (a car moving in the diegesis). Depending on the orientation of camera and character, the space that moves in the foreground or background of an active or passive follow shot may move left, move right, advance, recede, rise, or fall. Still more extreme would be to dissovle the center of interest.

Active and passive follow shots (numbers 7 and 8 in the text) are not entirely separate categories. One may have an *interactive* follow shot where, for example, the camera is being carried while an object is moving by itself, and vice versa, for example, a shot that shows the point of view of a passenger in a slow-moving car who is looking at someone walking beside the road, followed by a shot of the walking person's point of view of the passenger. Both shots include active and passive elements. That is, when the camera is being carried, the object moves by itself; when the camera moves by itself, the object is being carried.

Follow shots are common in classical narrative films, while a camera that is ahead or behind an action, or moving independently, is much less common. One reason for this preference for follow shots may be that a spectator can easily judge the *time* of, say, a person who is seen walking on screen (i.e., we instantly feel that time is being altered if a person's walk is seen to have been slowed or speeded up); thus, by moving a camera in time to a person's normal walk, a spectator will be able to quickly correlate the times of other objects seen in an image to the time in which they are being presented by a camera. (This reason is not the same as saying that an image is in the "present tense.") By contrast, there *may* be less certainty about time when a camera is moving independently, which may raise a question about how much time is passing in the diegesis, how fast, and whether the time of an unmoving object has "stopped."

50. In a fascinating empirical study Brian O'Leary has investigated the typical camera movements used in classical Hollywood cinema and also in the films of Howard Hawks. O'Leary is interested in the ways in which each of the three dimensions of space is narrativized in film. In order to measure the narrativization ("narrative informational content"), he draws on a "functional semiotics" derived from the linguistics of Michael Halliday. For O'Leary, a "pan" includes lateral tracks to the left and right; a "tilt" includes booming up and down; and a "zoom" includes dollying in and out. O'Leary found, in general, that pans outnumber tilts; pans outnumber zoom outs; pans toward

242

the right outnumber pans to the left; zoom ins outnumber zoom outs; and tilts that move downward as well as diagonal movements are relatively rare. He presents a number of reasons for these results. See Brian O'Leary, "Hollywood Camera Movements and the Films of Howard Hawks: A Functional Semiotic Approach," *New Review of Film and Television Studies* 1, 1 (November 2003): 7–30. See also O'Leary, "Camera Movements in Hollywood's Westering Genre: A Functional Semiotic Approach," *Criticism* 45, 2 (Spring 2003), 197–222; and Barry Salt, "A Note on 'Hollywood Camera Movements and the Films of Howard Hawks: A Functional Semiotic Approach' by Brian O'Leary," *New Review of Film and Television Studies* 3, 1 (May 2005), 101–103.

Raymond Durgnat mentions two additional tendencies of movements by a camera in classical narrative films:

1. "Whenever camera movements depart from 'natural' lines of sight or of movement, the spectator becomes vaguely conscious of a certain uneasiness, or of exhilaration."
2. "Until [Max] Ophuls, technicians' lore had it that one must never, never bring a pan back to its starting point."

Films and Feelings (Cambridge, Mass.: M.I.T. Press, 1967), 56.

51. Michael Snow has made a series of films that contain only movement and each film tests the limits of only one kind of movement: *Wavelength* (1967; zoom); *Back and Forth* (1969; pan); *La Région centrale* (1971; pan, tilt, rotation); and *Breakfast (Table-Top Dolly)* (1972 and 1976; dolly). The standard interpretation of Snow's films is that they literally and figuratively present aspects of "consciousness." The analytical concept of "anthropomorphism" that was discussed earlier does not license this interpretation, nor does its use inevitably lead to a "phenomenological" interpretation of texts. "Anthropomorphism" is meant not to make a claim about the reality of film or of a particular film or of an approach to criticism, but merely to draw attention to a possible (represented) feature of a film text in relation to the human body or, better, to draw attention to how we choose to sometimes *talk* about a film text. Why we choose to speak in this manner using the "grammars" of various film theories and engage in dialogue with certain institutions of film criticism are the real questions underlying "anthropomorphism." Which historical contexts encourage such talk? I will address some of these issues in chapters 4 and 5.

52. Lightman, "The Fluid Camera," 102 (original emphasis).

53. See "Current Problems of Film Theory: Christian Metz on Jean Mitry's L'Esthétique et Psychologie du Cinéma, Vol II," *Screen* 14, nn. 1/2 (Spring/ Summer 1973), sect. 2, "Subjective Images," 45–49.

54. For one view of classical narrative and the categories that are appropriate for analyzing the nature of a camera, see Stephen Heath, *Questions of Cinema* (New York: Macmillan, 1981), chap. 2, "Narrative Space," esp. 48–52.

55. Bordwell, *Narration in the Fiction Film*, 10 (my emphasis).

56. A stalking camera, for example, may be found in *Stalker* (Andrei Tarkovsky, 1979), *Man Bites Dog* (Rémy Belvaux, André Bonzel, and Benoît Poelvoorde, 1992), and the opening of *Psycho* (Hitchcock, 1960). The "wandering" camera and a camera's "unconscious optics" will be further addressed in chapter 4.

57. Dudley Andrew, "The Turn and Return of *Sunrise*," from *Film in the Aura of Art* (Princeton, N.J.: Princeton University Press, 1984), 35–36, revised from "The Gravity of 'Sunrise,'" *Quarterly Review of Film Studies* 2, 3 (August 1977), 362. This camera movement through the marsh in *Sunrise* has been much discussed. See, e.g., Bordwell's analysis in *Narration in the Fiction Film*, 121–25; Robin Wood, "The Couple and the Other," in *Sexual Politics and Narrative Film: Hollywood and Beyond* (New York: Columbia University Press, 1998), 33–34, 42; Jean-André Fieschi, "F. W. Murnau," in *Cinema — A Critical Dictionary: The Major Film-Makers* [vol. 2], ed. Richard Roud (New York: The Viking Press, 1980), 717–18.

58. André Bazin, *Jean Renoir*, trans. W. W. Halsey II and William H. Simon (New York: Simon & Schuster, 1973), chap. 5, "The French Renoir," 87.

59. See, e.g., A.H.C. Van der Heijden, "Attention," in *A Companion to Cognitive Science*, ed. William Bechtel and George Graham (Oxford: Blackwell, 1998), 121–28.

60. Although striving to be clear and distinct in the use of language is often an important goal in writing and speaking, certain methods of film analysis and certain kinds of 'analytic philosophy' within film theory lose track of what is significant in their attention to precise dissection. I believe that one of the sources of this misdirected effort lies with René Descartes, who used *attention* (the "eye's gaze") as an *analogy* for the proper use of the *intellect*, that is, for how concepts should be constructed so that the mind's eye can see clearly and distinctly. Descartes defines his notion of "clear" and "distinct" as follows:

> A perception which can serve as the basis for a certain and indubitable judgment needs to be not merely clear but also distinct. I call a perception 'clear' when it is present and accessible to the attentive mind — just as we say that we see something clearly when it is present to the eye's gaze and stimulates it with a sufficient degree of strength and accessibility. I call a perception "distinct" if, as well as being "clear," it is so sharply separated from all other perceptions that it contains within itself only what is clear.

Note that one might be tempted to say here that our "judgment" about a film is most "clear" *during an actual screening* when a film "is present and accessible to the attentive mind." This would be unfortunate because it would greatly limit the methods of textual analysis deemed appropriate as well as limit which 'judgments' might be taken to be important. Furthermore, the notion of a "distinct" perception that is "so sharply separated from all other perceptions" raises serious issues about 'sharpness' (see chapter 5 below) and 'separation' (i.e., 'framing,' see chapter 4 below, and cf. note 115 in chapter 4).

See *Principles of Philosophy in The Philosophical Writings of Descartes, Vol. I*, ed. John Cottingham, Robert Stoothoff, and Dugald Murdoch (Cambridge: Cambridge University Press, 1984), Part One, sect. 45, 207–08 (22); cf. *Meditations on First Philosophy* from *Vol. II*. For Descartes, 'forgetting' is due to a failure of *reason* to form *ideas* that are "clear" and "distinct" and not derived from either sense experience or the imagination.

On my approach to film "analysis," see the preceding chapter. For a new approach to "analytic philosophy," see *Post-Analytic Philosophy*, ed. John Rajchman and Cornel West (New York: Columbia University Press, 1985). Other alternatives to the "clear and distinct" paradigm derive from Freud, Nietzsche, Continental philosophy, post-structuralism, and the later work of Barthes, all of which in different ways have an interest in interminable, conflictual, and undecidable interpretation. See also chapter 4 below, section "Envoi: The Indefinite Boundary."

61. For Hugo Münsterberg, the mechanism of attention marshals our entire "bodily personality" in creating a sharp, focused impression that acts to generate our emotions while watching film. He says:

> We saw that the moving pictures give us the plastic world and the moving world, and that nevertheless the depth and the motion in it are not real, unlike the depth and motion of the [theater] stage. We find now that the reality of the action in the photoplay in still another respect lacks objective independence, because it yields to our subjective [mental] play of attention. Wherever our attention becomes focused on a special feature, the surrounding adjusts itself, eliminates everything in which we are not interested, and by [means of] the [camera's] close-up heightens the vividness of that on which our mind is concentrated. It is as if that outer world were woven into our mind and were shaped not through its own laws but by the acts of our attention.

Hugo Münsterberg on Film: The Photoplay — A Psychological Study and Other Writings, ed. Allan Langdale (New York: Routledge, 2002), chap. 4, "Attention," 85, 88; Münsterberg, *The Film — A Psychological Study: The Silent Photoplay in 1916* (New York: Dover Publications, 1970;

orig. 1916), chap. 4, "Attention," 37, 39. For three recent studies that bring psychological principles to bear on literary narrative, see *Narrative Theory and the Cognitive Sciences*, ed. David Herman (Stanford, Calif.: Center for the Study of Language and Information, 2003); Patrick Colm Hogan, *The Mind and Its Stories: Narrative Universals and Human Emotions* (Cambridge: Cambridge University Press, 2003); and *Narrative and Consciousness: Literature, Psychology and the Brain*, ed. Gary D. Fireman, Ted E. McVay, Jr., and Owen J. Flanagan (Oxford: Oxford University Press, 2003).

CHAPTER 3: WHAT IS A CAMERA?

This chapter is a thorough rewriting and expansion of my "What Is a Camera?" in *Cinema Histories, Cinema Practices*, ed. Patricia Mellencamp and Philip Rosen [The American Film Institute Monograph Series, vol. 4] (Frederick, Md.: University Publications of America, 1984), 87–107. The original version was translated into German as "Was ist eine Kamera?" in *Der Schnitt Das Filmmagazin* 8 (April 1997), 10–12, and into French as "Qu'est-ce qu'une caméra?" in *Champs Visuels: Revue interdisciplinaire de recherchessur l'image* 12–13 (Paris: L'Harmattan, Janvier 1999) (special issue edited by Guillaume Soulez on "Penser, cadrer: le *project du cadre*"), 33–55.

1. Jean-Pierre Geuens, *Film Production Theory* (Albany: State University of New York Press, 2000), 172 (my emphasis).

2. André Bazin, *What Is Cinema?*, vols. I and II, trans. Hugh Gray (Berkeley and Los Angeles: University of California Press, 1967 and 1971). To my knowledge, the first two authors to recognize that the nature of a camera raised interesting issues were Irving Pichel and David Bordwell. Pichel argues that a camera is a blend of several of the conceptions I describe in this chapter, while Bordwell demonstrates in a most instructive way the incompleteness of profilmic and perceptual accounts of the camera. Additional theories about the camera are discussed in chapter 5 below. Pichel, "Seeing with the Camera," *The Hollywood Quarterly of Film, Radio and Television* 1, 2 (Winter 1946), 138–45, reprinted in *Hollywood Directors 1941–1976*, ed. Richard Koszarski (New York: Oxford University Press, 1977), 69–81; also reprinted as "Change of Camera Viewpoint," in *The Movies as Medium*, ed. Lewis Jacobs (New York: Farrar, Straus & Giroux, 1970), 113–23. Bordwell, "Camera Movement and Cinematic Space" [orig. Summer 1977], in *Explorations in Film Theory: Selected Essays* from Ciné-Tracts, ed. Ron Burnett (Bloomington: Indiana University Press, 1991), 229–36. Bordwell also argues for a 'camera' that is immersed in problems of representation and ideology as opposed to 'other cameras' tied to technology, economics, and auteurs. See "Camera Movement, the Coming of Sound, and the Classical Hollywood Style," in *Film: Historical-Theoretical*

Speculations [The 1977 Film Studies Annual: Part Two] (Pleasantville, N.Y.: Redgrave, 1977), 27–31.

3. Cf. Edward Branigan, "'Here Is a Picture of No Revolver!': The Negation of Images and Methods for Analyzing the Structure of Pictorial Statements," *Wide Angle* 8, 3–4 (1986), 8–17.

4. Although in this chapter I will list eight major conceptions of a camera, I will try to avoid offering an objective or logical overview of the (real) nature of a camera. That is, I will try to avoid the kind of view that may be embodied by an eagle in a tree. In the next two chapters I will make my resistance to such an overview explicit by discussing the *radial* nature of certain theoretical terms (which prevents something from being contained or figured in an absolute way) combined with the *relative* nature of theoretical descriptions (which depend not only on defining a "what" but also on a *when*, i.e., on an occasion of language use). Wittgenstein's ideas about "language-games" will be one of my guiding principles in the next two chapters. There may also be a temptation to think that several of the eight conceptions of a camera might be gathered into a neat bundle. The links among such cameras would be forged by various modes of "causation." The problem, however, to be discussed in chapter 5, is that the notion of causality is not self-evident but is itself connected to modes of segmentation and our use of language. The question arises, Which sorts of causes for which occasions will be relevant for each link in the so-called bundle of cameras?

5. Interpreting behavior, like interpreting the meaning of an object or photograph, depends on weighing context. Psychologists have firmly demonstrated that neglect of context (situation, environment) in judging the meaning of a person's actions leads to a "fundamental attribution error."

6. In concentrating on the notion of a camera, I do not imply that it is the most important fact about film but merely that it is one fact about film and a convenient starting point. In addition, I will not address evaluative questions, such as what makes camerawork elegant, subtle, novel, complex, provocative, ineffective, mistaken, clumsy, etc. The eight conceptions of a camera that I do discuss are not meant to be an exhaustive list; consider, for example, Vivian Sobchack's work discussed in the next two chapters.

7. I am following Richard Wollheim's approach to the problem of meaning; see "Representation: The Philosophical Contribution to Psychology," *Critical Inquiry* 3, 4 (Summer 1977), 709–23.

8. Cf. O. K. Bouwsma, "What Is Meaning?" in *Toward a New Sensibility: Essays of O. K. Bouwsma*, ed. J. L. Craft and Ronald E. Hustwit (Lincoln and London: University of Nebraska Press, 1982), 33–59. See also Bryan Vescio, "Reading in the Dark: Cognitivism, Film Theory, and Radical Interpretation," *Style* 35, 4 (Winter 2001), 572–91; e.g., 574, 583, 589. It should be noted

that critics are seldom interested in an individual or idiosyncratic response to a film. Instead, critics discuss patterns or regularities of response within a particular group and/or declare what a person's response *ought* to have been. From the standpoint of Wittgenstein's approach to "meaning," which will be important in the next two chapters, there are delicate issues here. Wittgenstein focused on 'meaning as use,' but it is not immediately clear how to measure the "use" of a fictional text or what counts as "understanding" a fictional text. Wittgenstein strongly rejected various causal theories whereby a meaning would be determined by the effect on someone's thought, feeling, or action (as in behaviorism and communication theories). Thus, to build a Wittgensteinian approach, one would need to start by identifying interpretive communites and the institutions (and film theories) that set forth rules for making sense of texts. See generally Hans-Johann Glock, *A Wittgenstein Dictionary* (Oxford: Blackwell, 1996), "use," 376–81; cf. "intending and meaning something" and "intentionality," 179–89. With respect to the 'meaning' of a text and its relation to a person's 'response' to the text, consider Glock's comments on the "criteria" that may be used to ascribe intentional attitudes and on the potential applicability of Freud's notion of "unconscious" desires, 181, 186. Wittgenstein emphasizes that "understanding" is not a matter of "communication" but of how a person responds, explains, uses, and expands on what has been understood, that is, of being able to say, "Now I know how to go on." See *Philosophical Investigations*, trans. G.E.M. Anscombe (Oxford: Blackwell, 3rd ed. 1967), §§ 151, 154, 155, 179, 363, 525–34.

9. I will not undertake a definition of narrative. I offer a sketch of the nature of "narrative" in chapter 2 above and a more complete account in Branigan, *Narrative Comprehension and Film* (New York and London: Routledge, 1992).

10. See generally David Bordwell, *On the History of Film Style* (Cambridge, Mass.: Harvard University Press, 1997).

11. See note 4 above.

12. Figure 3.1 is taken from Ulric Neisser, "The Processes of Vision," in *Perception: Mechanisms and Models*, ed. Richard Held and Whitman Richards (San Francisco: W.H. Freeman, 1972), 252–59, reprinted from *Scientific American* 219, 3 (Sept. 1968), 210.

13. In saying that a camera is the "simplest" inference a spectator can make about certain perceptual arrays, I avoid saying it is a "necessary" inference. Not all movements ascribed to a camera are the result of movement by a camera, and, conversely, not all movements by a camera produce a perception of camera movement. Camerawork, like editing, involves the experience of form through successive, partial views, and such perception involves complex sensory processes. See, e.g., Julian Hochberg and Virginia Brooks, "Movies in the Mind's Eye," in *Post-Theory: Reconstructing Film Studies*, ed. by David Bordwell

and Noël Carroll (Madison, Wis.: University of Wisconsin Press, 1996), 368–87; Irvin Rock, "Anorthoscopic Perception," *Scientific American* 244, 3 (Sept. 1981), 145–53. I will discuss the problem of "movement" in chapter 5.

14. Percepts are fully "real" to an individual, and the perceptual processes on which they are based can be described scientifically. What is "illusory" is the fact that percepts are not reliable in all circumstances and can be produced artificially without guaranteeing the actual presence of that which is perceived. Typically the processes of interest to film theorists are more complex than the retinal image produced by an object but less complex than higher-order cognitive functions. It is well accepted that an accurate retinal image is neither necessary nor sufficient to explain visual perception. On the other hand, the appearance, say, of an optical illusion is usually not altered by the fact that we "know" it to be an illusion; it retains its power even in the face of disbelief and rational explanation. One seemingly cannot argue with an illusion. The irresistible nature of illusion combined with its unreliability contributes to the negative judgments of it by such writers as Plato and Brecht. Other writers celebrate illusion by tying it to primitive ritual, healing, myth, magic, and spirit. See, e.g, Rachel O. Moore, who draws on a mosaic of Jean Epstein, André Bazin, Georg Lukács, Walter Benjamin, and others in *Savage Theory: Cinema as Modern Magic* (Durham, N.C.: Duke University Press, 2000), chap. 6, "The Metal Brain," 84–95 ("The film image can be seen as the spirit double of the real thing it shows, always independent of that thing, an exact copy that is thoroughly autonomous and exists as part of the spirit world that is cinema," 87; cf. 94–95.).

15. E. H. Gombrich, "Illusion and Art," in *Illusion in Nature and Art*, ed. R. L. Gregory and E. H. Gombrich (New York: Charles Scribner's Sons, 1973), 192–243 (" . . . our problem is precisely to what extent art may elicit phantom perceptions," 212; see also 208); on cinema, see 240–41; Jean-Luis Baudry, "The Apparatus: Metapsychological Approaches to the Impression of Reality in the Cinema," in *Narrative, Apparatus, Ideology: A Film Theory Reader*, ed. Philip Rosen (New York: Columbia University Press, 1986), 299–318. Recent wrestling with illusion and film includes Richard Allen, *Projecting Illusion: Film Spectatorship and the Impression of Reality* (Cambridge, U.K.: Cambridge University Press, 1995); Richard Allen, "Looking at Motion Pictures," in *Film Theory and Philosophy*, ed. Richard Allen and Murray Smith (New York: Oxford University Press, 1997), 76–94; Gregory Currie, *Image and Mind: Film, Philosophy and Cognitive Science* (Cambridge, U.K.: Cambridge University Press, 1995); Joseph D. Anderson, *The Reality of Illusion: An Ecological Approach to Cognitive Film Theory* (Carbondale: Southern Illinois University Press, 1996); Trevor Ponech, "Visual Perception and Motion Picture Spectatorship," *Cinema Journal* 37, 1 (Fall 1997), 85–100.

16. Noël Burch, *To the Distant Observer: Form and Meaning in the Japanese Cinema* (Berkeley and Los Angeles: University of California Press, 1979), chap. 20, "Mizoguchi Kenji," 217–46, 222, passim; Noël Burch and Jorge Dana, "Propositions," *Afterimage* 5 (Spring 1974), 40–67. The notion of an unmotivated, or "gratuitous," movement of a camera refers to a movement that is not motivated by diegetic (i.e., "illusory") space, time, or narrative causality. I examined this notion in chapter 2.

17. Burch, "A Parenthesis on Film History," in *To the Distant Observer*, chap. 5, 61–66, and "Porter, or Ambivalence," *Screen* 19, 4 (1978/9), 91–105. It is often claimed that exploration of nonillusionist aspects of film falls to the avant-garde; see, e.g., Grahame Weinbren and Christine Brinckmann, "Selective Transparencies: Pat O'Neill's Recent Films," *Millennium Film Journal* 6 (Spring 1980), 50–72.

18. Charles Boultenhouse, "The Camera as a God" [orig. 1963], in *Film Culture Reader*, ed. P. Adams Sitney (New York: Cooper Square Press, 2000), 139.

19. Michael Baxandall, *Painting and Experience in Fifteenth Century Italy* (Oxford: Clarendon Press, 1972), 40–45. According to the Church, illusionist painting fostered piety because it was direct, emotional, and lasting. It also did not require literacy. Much has been written about the controversial relation of Renaissance perspective to cinema; see, e.g., William Wees, "The Cinematic Image as a Visualization of Sight," *Wide Angle* 4, 3 (1980): 28–37; Noël Carroll, *Mystifying Movies: Fads & Fallacies in Contemporary Film Theory* (New York: Columbia University Press, 1988), chap. 3, in "The Cinematic Image," 89–146.

20. Noël Burch, *Theory of Film Practice*, trans. Helen R. Lane (New York: Praeger, 1973), reprinted by Princeton University Press, Princeton, N.J., 1981.

21. On defamiliarization in film, see, e.g., Kristin Thompson, *Breaking the Glass Armor: Neoformalist Film Analysis* (Princeton, N.J.: Princeton University Press, 1988), chap. 1, "Neoformalist Film Analysis: One Approach, Many Methods," 3–46; Kristin Thompson, *Eisenstein's Ivan the Terrible: A Neoformalist Analysis* (Princeton, N.J.: Princeton University Press, 1981), chap. 1, "A Neoformalist Method of Film Criticism," 8–60.

22. On the role of the avant-garde in certain film histories, see Dana Polan, "Formalism and its Discontents," *Jump Cut*, no. 26 (1981), 65.

23. Sergei Eisenstein, "The Cinematographic Principle and the Ideogram," in *Film Form: Essays in Film Theory*, trans. Jay Leyda (New York: Harcourt, Brace & World, 1949), 41. Unmotivated camera movement is one instance of an obtrusive camera.

24. Bazin, "The Ontology of the Photographic Image" [orig. 1945], in *What Is Cinema?* [vol. I], 15.

25. Arthur C. Danto, "Moving Pictures," in *Philosophizing Art: Selected Essays* (Berkeley and Los Angeles: University of California Press, 1999), 205–32.

26. Roger Scruton, "Photography and Representation," *Critical Inquiry* 7, 3 (Spring 1981): 589, 598–603. Scruton claims that "The camera . . . is being used not to represent something but to point to it. The subject [i.e., the object being pointed to], once located, plays its own special part in an independent process of representation. The camera is not essential to that process: a gesturing finger would have served just as well." Scruton goes on to repeat the well-worn assertion that a camera may on occasion be used for interest, emphasis, and "peculiar effects of atmosphere." Again, the camera is deemed radically external to a dramatic mise-en-scène and, hence, for Scruton, incidental. Rudolf Arnheim argues that the cinema is truly art only insofar as it can escape photographic realism and create not an illusion but a "partial" illusion; *Film as Art* (Berkeley and Los Angeles: University of California Press, 1957), 26, 28; cf. 12, 59. For a recent examination of the claims of Scruton and Arnheim, see Berys Gaut, "Cinematic Art," *The Journal of Aesthetics and Art Criticism* 60, 4 (Fall 2002), 299–312. Although Roland Barthes argues that photography is a species of deixis, there are interesting complications. *Camera Lucida: Reflections on Photography*, trans. Richard Howard (New York: Hill and Wang, 1981), sect. 2 ("[T]he Photograph is never anything but an antiphon of 'Look,' 'See,' 'Here it is'; it points a finger at certain vis-à-vis, and cannot escape this pure deictic language.").

27. Scruton, "Photography and Representation," 594.

28. André Bazin, "William Wyler ou le janseniste de la mise-en-scène" from *Qu'est-ce que le cinéma?* [vol. I] (Paris: Éditions du Cerf, 1958), 157 (my emphasis). See also Dudley Andrew, "Realism and Reality in Cinema: The Film Theory of André Bazin and Its Source in Recent French Thought" (Ph.D. dissertation: University of Iowa, 1972), 82–93; and Andrew, *André Bazin* (1978; repr., New York: Columbia University Press; new preface, 1990).

29. André Bazin, *Orson Welles: A Critical View*, trans. Jonathan Rosenbaum (New York: Harper & Row, 1978), 77.

30. On editing and psychology, see Karel Reisz and Gavin Millar, *The Technique of Film Editing* (New York: Hastings House, 2nd ed. 1968), 249, 255. Cf. the debate among Bazin, Reisz and Millar, and Kristin Thompson involving the perceptual and aesthetic consequences of the long takes in Hitchcock's *Rope*; see note 10 in chapter 2 above. See generally *Hugo Münsterberg on Film: The Photoplay — A Psychological Study and Other Writings*, ed. Allan Langdale (1916; repr., New York: Routledge, 2002); Gerard Buckle, *The Mind and the Film* (1926; repr., New York: Arno, 1970).

31. Ernest Lindgren, *The Art of the Film* (New York: Collier Books, 1963), 158, 166.

32. Reisz and Millar, *The Technique of Film Editing*, 233–36.

33. Reisz and Millar, *The Technique of Film Editing*, 213, 215; Lindgren, *The Art of the Film*, 65–67. See also note 38 below.

34. André Bazin insists on the fundamental importance of "deep focus"; see, e.g., "The Evolution of the Language of Cinema," in *What Is Cinema?* [vol. I], 35–36, and "An Aesthetic of Reality: Neorealism" [vol. II], 28, 35–38.

   "Lateral depth of field" is a type of camera movement Bazin defined. He says that it results in the "almost total disappearance of montage." Lateral depth of field, to be discussed also in note 30 of the next chapter, is so important that I will quote Bazin's description at length.

> Since what we are shown is only significant in terms of what is hidden from us and since therefore the value of what we see is continually threatened, the *mise en scène* cannot limit itself to what is presented on the screen. The rest of the scene, while effectively hidden, should not cease to exist. The action is not bounded by the screen, but merely passes through it. And a person who enters the camera's field of vision is coming from other areas of the action, and not from some limbo, some imaginary "backstage." Likewise, the camera should be able to spin suddenly without picking up any holes or dead spots in the action.
>
> What all of this means is that the scene should be played independent of the camera in all its real dramatic expanse and that it is up to the cameraman to let his viewfinder play over the action. Reframing, then, is substituted as much as possible for a switching of points of view, which not only introduces spatial discontinuity, a phenomenon foreign to the nature of the human eye, but also sanctions the concept of the reality of a shot on a single plane, the idea of each shot as nothing more than a unit of place and action, an atom that joins with other atoms to make the scene and then the sequence. When a film is made in this way, with each shot lit and played separately, the screen hides nothing, because there is nothing to hide outside the action being filmed. And as cleverly as these separate bits are stitched together, they cannot fool the attentive spectator. The little moment of hesitation at the beginning of a first line, the little something in the fixed nature of the camera and above all in the framing, where nothing is left to chance — everything betrays the existence of a preconceived "shot."

Bazin, *Jean Renoir*, trans. W. W. Halsey II and William H. Simon (New York: Simon & Schuster, 1973), chap. 5, "The French Renoir," 89.

35. Bazin restricts the independence of a camera in a number of ways. Its vision and mobility in "lateral depth of field" are confined to what an invisible witness (who is curious but not perfect) *would see* under identical conditions. Thus, not all 'unmotivated' camera placements and movements will qualify. Also, not all 'motivated' camera placements and movements will qualify; see Bazin's comments on Hitchcock's *Rope*, quoted in chapter 2 above. See generally Bazin, *Jean Renoir*, 87–91, and "Theater and Cinema, Part Two," in *What Is Cinema?* [vol. I], 102–07.

36. A weaker claim is sometimes advanced that asserts that a film places the spectator only at a scene *as if* it were being played *on a stage*. This claim attempts to find a compromise between a film's apparent twin sources in real space and fictional space but only succeeds in postponing the problem: What is the nature of a stage play? There is no ontological halfway house. Note that these formulations of the nature of meaning involve statements in the subjunctive conditional mood. Some of the difficulties of analyzing statements in this mood are explored by A. J. Ayer, *Probability and Evidence* (New York: Macmillan, 1972), 111–39, and Nelson Goodman, *Fact, Fiction, and Forecast* (Cambridge, Mass.: Harvard University Press, 4th ed. 1983).

37. For Bazin, the 'facts' of reality are always prior to, and distinct from, 'meaning.' Thus, he shares the mystic's belief that there exists a kind of knowledge not expressible in a semantic system through words, pictures, gestures, etc. This sort of experience is either prior to language in the broadest sense or beyond language. See "An Aesthetic of Reality: Neorealism (Cinematic Realism and the Italian School of the Liberation)," in *What Is Cinema?* [vol. II], 28, 35–38; "Le Réalisme cinématographique et l'école italienne de la libération," in *Qu'est-ce que le cinéma?* [vol. IV], 34. Bazin argues that film responds to an individual's fear of death by promising to preserve life through film's unique power to "embalm" not just an instant of time in a single frame but also a continuous duration through a sequence of frames. In this way, as Philip Rosen points out, Bazin's theory of representation becomes immersed in theological values. See "The Ontology of the Photographic Image," in *What Is Cinema?* [vol. I], 9–16; and Rosen, *Change Mummified: Cinema, Historicity, Theory* (Minneapolis: University of Minnesota Press, 2001), chap. 1, "Subject, Ontology, and Historicity in Bazin," 3–41.

38. Kenneth Roberts and Win Sharples make the standard argument that camera movement must be unobtrusive in order to duplicate human perception:

> In the proper hands movement of the camera can be a powerful means of visual expression, but the secret to its success is in the ability to move without calling attention to the movement. This can be achieved by having the camera's movement resemble the physical and mental

> experiences of human vision. When the camera is moved so as to capture these experiences, the spectator will accept such movement because he is unaware of it.

A Primer for Filmmaking (Indianapolis, Ind.: Pegasus, 1971), 102; see also 102–07, 132–34.

39. On film history as a contest between realism and expressionism, see, e.g., Gerald Mast, "Kracauer's Two Tendencies and the Early History of Film Narrative," *Critical Inquiry* 6, 3 (Spring 1980): 475–76.

40. Bazin, *Jean Renoir*, 84–85, 105–06. See also Bazin's "The Evolution of the Language of Cinema," 23–40, and "Theater and Cinema, Part Two," 110, both in *What Is Cinema?* [vol. I].

41. See Bazin's analysis of *The River* (1951), a film that eschews the favored techniques yet, he affirms, is unsurpassed in its realism; *Jean Renoir*, chap. 8, "A Pure Masterpiece: *The River*," 104–19. See also "An Aesthetic of Reality," in *What Is Cinema?* [vol. II], 26 ("But realism in art can only be achieved in one way — through artifice."), 30 ("Some measure of reality must always be sacrificed in the effort of achieving it.").

42. On the "perfect view" convention and its varieties, see Edward Branigan, *Point of View in the Cinema: A Theory of Narration and Subjectivity in Classical Film* (Berlin and New York: Mouton, 1984); and *Narrative Comprehension and Film*.

43. Ernest Lindgren remarks that "Camera movement . . . very often carries with it a certain subjective impression. The movement of the camera draws attention to the *imaginary observer* whose movement it reproduces. The content of the shot is seen, not directly, but through the eyes, as it were, of someone who *is reacting to* that content in a certain way." *The Art of the Film*, 164 (my emphasis).

44. A useful summary of some issues involving expression theories is F. E. Sparshott, "Goodman on Expression," *The Monist* 58, 2 (April 1974): 187–202. On the ideology of Romanticism, see Tzvetan Todorov, "The Romantic Crisis," in *Theories of the Symbol*, trans. Catherine Porter (Oxford: Basil Blackwell, 1982), chap. 6, 147–221. William Rothman merges expression with "mystery" as follows:

> That we may know Hitchcock through his films may seem impossible, but it is no more impossible than that human beings are capable of expressing themselves in any other medium, are capable of expressing themselves at all. It is a fact that human beings are capable of revealing and declaring and creating themselves. Yet this fact is also a mystery.

The "I" of the Camera takes this mystery to be, historically, one of the central themes of film. Hitchcock's films, and the other films I write about, develop this theme by creating intimate, mysterious relationships between the camera and the camera's "subjects," the human beings who dwell within the world of the film (they are also the stars who present themselves to the camera and are revealed by it), and equally intimate and mysterious relationships between the camera and the author, the "I" the camera represents. (The camera also represents the viewer. Does it, then, always serve two masters?)

The "I" of the Camera: Essays in Film Criticism, History, and Aesthetics (Cambridge: Cambridge University Press, 2nd ed. 2004), xx.

45. The popular belief that film "reflects," "mirrors," or is a "window" onto the world or onto the soul is really little explanation. Related concepts such as likeness, similarity, resemblance, copy, and mimesis are scarcely better. See, e.g., Nelson Goodman, *Languages of Art: An Approach to a Theory of Symbols* (Indianapolis, Ind.: Hackett, 2nd ed. 1976), 3–19; Max Black, "How Do Pictures Represent?" in E.H. Gombrich, Julian Hochberg, and Max Black, *Art, Perception, and Reality* (Baltimore: Johns Hopkins University Press, 1972), 95–130. The above concepts, however, are suggestive of analogy and metaphor, which, combined with various schemata, will have an important explanatory role in the next chapter. The focus, however, will not be on the relation of film to the world or personal expression but, rather, on the relation of film to the particular language(s) we choose in describing a film's fit with our (multiple, incompatible) goals in the world. To modify a proverbial formula, beauty will be found not in the eye of a beholder but in a way of speaking (within a language-game) about how we choose to see. The "speaking" will often depend upon metaphor and projection.

46. On expression and innate brain fields, see Rudolf Arnheim, "The Gestalt Theory of Expression," in *Toward a Psychology of Art* (Berkeley and Los Angeles: University of California Press, 1966). Various expressive theories are combined by Béla Balázs, *Theory of the Film: Character and Growth of a New Art*, trans. Edith Bone (New York: Dover, 1970), esp. chap. 9, "Changing Set-up," 89–117. He says:

> The free, individual possibilities of the set-up bring about in the image the synthesis of subject and object which is the basic condition of all art. Every work of art must present not only objective reality but the subjective personality of the artist, and this personality includes his way of looking at things, his ideology and the limitations of the period. All this

is projected into the picture, even unintentionally. Every picture shows not only a piece of reality, but a point of view as well. The set-up of the camera betrays the inner attitude of the man behind the camera. (89–90)

47. Alexandre Astruc, "The Birth of a New Avant-garde: La Caméra–stylo," in *The New Wave*, ed. Peter Graham (New York: Doubleday, 1968), 17–23. The paintbrush metaphor for a camera is common. Because it is based on an expressive theory of meaning, it can lead, paradoxically, to the judgment that the camera is actually more of a machine than a creative instrument. See Virgil Aldrich, *Philosophy of Art* (Englewood Cliffs, N.J.: Prentice-Hall, 1963), 62–63.

48. Andrew Sarris, *The American Cinema: Directors and Directions*, 1929–1968 (New York: E. P. Dutton, 1968), 269–300; see also the introduction, "Toward a Theory of Film History," 19–37.

49. On narration as communication, see Hayden White, "The Value of Narrativity in the Representation of Reality," *Critical Inquiry* 7, 1 (Autumn 1980): 5; Victor Turner, "Social Dramas and Stories About Them," ibid., 167.

50. On the application of communication to language, literature, and film, see, e.g., Umberto Eco, *A Theory of Semiotics* (Bloomington: Indiana University Press, 1976), chap. 1, "Signification and Communication," 32–47; James Kinneavy, *A Theory of Discourse: The Aims of Discourse* (New York: W.W. Norton, 1971), sect. "Comprehensive Theory of the Field of English," 17–40; Seymour Chatman, *Story and Discourse: Narrative Structure in Fiction and Film* (Ithaca, N.Y.: Cornell University Press, 1978), 146–61.

51. On the phatic element in language, see Roman Jakobson, "Linguistics and Poetics," in *The Structuralists: From Marx to Lévi-Strauss*, ed. Richard and Fernande de George (Garden City, N.Y.: Anchor Books, 1972), 89, 92.

52. Nick Browne, "The Spectator-in-the-Text: The Rhetoric of *Stagecoach*," *Film Quarterly* 29, 2 (Winter 1975–76), 26, reprinted in *Narrative, Apparatus, Ideology: A Film Theory Reader*, ed. by Philip Rosen (New York: Columbia University Press, 1986), 102. See also Browne's "Film Form/Voice-Over: Bresson's *The Diary of a Country Priest*," *Yale French Studies* 60 (1980), 234–35; *The Rhetoric of Filmic Narration* (Ann Arbor, Mich.: UMI Research Press, 1976), 1, 25–27, 57–58. On the problems that arise with the concept of "voice," see, e.g., the special issue on "Voice and Human Experience," *New Literary History* 32, 3 (Summer 2001).

53. Some of the narrators found to be active in film: Dudley Andrew, "The Gravity of 'Sunrise,'" *Quarterly Review of Film Studies* 2, 3 (August 1977): 370 (village), revised as "The Turn and Return of *Sunrise*," in *Film in the Aura of Art* (Princeton, N.J.: Princeton University Press, 1984), 47; Bruce Kawin, *Mindscreen: Bergman, Godard, and First-Person Film* (Princeton,

N.J.: Princeton University Press, 1978), 173, 181, 183 (Paris); Browne, "The Spectator-in-the-Text," 35 (the character Lucy), also in *The Rhetoric of Filmic Narration*, 5; Browne, "Film Form/Voice-Over," 233, 237 (the priest); Tony Pipolo, "The Aptness of Terminology: Point of View, Consciousness and *Letter from An Unknown Woman*," *Film Reader* 4 (1979), 167, 169, 171 (the character Lisa); Browne, *The Rhetoric of Filmic Narration*, chap. 3, "Narration as Interpretation: The Rhetoric of *Au Hasard, Balthazar*," 73–77 (donkey), revised as "Narrative Point of View: The Rhetoric of *Au Hasard, Balthazar*," *Film Quarterly* 31, 1 (Fall 1977): 29–31; Kawin, *Mindscreen*, 93, 135, 139 (God); 56, 106 (arc rods of a projector); and 3, 17, 56, 92, passim (mind of the film text itself).

54. Some human traits that have been found to be possessed by the camera: Andrew, "The Gravity of 'Sunrise,'" 362, and "The Turn and Return of *Sunrise*," 35–36 (bold and exhibiting a sense of smell); Bazin, "The French Renoir," 87 (curious); James McLaughlin, "All in the Family: Alfred Hitchcock's 'Shadow of a Doubt,'" *Wide Angle* 4, 1 (1980): 13 (lewd); William Rothman, "Alfred Hitchcock's *Murder!*: Theater, Authorship and the Presence of the Camera," ibid., 60 (tactful); Danto, "Moving Pictures," 230 (lewd); Raymond Durgnat, "The Restless Camera," *Films and Filming* 15, 3 (Dec. 1968): 15–16 (impulsive; disorderly; smiling ironically).

    Tony Pipolo declares that "the correspondences between character and camera 'behavior' amount to this: the camera is personified to the degree that it acts in unison with, and often as a substitute for, the character consciousness which controls it." "The Aptness of Terminology," 172.

55. Kaja Silverman and Harun Farocki, *Speaking about Godard* (New York: New York University Press, 1998), 8, 9, 22, 57, 52, 55.

56. On film history as driven by new forms of authorial rhetoric, see David Bordwell, "The Art Cinema as a Mode of Film Practice," *Film Criticism* 4, 1 (Fall 1979), esp. 59–61; Steve Neale, "Art Cinema as Institution," *Screen* 22, 1 (1981), 11–39. A common idea is that overt authorial rhetoric is more 'honest' ('true' to itself) and so defeats 'illusionism.' For example, according to Robert Lapsley and Michael Westlake:

    In the case of films that do expose their discursive processes, that do move from the imaginary towards the symbolic, the spectator is no longer positioned in an illusory relation to the text but is actively involved in a process of reading that reveals the film's textuality. In this way the truth of cinema is allowed to unfold and reveal itself.

    Apparently, 'seeing is now believing' for any film that "is allowed to . . . reveal itself." It is as if truth had advanced into clearer view from behind a darkened glass because the author has come closer. Ideas about framing will be examined in the next chapter. Notice the figurative uses of "move" and "positioned" in the quote above; such uses will be examined in chapter 5. Note also that no film theory has ever proposed or advocated a spectator who is *not* "actively involved." Finally, it must be said that the fear of illusion and imitation, and of authors who hide themselves within a narrative, derives from numerous passages in Plato's *Republic*. Lapsley and Westlake, *Film Theory: An Introduction* (New York: St. Martin's Press, 1988), 87.

57. See, e.g., Freud's analysis of a primal enactment of presence and absence in the child's game of Fort/Da in *Beyond the Pleasure Principle*, trans. by James Strachey (1920; repr., New York: W.W. Norton & Co., 1961), 8–11.

58. Paul Willemen, "Through the Glass Darkly: Cinephilia Reconsidered," in *Looks and Frictions: Essays in Cultural Studies and Film Theory* (Bloomington: Indiana University Press, 1994), 241.

59. See, e.g., Laura Mulvey, "Visual Pleasure and Narrative Cinema," in *Visual and Other Pleasures* (Bloomington: Indiana University Press, 1989), 14–26; Jean-Louis Baudry, "Ideological Effects of the Basic Cinematographic Apparatus" and "The Apparatus: Metapsychological Approaches to the Impression of Reality in the Cinema," in *Narrative, Apparatus, Ideology: A Film Theory Reader*, ed. Philip Rosen (New York: Columbia University Press, 1986), 286–318.

60. The dream process in which the camera plays a direct role is known as "considerations of representability." See J. Laplanche and J.-B. Pontalis, *The Language of Psycho-Analysis*, trans. Donald Nicholson-Smith (New York: W.W. Norton, 1973), 389–90. Other processes of dream-work include condensation, displacement, and secondary revision; cf. phantasy. For an annotated bibliography, see Janet Jenks Casebier and Allan Casebier, "Selective Bibliography on Dream and Film," *Dreamworks* 1, 1 (Spring 1980): 88–93. "Identification" is another important psychological process and leads to the notion of a spectator's "identification with the camera." See, e.g., Christian Metz, "The Imaginary Signifier," in *The Imaginary Signifier: Psychoanalysis and the Cinema*, trans. Celia Britton, Annwyl Williams, Ben Brewster, and Alfred Guzzetti (Bloomington: Indiana University Press, 1982), sect. "Identification with the Camera," 49–52. Metz's detailed treatment of film and dream is "The Fiction Film and Its Spectator: A Metapsychological Study," in *The Imaginary Signifier*, 99–147. Susanne K. Langer offers an early theory of film and dream in *Feeling and Form: A Theory of Art* (New York: Charles Scribner's Sons, 1953), Appendix, "A Note on the Film," 411–15 (film's "artistic potentialities became evident only when the moving camera was introduced," 411). Another approach can be found in Robert T. Eberwein, *Film & The Dream Screen: A Sleep and a Forgetting* (Princeton, N.J.: Princeton University Press, 1984). O. K. Bouwsma,

however, raises many serious questions about how we use the words "dream" and "illusion" in "Failure I: Are Dreams Illusions?" in *Toward a New Sensibility*, 61–88.

61. Paul Willemen offers an example of how verbal language, camera movement, and the unconscious may intersect:

> This rigidity [of social conventions as depicted generally in films by Max Ophuls], this rigorous Order, transgression of which can bring death, is then depicted in the most fluid and flexible of ways, as if what was repressed by the rigorous social order re-emerges in the *mise en scène*. The most striking example of this is perhaps a structuring literalism in *Le Plaisir* (1952) [i.e., a literal production in the filmic text of a verbal metaphor]. As a joke — and it is interesting that he should have chosen to put it in this way — Ophuls explained that the reason for the convoluted crane movement along the walls of the brothel in the Maison Tellier episode, peering through windows but never cutting to the inside of the house, was that the Maison Tellier was, precisely, a *"maison close,"* literally "a closed house" but a common French phrase designating a private brothel. Behind its windows and doors is locked away what a rigorous social morality excludes from its legal order.
>
> So, the camera is on the side of the law (and of the people who cannot afford or pretend not to visit such places), *but what has been excluded and repressed* — in this case we see the repression and transformation of a verbal phrase [i.e., *"maison close"*] combined with the inscription of socio-sexual repression — *returns and energises the camera, moving it along* as it obsessively circles its object of fascination, tracing the outlines of the gaps in the social fabric, catching glimpses of the forbidden areas where desire reigns. The tracks, dolly shots and crane movements constantly hold out the promise that in passing, or in the move from one position or look to another, the look finally may find and possess its object of desire. . . . But the object of desire evades the look, never offering itself to a close-up, to detailed scrutiny. The look searches but is never allowed the illusion of possessing its object.

Willemen, "The Ophuls Text: A Thesis," from *Looks and Frictions*, 135 (footnote omitted; my emphases of last two phrases), revised from *Ophuls*, ed. Paul Willemen (London: British Film Institute, 1978), 70–71. Further details of what Willemen above terms a "structuring literalism" may be found in "Cinematic

Discourse: The Problem of Inner Speech," in *Looks and Frictions*, 27–55, and in his "Reflections on Eikhenbaum's Concept of Internal Speech in the Cinema," *Screen* 15, 4 (Winter 1974/75), 59–70, and "The Fugitive Subject," in *Raoul Walsh*, ed. Phil Hardy (Edinburgh: Edinburgh Film Festival, 1974), 62–89. For criticism, see Noël Carroll, "Language and Cinema: Preliminary Notes for a Theory of Verbal Images," *Millennium Film Journal* 7/8/9 (Fall/Winter 1980–1981), 186–217. See generally Roy Schafer, "Action and Narration in Psychoanalysis," *New Literary History* 12, 1 (Autumn 1980), 61–85.

62. On giving visual form to the unconscious of a patriarchal society, see, e.g., D. N. Rodowick, *The Crisis of Political Modernism: Criticism and Ideology in Contemporary Film Theory* (Urbana: University of Illinois Press, 1988), chap. 8, "Sexual Difference," 221–70. See generally Robert Stam, Robert Burgoyne, and Sandy Flitterman-Lewis, *New Vocabularies in Film Semiotics: Structuralism, Post-Structuralism and Beyond* (New York: Routledge, 1992), Part IV, "Psychoanalysis," 123–83.

Phallic aggression is depicted literally in *King Kong* (Merian C. Cooper, 1933). The heroine rehearses terrified reactions as the camera becomes King Kong by assuming in advance the creature's place. In Frank Borzage's *Liliom* (1930), the subordination of the female gaze is depicted literally when, in a scene involving a wedding portrait, a bride is told to look at her husband while he is told to look into the lens of the camera. The first example is from a lecture by Thierry Kuntzel at the University of Wisconsin, Madison, in Spring 1976.

On the "motionless voyage" of "imaginary presence," see Noël Burch, *Life to those Shadows*, trans. Ben Brewster (Berkeley and Los Angeles: University of California Press, 1990), 39, 59, 181, 202–33, 243, 250, 267–73. Cf. the Hitchcockian 'immobile camera' described by Slavoj Žižek in chapter 2 above. Burch's early work searched for sensory forms with which to defamiliarize the cinematic illusion. His later work focuses on a spectator's imaginary involvement with a diegesis that offers itself to touch. Movement of the camera is the device that joins the 'movement' of the psyche to the 'movement' of the hand (body) over a desired reality.

> However, if neither "primary identification" with the camera nor the constitution of a "haptic space" necessarily depend on camera movements, if they can ultimately be established without them, it is the case that [camera] movement represents the point of contact of two composite systems, one that centres the ubiquitous subject . . . and one that constitutes the effect of a "haptic" space. Here at one go we have both an analogue of the "motionless voyage" in diegetic space and the *tangible* proof of the three-dimensionality of "haptic" space. This is no doubt the source of the tendency to privilege [camera] movement in connection

with one or other of these basic functions when these are provided by far more complex means. (181; original emphasis)

63. Laura Mulvey, "Visual Pleasure and Narrative Cinema," in *Visual and Other Pleasures* (Bloomington: Indiana University Press, 1989), 21–22.

64. Metz, "The Imaginary Signifier," 17–19, 28–30, 52–53.

65. A starting point for thinking about film as language is the early work of Christian Metz. See *Language and Cinema*, trans. Donna Jean Umiker-Sebeok (The Hague: Mouton, 1974) and *Film Language: A Semiotics of the Cinema*, trans. Michael Taylor (New York: Oxford University Press, 1974). See generally Stam, Burgoyne, and Flitterman-Lewis, *New Vocabularies in Film Semiotics*, Parts I and II, "The Origins of Semiotics" and "Cine-semiology," 1–68.

66. Metz, "The Imaginary Signifier," 18.

67. On some implications of anthropomorphism, see, e.g., Alain Robbe-Grillet, "Nature, Humanism, Tragedy," in *For a New Novel: Essays on Fiction*, trans. Richard Howard (New York: Grove, 1965), 49–75. On some theoretical problems raised by anthropomorphism, see Branigan, *Narrative Comprehension and Film*, 109–10. See also the section on anthropomorphism in chapter 2 above.

68. See Roland Barthes, "The Structuralist Activity," in *Critical Essays*, trans. Richard Howard (Evanston, Ill.: Northwestern University Press, 1972), 219. On the history of critical institutions in film studies and canons of interpretation, see especially David Bordwell, *Making Meaning: Inference and Rhetoric in the Interpretation of Cinema* (Cambridge, Mass.: Harvard University Press, 1989).

69. Metz, "Problems of Denotation in the Fiction Film," in *Film Language*, 113, 143–45. For some of Metz's later views and refinements, see "The Imaginary Signifier" and his final book, *L'Énonciation impersonnelle, ou le site du film* (Paris: Méridiens Klincksieck, 1991). See generally the special issue on "Christian Metz & Film Theory," *Iris* 10, v. 6, n. 1 (April 1990).

70. Metz, "The Imaginary Signifier," 29 (my emphasis of "working conveniences" and "indefinite").

71. On Michael Snow's *La Région centrale* (1971), see David Bordwell, "Imploded Space: Film Style in *The Passion of Jeanne d'Arc*," in *Purdue Film Studies* [vol. 1] (Pleasantville, N.Y.: Redgrave, 1976), esp. 102–04. Hitchcock's description of the shot in *Vertigo* (1958) may be found in François Truffaut, *Hitchcock* (New York: Simon and Schuster, rev. ed. 1984), 246. The unusual camera movement in *Vertigo* that tracks back while zooming in may also be found in *Jaws* (Steven Spielberg, 1975), *GoodFellas* (Martin Scorsese, 1990), *The Mask* (Charles Russell, 1994), and other films. Examples of continuous camera movements that represent discontinuous narrative time may be found in Alain

Resnais's *Last Year in Marienbad* (1961), Miklós Jancsó's *The Red and the White* (1967), and Michelangelo Antonioni's *The Passenger* (1975). For additional unusual camera effects in mainstream films, see, e.g., Jeremy Vineyard, *Setting Up Your Shots: Great Camera Moves Every Filmmaker Should Know* (Studio City, Calif.: Michael Wiese Productions, 1999).

72. Raymond Durgnat, *A Long Hard Look at 'Psycho'* (London: British Film Institute, 2002), 235–36, n. 32 (original emphases). Durgnat emphasizes the role of a spectator's preconscious attention in watching a film. For Durgnat, this explains why rooms in *Psycho*, for example, take on different cinematic "shapes." See, e.g., 4–5, 124, 205, nn. 28, 38.

73. Rudolf Arnheim also makes stronger claims about the importance of gravity in the perception of forms. See *Art and Visual Perception: A Psychology of the Creative Eye* [The New Version] (Berkeley and Los Angeles: University of California Press, rev. ed. 1974), 23–24, 30–32, 101–03, 184–87. See also Arnheim, *The Dynamics of Architectural Form* (Berkeley and Los Angeles: University of California Press, 1977), chap. 2, 32–66; Irvin Rock, "The Perception of Disoriented Figures," *Scientific American* 230, 1 (July 1974): 78–85.

74. Another example: Because there is no "up" or "down" in outer space, astronomers are free to orient their images in a way that will produce a dramatic impact on the public. For instance, a digitally colored image of the Eagle Nebula may be presented as a thick and opaque, brownish mass at the bottom of an image, towering upward, becoming dark red as it rises (suggesting that it has come from a massive base), only to begin tapering off toward the center while becoming lighter with oranges, and then finally at the top bending over slightly, coming to a head outlined in glowing yellows that make space in the vicinity look transparent green and almost alive. The image has a very different appearance when rotated to another angle.

75. I have elaborated on the notion of the camera as viewing hypothesis in "The Spectator and Film Space — Two Theories," *Screen* 22, 1 (1981): 55–78; and in *Point of View in the Cinema*, 44, 53–54, 74, 179, 210.

76. On a type of literary point of view called "the camera," see, e.g., Norman Friedman, "Point of View in Fiction: The Development of a Critical Concept," *PMLA* 70, 5 (Dec. 1955): 1160–1184. On a type of verbal narration called "showing," see, e.g., Wayne C. Booth, "Distance and Point-of-View: An Essay in Classification," *Essays in Criticism* 11, 1 (Jan. 1961): 60–79; and *The Rhetoric of Fiction* (Chicago: University of Chicago Press, 2nd ed. 1983). See also Branigan, *Narrative Comprehension and Film*, sect. "A Synthesis: Telling/Showing/Summary/Scene," 146–49. For summaries of Friedman's and Booth's theories of literary point of view, see figures 2.1 and 2.2 in chapter 2 above.

77. Metz, "The Imaginary Signifier," 51.

CHAPTER 4: HOW FRAME LINES (AND FILM THEORY) FIGURE

I wish to thank Henry Bacon, Warren Buckland, John Kurten, Melinda Szaloky, and Charles Wolfe for their perceptive comments. This chapter is nearly four times the length of an earlier version that appeared in *Film Style and Story: A Tribute to Torben Grodal*, ed. Lennard Højbjerg and Peter Schepelern (Copenhagen: Museum Tusculanum Press, University of Copenhagen, 2003), 59–86. Preliminary accounts of some of the ideas in this chapter may be found in "*Quand* y a-t-il caméra?" *Champs Visuels: Revue interdisciplinaire de recherchessur l'image* 12–13 (Paris: L'Harmattan, January 1999), 18–32 (special issue edited by Guillaume Soulez on "Penser, cadrer: le *projet* du cadre") and in "How Frame Lines Figure," a paper presented at the Society for Cinema Studies conference, May 2002.

1. *Wittgenstein's Lectures, Cambridge, 1932–1935: From the Notes of Alice Ambrose and Margaret Macdonald*, ed. Alice Ambrose (Amherst, New York: Prometheus Books, 2001), Part I, § 29 (original emphasis). See also Part I, § 28, and Part II (The Yellow Book), §§ 2–3 (on the complicated grammar of such words as "good," "game," "kind," "concrete," "abstract," "mind," "thought," "soul," and "God"). Relevant also to the grammar of "good" is Wittgenstein's statement that "Ethics and aesthetics are one." O.K. Bouwsma, *Wittgenstein: Conversations*, 1949–1951, ed. J.L. Craft and Ronald E. Hustwit (Indianapolis: Hackett, 1986), 68; see also 40–42. Part of the problem, Wittgenstein says, is that we tend to "think of anything we mention as falling under one genus only; and we look on the qualities of things as comparable to the ingredients of a mixture." (§ 2) These issues are extensively discussed in Ludwig Wittgenstein, *Philosophical Investigations*, trans. G.E.M. Anscombe (1953; repr., Oxford: Blackwell, 3rd ed. 1967). The search for the "ingredients" of a thing is reminiscent of the method of 'vertical dissection' as opposed to 'horizontal intersection' discussed in chapter 1 above. For more on the analysis of "ingredients," see Ted Cohen, "The Philosophy of Taste: Thoughts on the Idea," in *The Blackwell Guide to Aesthetics*, ed. Peter Kivy (Oxford: Blackwell Publishing, 2004), 167–73.

One might also say that the word "good" acquires its meaning relative to a specific purpose or practical context, which is a larger theme in Wittgenstein's work on language. He says that when "you look for definitions corresponding to our concepts in aesthetics or ethics," you should "[i]n such a difficulty always ask yourself: How did we learn the meaning of this word ('good' for instance)? From what sort of examples? in what language-games? Then it will be easier for you to see that the word must have a family of meanings." *Philosophical Investigations*, § 77 (original emphasis). See also Wittgenstein's discussion of our "craving for generality" in *The Blue and Brown Books: Preliminary Studies for the "Philosophical Investigations"* (New York: Harper & Row, 2nd ed. 1960), 17–20.

O.K. Bouwsma provides a fine account of Wittgenstein's way of thinking about language in "The Blue Book" and brilliantly applies this way of thinking to untangle part of a sentence from Descartes's philosophy to reveal murky thought in "'On Many Occasions I Have in Sleep Been Deceived'"; both essays are in Bouwsma's *Philosophical Essays* (Lincoln: University of Nebraska Press, 1965). Note that film is sometimes compared to dream and illusion, as if to say, 'On many occasions I have in watching film been deceived.' I argue in this book that film theorists often pay insufficient attention to the language they deploy when making their claims (as in 'film is an illusion') and routinely ignore dangers uncovered byWittgenstein and Bouwsma.

2. James Elkins, *Visual Studies: A Skeptical Introduction* (New York: Routledge, 2003), 112 (footnote omitted). See also Elkins, "Preface to the Book *A Skeptical Introduction to Visual Culture*," *Journal of Visual Culture* 1, 1 (April 2002), 96; and 94–95.

3. David Bordwell, "The Art Cinema as a Mode of Film Practice," *Film Criticism* 4, 1 (Fall 1979), 60 (original emphases).

4. A worthy effort to overcome such distinctions as story/discourse and content/form in theorizing narrative may be found in David A. Black, "*Homo Confabulans*: A Study in Film, Narrative, and Compensation," *Literature and Psychology* 47, 3 (2001), 25–37. See also Black, *Law in Film: Resonance and Representation* (Urbana: University of Illinois Press, 1999).

5. F. Elizabeth Hart, "The Epistemology of Cognitive Literary Studies," *Philosophy and Literature* 25, 2 (October 2001), esp. 319–25. Mark Johnson makes a compelling argument for a middle-ground position between "Objectivism" or "foundationalism" and "relativism" in *The Body in the Mind: The Bodily Basis of Meaning, Imagination, and Reason* (Chicago: University of Chicago Press, 1987), 194–212. See generally, Norman N. Holland, "Where Is a Text? A Neurological View," *New Literary History* 33, 1 (Winter 2002), 21–38; Paul Hernadi, "Why Is Literature: A Coevolutionary Perspective on Imaginative Worldmaking," *Poetics Today* 23, 1 (Spring 2002), 21–42 (special issue on "Literature and the Cognitive Revolution"); Hernadi, *Cultural Transactions: Nature, Self, Society* (Ithaca, N.Y.: Cornell University Press, 1995); and, Richard A. Richards, who builds on an analogy with evolutionary fitness to examine aesthetic evaluations, "A Fitness Model of Evaluation," *The Journal of Aesthetics and Art Criticism* 62, 3 (Summer 2004), 263–75.

Richard Rorty offers another approach but states the problem in the same way as do Hart and Johnson:

Antirepresentationalists need to insist that "determinacy" is not what is in question — that neither does thought determine reality nor, in the sense intended by the realist, does reality determine thought. More precisely, it is no truer that "atoms are what they are because we use 'atom' as we do" than that "we use 'atom' as we do because atoms are as they are." *Both* of these claims, the antirepresentation[a]list says, are entirely empty. Both are pseudo-explanations.

Rorty, "Introduction: Antirepresentationalism, Ethnocentrism, and Liberalism," in *Objectivity, Relativism, and Truth: Philosophical Papers, Vol. I* (Cambridge: Cambridge University Press, 1991), 5 (original emphasis); see also p. 7.

6. On "ecological conventionalism," see Torben Grodal, *Moving Pictures: A New Theory of Film Genres, Feelings, and Cognition* (Oxford: Oxford University Press, 1997), index entry, 299; cf. "psychomimetic" representations of time, 139, 145. See also David Bordwell's middle-ground position between "sheer naturalism" and "radical conventionalism," which he terms a "moderate constructivism" based on "contingent cultural universals"; "Convention, Construction, and Cinematic Vision" in *Post-Theory: Reconstructing Film Studies*, ed. David Bordwell and Noël Carroll (Madison: University of Wisconsin Press, 1996), 87–107. Bordwell replies to criticism of "moderate constructivism" rather decisively in *Figures Traced in Light: On Cinematic Staging* (Berkeley and Los Angeles: University of California Press, 2005), 38–39, 258–265. See generally Steven Pinker, *The Blank Slate: The Modern Denial of Human Nature* (New York: Viking Penguin, 2002), Appendix, "Donald E. Brown's List of Human Universals," 435–439.

   For two recent and sophisticated appraisals of cognitive film theory, see Carl Plantinga, "Cognitive Film Theory: An Insider's Appraisal," pp. 15–37, in the special issue on "cinema and cognition" of *CiNéMAS* 12, 2 (Winter 2002); and Laurent Jullier, *Cinéma et cognition* (Paris: L'Harmattan, 2002). See also David Bordwell, "A Case for Cognitivism," *Iris* 9 (Spring 1989), 11–40 (special issue on "Cinema and Cognitive Psychology"); and Bordwell, "A Case for Cognitivism: Further Reflections," *Iris* 11 (Summer 1990), 107–112.

7. Torben Grodal, "The Experience of Realism in Audiovisual Representation," in Northern Lights Film and Media Studies Yearbook 2002, *Realism and "Reality" in Film and Media*, ed. Anne Jerslev (Copenhagen: Museum Tusculanum Press, University of Copenhagen, 2002), 67–68. Roughly speaking, the eleven types of realism identified by Grodal are as follows: perceptual, emotional, magic, poetic, psychological, social, categorical/cognitive, Dogme 95, extreme, imperfect perceptual, and postmodern reflexive.

8. Grodal, *Moving Pictures*, 209–10; and see index entry on "frame," 300. The five main cognitive processes of framing that are discussed by Grodal are as follows: picture-frame as container; window/camera as both mask and

source of vision; focus of attention; frame-system for organizing hypotheses; and emotional filter.

9. See, e.g., Ellen Spolsky, "Darwin and Derrida: Cognitive Literary Theory as a Species of Post-Structuralism," *Poetics Today* 23, 1 (Spring 2002), 43–62. Spolsky asserts,

> Since the study of just about everything is conducted in words, these inherent instabilities or ambiguities [in language], previously described as "literary" phenomena parasitic on "normal" language . . ., [are] now understood as a general condition of language use, including language used to conduct scholarly debate. (50)

Bryan Vescio goes even further by arguing that there is no important distinction between image and word, perceiving and reading; "Reading in the Dark: Cognitivism, Film Theory, and Radical Interpretation," *Style* 35, 4 (Winter 2001), 572–91.

10. Two approaches to the question of why we watch films may be found in Noël Carroll's "The Power of Movies," in *Theorizing the Moving Image* (Cambridge: Cambridge University Press, 1996), 78–93, and in Christian Metz's "The Imaginary Signifier" [orig. 1975], in *The Imaginary Signifier: Psychoanalysis and the Cinema*, trans. Celia Britton, Annwyl Williams, Ben Brewster and Alfred Guzzetti (Bloomington: Indiana University Press, 1982), sects. "'Going to the Cinema,'" "'Talking about the Cinema,'" and "'Seeing a Film,'" 6–13, 56–57. Consider a comment by Stanley Cavell:

> Film studies has recently declared itself in need of reconception, and I hope part of this reconception will take the form of a wish to understand how it got to its present form. Part of seeking that understanding, were I to attempt to trace it, would be to follow out my impression that the wholesale attack of film studies upon a large portion of its subject was driven by a moralism as intense as Plato's obsession with poetry. I cannot avoid the feeling that a fear of the power of film remains insufficiently analyzed.

Cities of Words: Pedagogical Letters on a Register of the Moral Life (Cambridge, Mass.: Harvard University Press, 2004), 319.

11. See generally, David Bordwell, *Making Meaning: Inference and Rhetoric in the Interpretation of Cinema* (Cambridge, Mass.: Harvard University Press, 1989), and James Elkins, *Our Beautiful, Dry, and Distant Texts: Art History as Writing* (New York: Routledge, 2000).

12. On the advantages of ambiguity in film theory, see Edward Branigan, "To Zero and Beyond: Noël Burch's *Theory of Film Practice*," in *Defining Cinema*, ed. Peter Lehman (New Brunswick, N.J.: Rutgers University Press, 1997), 149–68. In this essay on Burch's theory, I trace out a sequence of radial meanings of the concepts "zero" and "clumps of fuzziness" in an image. I will return to the problem of ambiguity in film theory in the last four sections of this chapter.

13. In this book I will concentrate on the "frame" as it is used in critical discourse in film studies. For works that consider the "frame" in painting, see, e.g., *The Rhetoric of the Frame: Essays on the Boundaries of the Artwork*, ed. Paul Duro (Cambridge: Cambridge University Press, 1996); Jacques Derrida, *The Truth in Painting*, trans. Geoff Bennington and Ian McLeod (Chicago: University of Chicago Press, 1987); and Barbara E. Savedoff, "Frames," *The Journal of Aesthetics and Art Criticism* 57, 3 (Summer 1999), 345–56.

14. I am setting aside the considerable, and still unresolved, theoretical difficulties that arise in attempting to make distinctions among homonymy, polysemy, vagueness, scope ambiguity, and univocality. See, e.g., Michael V. Antony, "Is 'Consciousness' Ambiguous?," *Journal of Consciousness Studies* 8, 2 (February 2001), 19–44.

15. See esp. George Lakoff, *Women, Fire, and Dangerous Things: What Categories Reveal about the Mind* (Chicago: University of Chicago Press, 1987), chap. 6, "Radial Categories," 91–114, and 146–47, 290, 346–48, 537–40, passim. For a summary of Lakoff's approach, see 153–54, 334–37. See also George Lakoff and Mark Johnson, *Metaphors We Live By* (Chicago: University of Chicago Press, 1980), chap. 18, "Some Consequences for Theories of Conceptual Structure," 106–114. For Wittgenstein, see the epigraph. Jeffrey T. Dean applies Lakoff's methods to argue that the word "Art" is radial in meaning; "The Nature of Concepts and the Definition of Art," *The Journal of Aesthetics and Art Criticism* 61, 1 (Winter 2003), 29–35. A contrary view is offered by Thomas Adajian, who presumes that metaphysical conditions will be discovered to ground radical categories as well as, presumably, those messy language-games; "On the Prototype Theory of Concepts and the Definition of Art," *The Journal of Aesthetics and Art Criticism* 63, 3 (Summer 2005), 231–36. In the same journal issue, Amie L. Thomasson offers support for Dean from another direction, "The Ontology of Art and Knowledge in Aesthetics," 221–29. See generally the special issue on "Art, Mind, and Cognitive Science," *The Journal of Aesthetics and Art Criticism* 62, 2 (Spring 2004).

16. I offer the following analogy for the "motivated conventions" (Lakoff) underlying radial meaning. Imagine a painter who fills a brush with paint

and snaps it at a canvas. The painter can expect a certain (core) splat to appear in a certain place and even expect certain (radial) streaks to appear, but he or she cannot predict the entire distribution of the pattern and where gaps will be. The overall pattern is neither arbitrary nor fully determined, nor does the pattern grow logically or organically like a tree and its branches. The "lumpiness" of the pattern cannot be explained by its intrinsic properties but only in reference to several kinds of causation, i.e., only in relation to larger patterns that — especially in the case of radial meaning — are adaptive, contingent, ecological, and perhaps unpredictable.

17. See Johnson, *The Body in the Mind*, "Preface," ix–xvi. The seven challenges to Objectivism discussed in Johnson's book are categorization, the framing of concepts, metaphor, polysemy, historical semantic change, non-Western conceptual systems, and the growth of knowledge.

18. Real edges on the screen have real effects. Consider such optical effects as the split screen and wipe; the vertical "blend lines" and horizontal synchronization that is required moment-by-moment for the three images projected in Cinerama; and the need for double interlock projection and precise registration in non-anaglyphic 3-D films. Not far away is the physicality of the "jump cut," because the "jump" onscreen becomes salient only when we believe that it interrupts *a single shot* as opposed to, say, the fragmentation of a montage sequence.

19. On the frame as a line that produces edge contrast, see Jacques Aumont, *The Image*, trans. Claire Pajackowska (London: British Film Institute, 1997), 14–16, 40–44; on framing, 106–18. In chapter 2, I defined four varieties of active and passive follow shots. In effect, *motion* on the screen (in the background or else in the foreground) is being used to continuously frame a character or object that is held steady for our contemplation. The disjunction between motion and immobility marks the "line" of this kind of "frame."

20. On composition and film framing, see generally, David Bordwell and Kristin Thompson, *Film Art: An Introduction* (New York: McGraw-Hill, 7th ed. 2004), chap. 7, "The Shot: Cinematography," 229–93. Many clever examples of framing inside a composition can be found in Jean Cocteau's *Beauty and the Beast* (1946) and Rainer Werner Fassbinder's *Veronika Voss* (1982). For relentless mirror imagery, see Fassbinder's *Effi Briest* (1974). I discuss some theoretical issues of composition in *Narrative Comprehension and Film* (New York and London: Routledge, 1992), chap. 2, "Story World and Screen," sect. "Screen Space and Stylistic Metaphors," 56–62 (on Hitchcock's *The 39 Steps*).

 A few interesting books on the principles of composition: Arthur Wesley Dow, *Composition: A Series of Exercises in Art Structure for the Use of Students and Teachers* (Berkeley and Los Angeles: University of California

Press, 13th ed. 1997; orig. 1899); Victor Oscar Freeburg, *Pictorial Beauty on the Screen* (1923; repr., New York: Arno Press, 1970); Vladimir Nilsen, *The Cinema as a Graphic Art (On a Theory of Representation in the Cinema)*, trans. Stephen Garry (1937; repr., New York: Hill and Wang, 1959) (reprinted by Garland Publishing, New York, 1985); Gyorgy Kepes, *Language of Vision* (Chicago: Paul Theobald, 1944); Rudolf Arnheim, *Art and Visual Perception: A Psychology of the Creative Eye — The New Version* (Berkeley and Los Angeles: University of California Press, rev. ed. 1974); Rudolf Arnheim, *The Power of the Center: A Study of Composition in the Visual Arts — The New Version* (Berkeley and Los Angeles: University of California Press, 1988), and see chap. 4, "Limits and Frames," 51–71; Maureen Turim, "Symmetry/ Asymmetry and Visual Fascination," *Wide Angle* 4, n. 3 (1980), 38–47.

21. Sergei Eisenstein argues that in certain situations "colour veils its self-asserting power and acts as a frame which, in the interests of the close-up, excludes all that is not essential, all that, given in a long shot, might draw our attention away from the object presented in the close-up." "Colour Film," in *Movies and Methods: An Anthology* [vol. I], ed. Bill Nichols (Berkeley and Los Angeles: University of California Press, 1976), 384.

22. On walking as the core metaphor, see Giuliana Bruno, "Collection and Recollection: On Film Itineraries and Museum Walks" in *Camera Obscura, Camera Lucida: Essays in Honor of Annette Michelson*, ed. by Richard Allen and Malcolm Turvey (Amsterdam: Amsterdam University Press, 2003), 231–60. On metaphors involving film framing and the *flâneur*, see, e.g., Siegfried Kracauer, *Theory of Film: The Redemption of Physical Reality* (with an introduction by Miriam Bratu Hansen) (1960; repr., Princeton, N.J.: Princeton University Press, 1997), 72–73, 17071; cf. 52; Walter Benjamin, *The Arcades Project*, trans. Howard Eiland and Kevin McLaughlin (Cambridge, Mass.: Harvard University Press, 1999), 83, 416–55; and *Cinema and the Invention of Modern Life*, ed. Leo Charney and Vanessa R. Schwartz (Berkeley and Los Angeles: University of California Press, 1995), "Introduction," 5–6. On metaphors involving film framing and the train window, see Lynne Kirby, *Parallel Tracks: The Railroad and Silent Cinema* (Durham, N.C.: Duke University Press, 1996). On metaphors for film framing derived from trains and amusement park rides, see, e.g., Peter Wollen, "*Rope*: Three Hypotheses," in *Alfred Hitchcock: Centenary Essays*, ed. Richard Allen and S. Ishii-Gonzalès (London: British Film Institute, 1999), esp. sect. "Mobility and Claustrophobia," 81–83.

23. On the three standard metaphors of "window," "window frame," and "mirror," see, e.g., Dudley Andrew, *Concepts in Film Theory* (Oxford: Oxford University Press, 1984), 134–35, and Vivian Sobchack, *The Address of the Eye: A Phenomenology of Film Experience* (Princeton, N.J.: Princeton

University Press, 1992), 14–20. One might wonder about the status of film sound in these standard metaphors: Is it unheard, muffled, secondary, incidental? Also, "mirror" imagery may be taken as a "second-degree" window where "reflective" becomes "reflexive"; cf. the notion of a camera as a "channel for communication" in chapter 3 above. The "window" metaphor is obviously a deeply rooted metaphor because it purports to represent what it means simply "to see" (i.e., normally the glass is transparent). I will defer a detailed analysis of the "window" to later sections of this chapter on "A Role for the Body — The Container Schema" and "Color as Container."

Sobchack avoids the standard metaphors while still using everyday, embodied perception to create a radically new conception of the frame and the activity of framing. She denies the usual distinction between animate and inanimate and argues that film itself is a conscious and experiencing entity, not merely an inanimate thing that is subject to anthropomorphism. "Along with its objective existence for us as its spectators, a film possesses its own being. That is, it *has being* in the sense that it *behaves*." (61, original emphases) The result is that the frame acquires a special role: "The frame provides the *synoptic center* of the *film's experience* of the world it sees; it functions for the film as the field of our bodies does for us." (134, my emphasis of the second pair of words; see also 131, 135, 211)

It should be noted that the window metaphor is so pervasive in our thinking that it applies to language generally. In analyzing this metaphor, O. K. Bouwsma says, "The sentence is the window. And the meaning is on the other side of the window." He elaborates,

> A sentence is like a window through which one sees the meaning, and a good sentence is like a window through which one sees without seeing it. This is, of course, only a part of a much worn extensive figure involving light and darkness and distinctions involved in seeing.

What is important in Bouwsma's remark is the idea that a visual metaphor such as a window has not been designed to explain film but is used to facilitate (frame) our thinking generally about knowledge and belief. Bouwsma goes on to point out the severe limitations of the window metaphor. This could suggest a degree of caution in supposing that there is a necessary or natural link between the visibility of film and a metaphor for visibility such as "window." "What Is Meaning?" in *Toward a New Sensibility: Essays of O. K. Bouwsma*, ed. J. L. Craft and Ronald E. Hustwit (Lincoln: University of Nebraska Press, 1982), 40, 39. Cf. the aesthetic principle of "unobtrusiveness" discussed in connection with "profilmic" and "postfilmic" theories of a camera in chapter 3 above.

24. Wittgenstein's entire statement is as follows:

> To observe is not the same thing as to look at or to view.
>
> "Look at this colour and say what it reminds you of." If the colour changes you are no longer looking at the one I meant.
>
> One observes in order to see what one would not see if one did not observe.

Remarks on Colour, ed. G.E.M. Anscombe, trans. Linda L. McAlister and Margarete Schättle (Berkeley and Los Angeles: University of California Press, 1977), Part III, § 326. In the text above I have used the word "inspection" to characterize the fourth variation of a standard metaphor for framing (involving a viewer in front of a window) in order to suggest that for Kracauer, Benjamin, and Freud the observing depends on a 'specialized way' of observing that goes beyond mere looking or viewing, yet it is tied to the objective world (and to the image as an objectification of the world) and therefore is less than a free association or individual 'memory.' On 'excess' and 'aura,' see note 26 below.

25. Kracauer, *Theory of Film*, 52–57. See also the special issue on Kracauer, *New German Critique* 54 (Fall 1991) and Gertrud Koch, *Siegfried Kracauer: An Introduction*, trans. Jeremy Gaines (Princeton, N.J.: Princeton University Press, 2000). Noël Carroll is unsympathetic in "Kracauer's *Theory of Film*," *Defining Cinema*, 111–31.

26. Sigmund Freud, *The Psychopathology of Everyday Life*, trans. Alan Tyson, ed. James Strachey (New York: W.W. Norton & Co., 1965). Benjamin, "The Work of Art in the Age of Mechanical Reproduction" [orig. 1936], from *Illuminations*, ed. Hannah Arendt, trans. Harry Zohn (New York: Schocken, 1969), sect. 13, 235–37. See generally, Rosalind E. Krauss, *The Optical Unconscious* (Cambridge, Mass.: MIT Press, 1993), 178–80. The one-way glass analogy for inspecting everyday life remains the same when the glass is removed and the frame shrunk and changed into the shape of a keyhole allowing the observer to remain hidden (e.g., in the viewing of the "primal scene" and certain other phantasies described by Freud). Note that the one-way glass/keyhole analogy does *not* provide the foundation for a general psychoanalytic approach to framing in film (for which see definition 14 in the text above). One-way glass, for example, would not allow "transference" nor protect the analyst from "countertransference," and there are many aspects of therapy that do not depend on observing a patient during "everyday life." Benjamin, too, distinguishes between an unconscious that is "optical" — introduced by the camera — and one that is characterized by fluctuating "moods" and "impulses," invisible drives and instincts — introduced by psychoanalysis.

One step beyond the ideas of Kracauer and Benjamin/Freud is perhaps Barthes's idea of a photographic and filmic "excess," which is a detail that becomes 'paradoxical,' 'odd,' and "indescribable," due to a spectator's intense scrutiny of an image. Barthes's notion of "excess" retains a link to the definition of the frame as a window because of its grounding in the still image or shot. If this grounding, however, were loosened, then the notion of excess would shift more toward the frame as a psychic state (i.e., toward the specific psychic state that causes the 'intense scrutiny' of the image; see definition 14 in the text above). At the same time, the status of "things normally unseen" in the image (Kracauer; definition 8 [iv]) would shift toward abstract things — 'things seen in an image as if it were a Rorschach-like inkblot.' It is also possible that if the grounding for the notion of excess were loosened, then excess could shift in the other direction (downstream) toward the frame as a *material* aspect of the film medium, or as a *sensation*, out of which narrative meaning is made (i.e., "excess" would reveal some object or thing *in itself* prior to its assigned meaning in a rhetorical context; see, for example, definition 4). A special case of "excess," perhaps, is Benjamin's notion of the "aura" of an artwork. "Aura" seems to have both a physical aspect (as definition 1) and a dependence on historical context (as definition 15). See generally, Kristin Thompson, "The Concept of Cinematic Excess," in *Narrative, Apparatus, Ideology: A Film Theory Reader*, ed. Philip Rosen (New York: Columbia University Press, 1986), 130–42; James Elkins, *On Pictures and the Words That Fail Them* (Cambridge: Cambridge University Press, 1998). See also Roland Barthes, "The Third Meaning: Research Notes on Some Eisenstein Stills," in *Image, Music, Text*, trans. Stephen Heath (New York: Hill and Wang, 1977), 52–68, 61, 64, 65, 68, as well as his notion of the *punctum* in *Camera Lucida: Reflections on Photography*, trans. Richard Howard (New York: Hill and Wang, 1981).

Dudley Andrew weaves together several notions of framing to produce a remarkable, holistic analysis of a text's use of excess or "surplus." He ultimately links "surplus" to a spectator's feeling of awe (of the awesome, of the "eerie, unpredictable power of the frame," of the sublime) that is generated only by the greatest of artworks (58). For Andrew, a fundamental "opposition between framing and being framed" becomes evident in the effort both to make a film and to watch it (55). See "The Turn and Return of *Sunrise*," from *Film in the Aura of Art* (Princeton, N.J.: Princeton University Press, 1984), 28–58. More recently, Andrew has drawn on Deleuze to propose that the frame is a "mesh screen" (as on a window?) that *filters* the world with wider or narrower meshwork (28). Andrew agrees with Žižek, who

> imagines the screen to be part of a three-dimensional model where the gap [in the mesh screen] affords a glimpse of what lies beyond the

screen, what allows the substance of another layer to leak or pour into the screen from beyond, or what lures us to move beyond the apparent narrative problem to reformulate it in another dimension. Žižek believes (and I with him) that this process by which the spectator finds the screen suddenly raised to a higher dimension occurs in every film we are apt to care deeply about. (31; cf. 32)

Andrew says that things in the world "can suddenly bubble into and color the frame" or "leak or pour into the screen from beyond" (31). I begin to analyze such metaphors in a section of the present chapter below, "Color as Container," where the "mesh screen" appears in the form of a 'color filter.' Note that the idea of a "mesh screen," or 'color filter,' is especially important if one wishes to emphasize (as does Andrew) the *continuity*, or continuous transition, between two frames, such as the purported continuity between what is framed by a profilmic camera and what appears framed on the screen. Andrew is able to speak of "a higher dimension" in our response to film because he allows a more expansive definition of the frame to intrude (i.e., he envisions the appearance of still another kind of frame): "Let us consider the screen as a metaphor for metaphor, that is, as a site of transit where one space takes us into another space." (25) Andrew, "The Frame-Mobile and the Age of Cinema," in *Limina/le soglie del film — Film's Thresholds, X International Film Studies Conference*, ed. by Veronica Innocenti and Valentina Re (Italy: University of Udine, 2004). If, on the other hand, one wishes to emphasize a discontinuity or distortion between two frames (e.g., what is framed by a profilmic camera and what appears framed on the screen), one might summon the analogy of a design that has been drawn or scratched on the window through which one looks. Moreover, one may be completely unaware of the design. What sort of "design" could this be? One possibility would be an embodied or "submerged" analogy that exists in a 'language-game' — a game we presume while watching. Another possibility would be to emphasize the importance of mental schemata and heuristics while watching. See Bouwsma, "'On Many Occasions I Have in Sleep Been Deceived,'" 161–162.

Lying beneath the concept of excess and Andrew's higher 'other dimensions' may well be the vexed issue of cinephilia. See esp. Metz, "The Imaginary Signifier," sects. "'Loving the Cinema'" and "'Theorise,' he says ... (Provisional Conclusion)," 14–16, 79–80; and Paul Willemen, "*Photogénie* and Epstein" and "Through the Glass Darkly: Cinephilia Reconsidered," in *Looks and Frictions: Essays in Cultural Studies and Film Theory* (Bloomington: Indiana University Press, 1994), pp. 124–33, 223–57. In thinking about the feelings associated with cinephilia, which are most intense at certain moments of a film (moments of close inspection that create "excess" or "surplus"), one might also consider recent theories of the emotions; see *Passionate Views: Film, Cognition, and Emotion*, ed. Carl Plantinga and Greg M. Smith (Baltimore: Johns Hopkins University Press, 1999). Notice in the text that I discuss the "frame" mainly in perceptual and cognitive terms, and leave implicit or unexamined how emotions (body preferences, action tendencies) might "frame" or "reframe" what we see.

27. *S. M. Eisenstein: Selected Works, Vol. I Writings, 1922–34*, ed. and trans. Richard Taylor (London: BFI Publishing; Bloomington and Indianapolis: Indiana University Press, 1988), "The Dramaturgy of Film Form (The Dialectical Approach to Film Form)" [orig. 1929], 164; Sergei Eisenstein, "A Dialectic Approach to Film Form," in *Film Form: Essays in Film Theory*, ed. and trans. Jay Leyda (New York: Harcourt, Brace & World, 1949), 49. Though Eisenstein does not mention the stereoscope, he does draw a parallel between images in dialectical collision and stereoscopy. See also *S. M. Eisenstein: Selected Works, Vol. II, Towards a Theory of Montage*, ed. and trans. Michael Glenny and Richard Taylor (London: BFI Publishing, 1991), "Vertical Montage" [orig. 1940], 332, 392–93, translated as "Synchronization of Senses" and "Form and Content: Practice" in Sergei M. Eisenstein, *The Film Sense*, ed. and trans. Jay Leyda (New York: Harcourt, Brace & World, 1942), 78–80, 201–05. Another way of displacing the ocular perspective in film theory may be found in the intuitive aesthetics of Kant; see Melinda Szaloky, "Making New Sense of Film Theory through Kant: A Novel Teaching Approach," *New Review of Film and Television Studies* 3, 1 (May 2005), pp. 33–58.

28. Gerald Mast, "On Framing," *Critical Inquiry* 11, 1 (September 1984): 109. Note that Mast's comparison of the cinema frame to the "fun house mirror" merges two rationales for seeing an image, namely, the 'view from an amusement park ride' and the 'window as a mirror.' See the preceding discussion of the word "frame" (definition 8) in the text above. I will analyze Mast's example in more detail in the next chapter.

29. Jean Mitry, *The Aesthetics and Psychology of the Cinema*, trans. Christopher King (1963; repr., Bloomington: Indiana University Press, 1997), 190.

30. André Bazin's notion of a distinctive mobile framing that creates a "lateral depth of field" may rest upon a real-world analogy: Just as an object in the world conceals what is behind it, so a static framing in film conceals what lies at a distance laterally from the sides of an object. Certain points of view are denied the spectator, and limits are placed on attention. To this analogy Bazin, in effect, adds the imperative that film art must discover the 'telling details' hidden in the world behind and to the sides of an object, hence causing the need for a special kind of mobile framing that reveals the world

through its shifts. Ideally, a camera through its movements will act for the spectator. Put another way, one could say that for Bazin *narrative* exposition should emerge from a mobile framing that is not omniscient, but merely inquisitive, and that seeks to disclose the mysterious relations among concrete objects in the way that a spectator might naturally discover the qualities of a locale, including the discovery of what he or she cannot know. Bazin does not advocate a framing that instantly reveals all and only the important details. See also Bazin's famous contrast between the theater's self-sufficient and brilliant "crystal chandelier" that "holds us prisoners" and the cinema's "little flashlight of the usher, moving like an uncertain comet across the night of our waking dream, the diffuse space without shape or frontiers that surrounds the screen." "Theater and Cinema: Part Two" [orig. 1951], in *What Is Cinema?* [vol. I], trans. Hugh Gray (Berkeley and Los Angeles: University of California Press, 1967), 107; and see "Painting and Cinema" [n.d. for orig.], 165–66. On "lateral depth of field," see Bazin, *Jean Renoir*, trans. W. W. Halsey II and William H. Simon (New York: Simon & Schuster, 1973; orig. unpub. ms. 1958), chap. 5, "The French Renoir," 86–91. Bazin's concept of "lateral depth of field" is discussed in the preceding chapter in note 34. Cf. Kracauer, *Theory of Film*, "Affinities," 18–20 (i.e., the inherent affinities of photography with reality); see also 37–39, 60–74. For a detailed treatment of the properties of narrative and style that influenced Bazin's notion of "lateral depth of field," see Alexander Sesonske, *Jean Renoir: The French Films, 1924–1939* (Cambridge, Mass.: Harvard University Press, 1980).

31. See, e.g., *Eisenstein: Selected Works, Vol. I*, "Beyond the Shot" [orig. 1929], 146–48. In a different translation of this passage, framing is described as "Hewing out a piece of actuality with the ax of the lens." Eisenstein, *Film Form*, "The Cinematographic Principle and the Ideogram," 41; Noël Burch, *Theory of Film Practice*, trans. Helen R. Lane (1969; repr., Princeton, N.J.: Princeton University Press, 1981). See also Rudolf Arnheim, *Film as Art* (Berkeley and Los Angeles: University of California Press, 1957), "Selections Adapted from *Film*" [orig. 1933], sect. 1 "Film and Reality," subsect. "Delimitation of the Image and Distance from the Object," 16–20, and esp. "Artistic Use of the Delimitation of the Picture and of the Distance from the Object," 73–87. Arnheim asserts that "[t]he limitations of the picture are felt immediately. The pictured space is visible to a certain extent, but then comes the edge which cuts off what lies beyond. It is a mistake to deplore this restriction as a drawback. I shall show later that on the contrary it is just such restrictions which give film its right to be called an art." (17) Early film theorists usually discussed the topic of "framing" in terms of the "close-up" shot.

32. Consider, for example, the difficult subjectivities produced by such art cinema directors as Chantal Akerman, Michelangelo Antonioni, Ingmar

Bergman, Bernardo Bertolucci, Robert Bresson, Luis Buñuel, Atom Egoyan, Rainer Werner Fassbinder, Federico Fellini, Peter Greenaway, Werner Herzog, Shohei Imamura, Krzysztof Kieślowski, Emir Kusturica, David Lynch, Dusan Makavejev, Chris Marker, Nagisa Oshima, Pier Paolo Pasolini, Yvonne Rainer, Alain Resnais, Jacques Rivette, Raúl Ruiz, Andrei Tarkovsky, Béla Tarr, François Truffaut, Lars von Trier, and Wong Kar-Wai.

33. See Bordwell's "The Art Cinema," 56–64, and his *Narration in the Fiction Film* (Madison: University of Wisconsin Press, 1985), chap. 10, "Art-Cinema Narration," 205–33. Cf. Gilles Deleuze, *Cinema 2: The Time-Image*, trans. Hugh Tomlinson and Robert Galeta (Minneapolis: University of Minnesota Press, 1989), 8. See generally Roy Armes, *The Ambiguous Image: Narrative Style in Modern European Cinema* (Bloomington: Indiana University Press, 1976). I analyze a spectrum of possibilities that lie between a character's point-of-view shot and a shot that represents no character's point of view in *Narrative Comprehension and Film*, chap. 6, "Objectivity and Uncertainty," 161–91.

34. See Torben Grodal, "Art Film, the Transient Body, and the Permanent Soul," *Aura* 6, 3 (2000): 33–53. Casper Tybjerg contrasts Grodal's approach with other interpretive strategies by applying them to Carl Dreyer's *Ordet* (1954); "The Sense of *The Word*," in *Film Style and Story: A Tribute to Torben Grodal*, ed. Lennard Højbjerg and Peter Schepelern (Copenhagen: Museum Tusculanum Press, University of Copenhagen, 2003), 171–213.

35. A metaphorical image need not be specially marked in a film (e.g., by making it a nondiegetic insert); a given image may be both literally and metaphorically true of an element in the plot. Thus, in general, the "framing" accomplished by a rhetorical figure is not so much *on* the screen as *within a pattern* of images or in a way of looking at what is on the screen. An interesting example of mobile framing used to evoke the rhetorical figure of prosopopoeia (which Comolli may be saying is intrinsic to film) is analyzed by Jean-Louis Comolli in "Mechanical Bodies, Ever More Heavenly," *October* 83 (Winter 1998), 23–24. Gilles Fauconnier and Mark Turner posit four basic types of "framing networks" (simplex, mirror, single-scope, and double-scope) akin to metaphorical thinking in *The Way We Think: Conceptual Blending and the Mind's Hidden Complexities* (New York: Basic Books, 2002), especially chapters 3 and 7.

36. On the dynamic interplay of onscreen and offscreen space, see Burch, *Theory of Film Practice*, chap. 2, "*Nana*, or the Two Kinds of Space," 17–31. Raymond Durgnat finds a general principle at work in a Hitchcock shot that starts with a character looking downward toward the camera and then turning away. The camera then tilts down, following the character's glance, to reveal a surprise: an envelope lying nearby stuffed with money.

In general principle, it's akin to the famous trope in *Stagecoach*, where the camera pulls back from the stage coach *far away down there* and reveals the Red Indians *back here* — waiting to attack . . . . In theorizing offscreen space, it's easy to overlook the fact that, even when the camera is "in" the scene, it's almost always *back from the* shot: the edge of the frame is varying distances from the camera, with an "apron" of hidden space between camera and picture.

A Long Hard Look at 'Psycho' (London: BFI Publishing, 2002), 232 n. 12 (original emphases and ellipsis points). In the remake of *Psycho* by Gus Van Sant in 1998, the character does not look toward the camera, so both the subsequent camera movement and the sight of the money are surprises. The surprises are motivated but not by a character. Here's another example of the interplay between onscreen and offscreen space. A scene in Godard's *Weekend* (1967) is done in a single shot, as follows.

> We fade in on many wrecked cars mysteriously burning alongside a road. The camera booms upward, stops, moves right, and finds two characters emerging out of the smoke walking on the road toward the camera. The camera follows the characters to the right as they are asking dead people lying on the pavement for directions. The camera stops; the characters exit right. The camera booms down, then moves back left to its starting point where it stops. The shot is held; nothing happens. Fade out.

The camera, by its geometric movements, has carefully traced a large rectangle as a "frame" for the scene. My description of the "framing" draws on both *gestalt form* (definition 3) and the notion of a *scene* (definition 11); different descriptions, of course, might have been constructed using other definitions of the "frame." With respect to the "scene" (definition 11), one may see the camera movement as being conventional in that it has three parts, a beginning, middle, and end. It establishes a locale, discovers and follows an action, and, when the action is lost, reestablishes the locale at the end. As is typical, a spectator is given time at the end of the scene to reflect on the significance of what has happened. Nonetheless, one has the feeling of a visual non sequitur (definition 10). Although the camera movement has created a perceptual whole (the gestalt rectangle and a closed action), it has apparently been unable to elucidate or hold together the "world" of *Weekend*: The world has been cut into parts (actions in a locale) that don't otherwise make a whole. The point is that a familiar segmentation no longer makes sense.

37. On the fascinating concept of a "retrospective match" along with its varieties, see Branigan, "To Zero and Beyond: Noël Burch's *Theory of Film Practice*,"

149–68, 157 n. 10. Cf. the linguistic notions of "scope ambiguity," "sylleptic ambiguity" (e.g., "*blue* moods and pictures," "*deep* rivers and thoughts"), and "frame-rejecting negation." On the latter, see Lakoff, *Women, Fire, and Dangerous Things*, pp. 21, 68, 116–17, 131–33, 331.

38. On narration as a form of 'searching,' see, e.g., Kenneth Johnson, "The Point of View of the Wandering Camera," *Cinema Journal* 32, 2 (Winter 1993): 49–56. See also David Bordwell, "Intensified Continuity: Visual Style in Contemporary American Film," *Film Quarterly* 55, 3 (Spring 2002): subsect. "A free-ranging camera," 20, and 24, 25. Vivian Sobchack states, "If the camera moves erratically in its interest or seems bored with its previous objects (following, for example, a wire up a wall or moving out a window when something more central to the narrative it has been expressing is happening elsewhere), we become aware of its *bodily*, perspectival difference from ourselves." Sobchack, "Toward Inhabited Space: The Semiotic Structure of Camera Movement in the Cinema," *Semiotica* 41, 1/4 (1982): 329–30 (my emphasis; footnote omitted). Both camera movements mentioned by Sobchack are from Antonioni's *The Passenger* (1975).

In effect, the 'wandering' of a wandering camera offers the spectator 'a shot within a shot.' That is, we may imagine that the camera presents a locale and details while at the same time — somehow *within* the shot — the camera also 'wanders' and seeks something else, a new or better 'shot,' as if it were unsatisfied with what was being shown. This formulation raises a deeper question: "What constitutes a 'shot'?" I am suggesting here that the meaning of "shot" is radial. In the present context (definition 13), "shot" is being defined in relation to the movement of narration (i.e., a wandering camera movement as it relates to other, more stable levels of narration). In other contexts, the concept of "shot" (and, thus, of "editing") will be quite different. In the context of definition 1, for example, the shot will be defined as a continuous run of the camera, and editing will be defined as "splicing celluloid." That is, for definition 1, editing will involve adjacent shots, whereas for definition 13, a group of narrational elements may be assembled within a single shot or in nonadjacent shots and still count as an effect of "editing."

39. I use the concept of "frame" as one of six general elements that define narration in *Point of View in the Cinema: A Theory of Narration and Subjectivity in Classical Film* (Berlin and New York: Mouton, 1984). The six elements are analogous to a generative case grammar (a slot and filler mental model) and are meant to account for important top-down effects in our comprehension of narrative. The approach is further refined in "'Here Is a Picture of No Revolver!': The Negation of Images and Methods for Analyzing the Structure of Pictorial Statements," *Wide Angle* 8, nos. 3–4 (1986), esp. 13–14. Jan Simons correctly notes that the term "frame" in *Point of View in the Cinema*

is "used rather ambiguously." Perhaps the same may also be said of the five other elements. The present chapter is meant to delve further into this issue of "ambiguity" while raising the general issue of how film theories frame. See Simons, "'Enunciation': From Code to Interpretation," in *The Film Spectator: From Sign to Mind*, ed. Warren Buckland (Amsterdam: Amsterdam University Press, 1995), 200–02. With respect to the definition in the text above of narration as a set of principles, cf. Nelson Goodman, *Ways of Worldmaking* (Indianapolis: Hackett Publishing Co., 1978), chap. 1, "Words, Works, Worlds," sect. 4, "Ways of Worldmaking," 7–17.

40. The ever-present restrictions of narration are made quite palpable in, for example, Abbas Kiarostami's *Through the Olive Trees* (1994). On some of the techniques employed by narration to mislead and lie, see, e.g., Roland Barthes, *S/Z*, trans. Richard Miller (New York: Hill and Wang, 1974). A self-conscious form of the "perfect" view is the so-called "impossible" camera position (e.g., a framing from within a refrigerator or fireplace, or from under a train). This type of narration is something like a view from inside the mind of an object, if objects had minds. It may also represent a clever aside to the audience that carries an overtone of detached irony, or even parody. Barthes argues that irony, in general, reaffirms, rather than disturbs, the classic narrative; *S/Z*, sect. 21, 59.

41. On the components of one common type of invisible observation, that of an "invisible observer," see Branigan, *Narrative Comprehension and Film*, 95–96, 164–72. In the text above I refer to the invisible observer as a "downstream" metaphor because the projection from 13 onto 8 or 9 is in the direction of basic-level and subordinate categorization, to be discussed later in this chapter. For more on invisible observation without an observer (what George M. Wilson calls "an unoccupied perspective"), see "*Le Grand Imagier* Steps Out: The Primitive Basis of Film Narration," *Philosophical Topics* 25, 1 (Spring 1997), 295–318. Notice that the 'frame' for Wilson's thinking about "perspective" must be superordinate (10–15) in order to be compatible with "unoccupied." See also Warren Buckland's discussion of invisible observation in "Orientation in Film Space: A Cognitive Semiotic Approach," *Recherches en communication* 19 (2003), pp. 87–102. Theories of suture, to be discussed later in this chapter, work to anchor an invisible observer (the Absent One) in definitions 14 or 15 as an "upstream" metaphor projected from definitions 1, 3, 5, 8, 9, or 13.

  The debate on these issues continues. Wilson (and others) are taken to task by Andrew Kania for introducing too many generalized fictional narrators, especially those offering a spectator or reader some form of 'invisible observation.' Kania believes that sometimes only the actual author is needed to explain 'invisible observation.' Hemingway, however, is not a good example of invisible observation "because somehow his prose retains a forceful personal style despite his complete narratorial self-effacement. . . . [Graham] Greene seems the ideal transparent stylist." But what is the grammar of the word "transparent"? I believe that the grammar used by Kania lies within the theories of framing outlined in definitions 8 and 9. Kania, "Against the Ubiquity of Fictional Narrators," *The Journal of Aesthetics and Art Criticism* 63, 1 (Winter 2005), 50.

42. Thomas Elsaesser argues that certain psychic conditions of spectators as well as characters may be *displaced* onto the composition of an image in "Tales of Sound and Fury: Observations on the Family Melodrama," in *Movies and Methods: An Anthology, Vol. II*, ed. Bill Nichols (Berkeley and Los Angeles: University of California Press, 1985), 165–89. On identification, misrecognition, and other psychoanalytic concepts, see generally, Robert Stam, Robert Burgoyne, and Sandy Flitterman-Lewis, *New Vocabularies in Film Semiotics: Structuralism, Post-Structuralism and Beyond* (New York: Routledge, 1992); and *Endless Night: Cinema and Psychoanalysis, Parallel Histories*, ed. Janet Bergstrom (Berkeley and Los Angeles: University of California Press, 1999). On fetishistic scopophilia, see Laura Mulvey, "Visual Pleasure and Narrative Cinema," in *Visual and Other Pleasures* (Bloomington: Indiana University Press, 1989), 14–26. On reflexive framing, see Robert Stam, *Reflexivity in Film and Literature: From Don Quixote to Jean-Luc Godard* (New York: Columbia University Press, 1992); and Bruce F. Kawin, *Mindscreen: Bergman, Godard, and First-Person Film* (Princeton, N.J.: Princeton University Press, 1978). On the relation of fantasy to other psychoanalytic theories of cinema, see Constance Penley, "Feminism, Film Theory, and the Bachelor Machines," in *The Future of an Illusion: Film, Feminism, and Psychoanalysis* (Minneapolis: University of Minnesota Press, 1989), 56–80. On masquerade as a reaction to patriarchy, see Mary Ann Doane, *Femmes Fatales: Feminism, Film Theory, Psychoanalysis* (New York: Routledge, 1991). On dream framing, see Vlada Petric, "Tarkovsky's Dream Imagery," *Film Quarterly* 43, 2 (Winter 1989–90), 29 (on *Mirror*, 1975, and *Stalker*, 1979); Robert T. Eberwein, *Film & The Dream Screen: A Sleep and a Forgetting* (Princeton, N.J.: Princeton University Press, 1984); and Janet Jenks Casebier and Allan Casebier, "Selective Bibliography on Dream and Film," *Dreamworks* 1, 1 (Spring 1980), 88–93. On "emotional buffer frames," see Grodal, *Moving Pictures*, 178–79.

An example of "disframing" in Hitchcock's *Suspicion* (1941) is analyzed at length by Stephen Heath, *Questions of Cinema* (New York: Macmillan, 1981), chap. 2, "Narrative Space" [orig. 1976], 19–24, 63; see also "On Screen, in Frame: Film and Ideology" [orig. 1976], 1–18. "Disframing" involves a return of unconscious and repressed "excess" textual material that must be repressed anew by the narrative. The double framing of Žižek's "blot" is discussed in chapter 2 above in relation to schemes for analyzing the subjectivity of camera movement. The notion of the "blot" should be compared to Derrida's "parergon" in *The Truth in Painting* and to Freud's "uncanny" in "The 'Uncanny'" from *The Standard Edition of the Complete Psychological Works of Sigmund Freud, Vol. XVII (1917–1919)*, ed. James Strachey (London: The Hogarth Press, 1955), 219–52. On the fetishistic pleasure of framing-deframing, see Christian Metz, "Photography and Fetish," *October* 34 (Fall 1985), 86, 89. He states,

> More generally, the play of framings and the play with framings, in all sorts of films, work like a striptease of the space itself. . . . The moving camera caresses the space, and the whole of cinematic fetishism consists in the constant and teasing displacement of the cutting line which separates the seen from the unseen. But this game has no end. (88)

See also Metz, "The Imaginary Signifier," from *The Imaginary Signifier*, sect. "Fetish and Frame," 77–78.

In psychoanalytic theory, certain states of being (desire, guilt, dread, etc.) are able to cross the boundary between animate and inanimate in order to infuse and animate an object for a person. Thus, it may make sense within this framework to speak of the point of view of an inanimate object, for example, the point of view of an envelope containing $40,000 in Hitchcock's *Psycho* (1960). See Kaja Silverman, *The Subject of Semiotics* (New York: Oxford University Press, 1983), 208; cf. 211 (the point of view of a showerhead in *Psycho*). See also the discussion of a camera as a "channel for communication" in chapter 3 above.

43. On the problem of deciding which inferences are relevant for an occasion, see, e.g., Dan Sperber and Deirdre Wilson, *Relevance: Communication and Cognition* (Oxford: Blackwell, 2nd ed. 1995). See generally, Daniel Dennett, "Cognitive Wheels: The Frame Problem of AI," in *The Robot's Dilemma: The Frame Problem in Artificial Intelligence*, ed. Zenon W. Pylyshyn (Norwood, N.J.: Ablex Publishing, 1987), 41–64. The "frame problem," in general, is a problem about how the mind represents knowledge of the invariants of a situation, such as the fact that walking into a room does not change the color of objects. This problem is related to the problem of "sustaining" causes that I will discuss in the next chapter.

44. On possible worlds semantics and "frames of reference," see David Herman, *Universal Grammar and Narrative Form* (Durham, N.C.: Duke University Press, 1995), chap. 5, "Modes of Meaning in Film," 203–24.

45. Daniel C. Dennett, "Real Patterns," *The Journal of Philosophy* 88, 1 (Jan. 1991), 31.

46. Dennett discusses five "different grades or kinds of realism," the middle one of which is his own "mild realism," in "Real Patterns," 30, 49–51. I believe that Dennett's approach to thinking about *patterns* may be usefully applied to the hierarchy of levels (patterns, frames) of narration sketched in my *Narrative Comprehension and Film*, chapter 4, 86–124. A spectator's interpretive statement about a film would be understood as a projection through a particular level or pattern of narration.

47. Rorty, "Inquiry as Recontextualization: An Anti-Dualist Account of Interpretation," in *Objectivity, Relativism, and Truth*, 110 (footnotes omitted; original emphasis); partly quoted in Vescio, "Reading in the Dark," 589.

48. Stan Brakhage, "Metaphors on Vision," *Film Culture* 30 (1963), opening para. (n.p.). Brakhage's reverie should be compared with the two kinds of knowledge posited by Schopenhauer, for which see, e.g., Monroe C. Beardsley, *Aesthetics from Classical Greece to the Present: A Short History* (New York: Macmillan, 1966), 267–70. One might even include Alain Robbe-Grillet in the reverie; see, e.g., "A Future for the Novel," in *For a New Novel: Essays on Fiction*, trans. Richard Howard (New York: Grove Press, 1965), 20–22. For an informative application of cognitive theory to the films of Brakhage and to experimental film generally, see James Peterson, *Dreams of Chaos, Visions of Order: Understanding the American Avant-Garde Cinema* (Detroit: Wayne State University Press, 1994).

Jens Brockmeier offers a quite different view of 'world knowledge' in which language is constitutive of ineffable experience; see "Ineffable Experience," *Journal of Consciousness Studies* 9, nn. 9–10 (Sept./Oct. 2002), 79–95. The alternatives mentioned by Rorty and Brakhage might be visualized by contrasting Peter Greenaway's *The Falls* (1980) with Godfrey Reggio's *Koyaanisqatsi* (1983), respectively.

49. Cf. *Wittgenstein's Lectures*, Part I, § 28 ("Luther said that theology is the grammar of the word 'God.'"). My doubts about the existence of an immutable "medium" of film parallel those of Richard Rorty and Donald Davidson about the "medium" of language; see Richard Rorty, *Contingency, Irony, and Solidarity* (Cambridge: Cambridge University Press, 1989), chap. 1, "The Contingency of Language," esp. 10–16, 19.

50. For a recent, detailed review of solutions that have been offered to the problem of agency in film, see David A. Gerstner, "The Practices of Authorship," and Janet Staiger, "Authorship Approaches," in *Authorship and Film*, ed. David A. Gerstner and Janet Staiger (New York: Routledge, 2003), 3–57. Dudley Andrew offers a brief survey of conceptions of authorship and discusses the

economic sign that the author has become today; see "The Unauthorized Auteur Today," in *Film and Theory: An Anthology*, ed. Robert Stam and Toby Miller (Oxford, U.K.: Blackwell, 2000), 20–29. See generally, *The Death and Resurrection of the Author?*, ed. William Irwin (Westport, Conn.: Greenwood Press, 2002). Cognitive accounts of the problem of authorship may be found in *Visual Authorship: Creativity and Intentionality in Media*, ed. Torben Grodal, Bente Larsen, and Iben Thorving Laursen (University of Copenhagen: Museum Tusculanum Press, 2005).

51. I apply such concepts as schema, top-down and bottom-up perception, the pragmatics of a middle world, and basic-level categorization to a theory of film sound in "Sound, Epistemology, Film," in *Film Theory and Philosophy*, ed. Richard Allen and Murray Smith (New York: Oxford University Press, 1997), 95–125. Even a silent film will provide a rationale to justify how sound can be heard, because a spectator does not presume characters to be deaf nor the world mute. See, e.g., Melinda Szaloky, "Sounding Images in Silent Film: Visual Acoustics in Murnau's *Sunrise*," *Cinema Journal* 41, 2 (Winter 2002), 109–31.

52. The distinction between bottom-up and top-down perception is not based on whether visual illusions and constancies, which are usually thought of as bottom-up phenomena, are present or not. The reason is that top-down perception is subject to many kinds of cognitive illusions, biases, and fallible heuristics (e.g., the fundamental attribution error, belief perseverance, and dilution). Bottom-up perception is stimulus driven. It is involuntary, serial, rapid, atomistic, computational, highly specialized, and inaccessible to memory and consciousness. Bottom-up perception operates directly upon the visible and audible data of film by organizing it automatically into such features as aural pitch, loudness, timbre, edge, slant, corner, depth, volume, orientation, motion, speed, direction, size, shape, surface, color, and texture. By contrast, top-down perception is task driven and alert to situational factors. It enables one to perceive narrative patterns in novels and films, and to construct a cognitive map of a locale on the basis of seeing a few shots or reading a few sentences. Top-down perception is based on acquired knowledge, memory, predisposition, inference, practical postulates, and schemata and, hence, is "context-sensitive." Top-down perception is not constrained by stimulus time and operates indirectly, often abductively, on the visible and audible data of film using a spectator's expectations and goals as principles by which to organize knowledge and, especially, to project hypotheses. As the Queen remarks to Alice in Lewis Carroll's *Through the Looking-Glass* (chap. 5), "It's a poor sort of memory that only works backwards."

Separating "bottom-up" from "top-down" perception has theoretical implications for the debate over the existence of "computational algorithms" in the mind as opposed to more flexible, "context-sensitive" processes. See, e.g., the "Dialogue" among John Tooby, Leda Cosmides, and Ellen Spolsky, *SubStance* 94/95, v. 30, nos. 1/2 (2001), 199–202 (special issue "On the Origin of Fictions: Interdisciplinary Perspectives"). There is also a question how far to carry the idea of a perceptual 'illusion' into the core tenets of a theory of film. Compare Richard Allen, *Projecting Illusion: Film Spectatorship and the Impression of Reality* (Cambridge: Cambridge University Press, 1995) with *Journal of Consciousness Studies* 9, nn. 5–6 (2002) (special issue on "Is the Visual World a Grand Illusion?").

A diagram of the hierarchical arrangement of 47 "modules" (areas, stages) of the visual system based on forward (bottom-up) and backward (top-down) neuronal projections may be found in Francis Crick, *The Astonishing Hypothesis: The Scientific Search for the Soul* (London: Simon & Schuster, 1994), 156. For a recent introduction and bibliography, see Steven Pinker, *How the Mind Works* (New York: W.W. Norton & Co., 1997). For a brief comment on the crucial role of top-down effects in the perception of art, see Erich Harth, "Art and Reductionism," *Journal of Consciousness Studies* 11, nn. 3–4 (March/April 2004), 111–16. In addition to bottom-up and top-down, there are also "lateral" interactions in the brain and mind.

53. On the philosophical significance of embodied basic-level categories and their relation to imagery, knowledge structure, and "realism," see esp. George Lakoff and Mark Johnson, *Philosophy in the Flesh: The Embodied Mind and Its Challenge to Western Thought* (New York: Basic Books, 1999), 26–30, and Lakoff, *Women, Fire, and Dangerous Things*, 12–57. See also Antonio Damasio, *The Feeling of What Happens: Body and Emotion in the Making of Consciousness* (New York: Harcourt Brace, 1999), and Robert F. Port and Timothy van Gelder, eds., *Mind as Motion: Explorations in the Dynamics of Cognition* (Cambridge, Mass.: MIT Press, 1995). Also, it is important to consider the "person schema" in understanding the embodiment of characters within a basic-level fictional world; see, e.g., Murray Smith, *Engaging Characters: Fiction, Emotion, and the Cinema* (Oxford: Oxford University Press, 1995), 17–39, 113–16.

54. See Grodal, "Art Film, the Transient Body, and the Permanent Soul," pp. 35–38, 46–50. I believe that within a single sentence Vlada Petric is referring to basic-level, subordinate, and superordinate categories when he asserts that "[Andrei] Tarkovsky finds a balance between the ontological authenticity of the film's image [basic-level; the frame as a window] and its phenomenological obliqueness [subordinate], which helps his dream imagery transcend [superordinate] the film 'language' as a system of signs, reaching the level of audiovisual abstraction [super-superordinate]." Note also the order in which these types of categories are presented in the sentence. The aim is to reach

the supersensible below and above mere basic-level embodied existence; the truly important truths are the 'highest.' "Tarkovsky's Dream Imagery," *Film Quarterly*: 29.

55. Eisenstein asks, "Now why should the cinema follow the forms of theater and painting rather than the methodology of language, which allows wholly new concepts of ideas to arise from the combination of two concrete denotations of two concrete objects? Language is much closer to film than painting is." Eisenstein, "A Dialectic Approach to Film Form," in *Film Form*, 60; *Eisenstein: Selected Works, Vol. I*, "The Dramaturgy of Film Form (The Dialectical Approach to Film Form)," 178.

56. Wittgenstein, *Philosophical Investigations*, § 114; cf. §§ 104, 122.

57. Deleuze, *Cinema 2*, chap. 8, "Cinema, Body and Brain, Thought," 189. In this passage Deleuze may be seeking to partially reverse René Descartes's famous dictum, "I am thinking, therefore I exist" into something like 'I exist, therefore I am thinking with my body'; that is, for Deleuze, thinking is corporeal. See Descartes, "Discourse on the Method," in *The Philosophical Writings of Descartes, Vol. I*, ed. John Cottingham, Robert Stoothoff, and Dugald Murdoch (Cambridge: Cambridge University Press, 1984), Part Four, 127; cf. *Meditations on First Philosophy* in *Vol. II*, "Second Meditation," third paragraph, 17. Further thoughts by Deleuze on framing may be found in *Cinema 1: The Movement-Image*, trans. Hugh Tomlinson and Barbara Habberjam (Minneapolis: University of Minnesota Press, 1986), 12–18.

58. See, e.g., Johnson, *The Body in the Mind*, 205–12. See generally Ziva Kunda, *Social Cognition: Making Sense of People* (Cambridge, Mass.: MIT Press, 1999); Susan T. Fiske and Shelley E. Taylor, *Social Cognition* (New York: McGraw-Hill, 2nd ed. 1991); David Martel Johnson, *How History Made the Mind: The Cultural Origins of Objective Thinking* (Chicago: Open Court, 2003).

59. Charles Forceville examines how a folk theory of anger is based on a projection from the container schema; see "Visual Representations of the Idealized Cognitive Model of Anger in the Asterix Album *La Zizanie*," *Journal of Pragmatics* 37, 1 (2005), 69–88.

60. On the container schema and other embodied image schemata, see, e.g., Johnson, *The Body in the Mind*, chap. 2, "The Emergence of Meaning through Schematic Structure," 18–40, and chap. 4, "Metaphorical Projections of Image Schemata," 65–100; on schematic constraints, 112–26; on polysemy and schemata, 107. A classic statement of the relation of metaphor and mind is George Lakoff and Mark Johnson's *Metaphors We Live By* (Chicago: University of Chicago Press, 1980). See also Lakoff, *Women, Fire, and Dangerous Things*, pp. 269–78. On schematic structure (an "adaptive representational network"), see generally, Peggy La Cerra and Roger Bingham, *The Origin of*

Minds: Evolution, Uniqueness, and the New Science of the Self (New York: Harmony Books, 2002). Warren Buckland discusses the container schema and other embodied schemata in *The Cognitive Semiotics of Film* (Cambridge: Cambridge University Press, 2000), chap. 2, "The Body on Screen and in Frame: Film and Cognitive Semantics," esp. 39–51. See generally Maureen Turim, "Postmodern Metaphors and the Images of Thought," *Polygraph* 13 (2001), 112–19.

Embodied image schemata are similar to so-called "mental models," which are diagrammatic pictures in working memory that are connected to perception and imagination as well as to an interpretation of the propositional content of a sentence. Also, there exist alternative ways to conceptualize a schema besides as an embodied image schema. A notable alternative is an approach in which a schema is seen as a "frame" for procedural and generic knowledge that contains "slots" that can accept a limited range of "values," including "default values," e.g., a schema for a "living room" or a "birthday party." In addition, there are other important kinds of knowledge structures besides schemata, e.g., folk models and judgment heuristics. The notion of "mental models" should be compared with Venn diagrams and Euler diagrams. On various methods and concepts of cognitive science, see generally *The MIT Encyclopedia of the Cognitive Sciences*, ed. Robert A. Wilson and Frank C. Keil (Cambridge, Mass.: MIT Press, 1999).

61. I would like to mention a technical point. When figure 4.1 is construed as a representation of Wittgenstein's notion of "family resemblance," the "resemblances" (i.e., the relations among the boxes) may be more 'open' than is usually allowed by commentators on Wittgenstein. That is, Wittgenstein's notion of a "continuous transition" (see epigraph) from one use of a word in one context to another use of the same word in a different context may appear in my diagram in some places as a 'discontinuity,' or gap, between one group of things referred to by a word (one box) and another group of things referred to by the same word (another box). That is, an empty space may appear between two boxes (two contexts). The reason for this slightly expanded 'openness' in my representation of "family resemblance" is that I wonder whether the "continuous transition" is always of the same type. Do all "continuous transitions" have something in common? Or are some links and 'small jumps' instead based on 'proximity,' 'associations,' or 'analogies'? (Rhetoric has many ways of figuring.) I prefer a somewhat more open notion for the "resemblances" of "family resemblance" because this avoids having to identify a strict set of 'features' that characterize either the "family" or the overall set of "resemblances" among family members. (This makes "resemblance" a "family resemblance" concept.) Isolating such absolute 'features' would amount to locating the features within some context superordinate

to the individual "resemblances" among the groups of things referred to by the same word. I believe that attempting to isolate such a priori features would fail to account for the behavior, practice, and circumstance in which each "resemblance" acquires a pertinence that may be projected in *unanticipated* ways at some future time. In sum, I am trying to avoid in figure 4.1 the presumption that "transitions" have a single nature: either continuous, continuous with boundaries, continuous with temporal parts, adjacent, or discontinuous. The heterogeneity of figure 4.1 may be taken to represent the breaks within a culture brought about through changing circumstances and in defiance of an origin or essence. Also a somewhat more open account of "family resemblance" better accords with the notions of ecological conventions (Grodal), motivated conventions (Lakoff), moderate constructivism (Bordwell), and mild realism (Dennett). A slightly more conservative view of "family resemblance" is offered by Hans-Johann Glock in *A Wittgenstein Dictionary* (Oxford: Blackwell, 1996), "family resemblance," 121. One should not become over confident about one's ability to identify a family resemblance within a group of simple elements, even when the group numbers only four. See Mary M. Smyth and Steven E. Clark, "My Half-Sister is a THOG: Strategic Processes in a Reasoning Task," *The British Journal of Psychology* 77 (May 1986), 275–87.

62. On levels of narration and their organization in terms of dependency (hypotaxis) or relative autonomy (parataxis), see Branigan, *Narrative Comprehension and Film*, chap. 4, "Levels of Narration," esp. 113–14. The term "heterarchy" comes from Marvin Minsky's classic study of intelligence, *The Society of Mind* (New York: Simon and Schuster, 1985), 35. Figure 4.1 in the text above may also be used to represent dynamic framings in a film, for example, temporal articulations and camera movements; cf. *Narrative Comprehension and Film*, figure 3, page 41. Indeed the word "movement" is radial; see chapters 2 and 5 in the present book. Notice that I am using the concept of heterarchy to oppose both a hierarchy and a simple chain or loop structure; a heterarchy need not have a preferred "direction" and may contain partial and multiple overlaps as well as "gaps" or "blanks." Strong examples of the links, jumps, and tangents of multiple heterarchies may be found in music sampling and James Joyce's *Ulysses* as well as in films by Jean-Luc Godard, Peter Greenaway, Chris Marker, Raúl Ruiz, Wim Wenders, Wong Kar-Wai, Atom Egoyan, and Jean-Marie Straub and Danièle Huillet. One might contrast Carlos Saura's vertical hierarchy in *Carmen* (1983) with Godard's horizontal dispersion in a heterarchy of the elements of the same story in *First Name: Carmen* (1983).

63. I discuss an example of nonlocal editing, hyperdiegetic narration, in *Narrative Comprehension and Film*, 187–90; see also index entry, 313, and chap. 2, n. 25.

Hyperdiegetic narration is not concerned with repeated motifs but, rather, with a spectator's assembly of nonadjacent shots to create a significant new order. A similar notion is discussed by Peter Wuss, "The Documentary Style of Fiction Film in Eastern Europe: Narration and Visual Style," in *Film Style and Story*, 231 ("distance montage," "montage of the contexts"). Cf. David Bordwell, "Cognition and Comprehension: Viewing and Forgetting in *Mildred Pierce*," *Journal of Dramatic Theory and Criticism* 6, 2 (Spring 1992), 183–98.

64. On a character's look at the camera that breaks, but sometimes does not break, the frame, see Marc Vernet, "The Look at the Camera," *Cinema Journal* 28, 2 (Winter 1989), 48–63. A theorist may take any of the 15 definitions of frame and imagine a distinctive kind of "breaking" of that frame. For example, if a shot is viewed as being "broken off" at its four edges, then an off-center composition or certain uses of diagonal lines, etc., may serve to "disconnect" the composition, leaving the shot incomplete (cf. definition 5). Another way of breaking the frame is by "passing through" to a world that has new laws (cf. definition 15). Consider, for example, such explicit dramatizations of "passing through" as Lewis Carroll's *Through the Looking-Glass and What Alice Found There*, *Orpheus* (Jean Cocteau, 1950), *Bram Stoker's Dracula* (Francis Ford Coppola, 1992), *The Matrix* (Andy and Larry Wachowski, 1999), and *The Sixth Sense* (M. Night Shyamalan, 1999).

65. The Deleuze quote appears in the text at note 57. On the nonobjective (mixed) status of film theory, see Branigan, "To Zero and Beyond," 150, 159. Cf. the use of simple, available, and mostly transparent analogies when constructing a film theory: Peter Larsen, "Urban Legends: Notes on a Theme in Early Film Theory," in *City Flicks: Indian Cinema and the Urban Experience*, ed. Preben Kaarsholm (Calcutta: Seagull Books, 2004); Malcolm Turvey, "Can the Camera See? Mimesis in *Man with a Movie Camera*," *October* 89 (Summer 1999), 25–50; and David Bordwell, "The Musical Analogy," *Yale French Studies* 60 (1980), 141–156.

66. On the lack of a relationship between film theory and film criticism, see esp. Bordwell, *Making Meaning*, 4–7, 26–27, 28, 104, 107, 122, 144, 211–12, 250–53.

67. Cf. Inez Hedges, *Breaking the Frame: Film Language and the Experience of Limits* (Bloomington, Ind.: Indiana University Press, 1991).

68. The source-path-goal schema may even be used to *model* a theoretical paradigm. Francesco Casetti describes his film theory in the following way: "Thus, the themes identified earlier — that the text opens itself to a spectator's *presence*, that it gives to this spectator a well-defined *place* and requires that this spectator accomplish a true *journey* — no longer appear as simple metaphors but rather as parameters that enable an appreciation of the film's 'self-offering' to vision and hearing. . . . We have an outline here

of the frame in which we have conducted our research, without omitting its foundations and limits." *Inside the Gaze: The Fiction Film and Its Spectator*, trans. Nell Andrew with Charles O'Brien (Bloomington: Indiana University Press, 1998), 126 (original emphases). Gilles Deleuze begins to address the problem of a *time* span or time frame by employing set theory and invoking Bergson's notion of a relation among "time," the "whole," and "openness." Deleuze states that Bergson's notion of time can be found by considering:

> three coexisting levels in cinematography: framing, which defines a provisional artificially limited set of things; cutting, which defines the distribution of movement or movements among the elements of the set; and then this movement reflects a change or variation in the whole, which is the realm of *montage*.

Deleuze, "On *The Movement—Image*," in *Negotiations, 1972–1990*, trans. Martin Joughin (New York: Columbia University Press, 1995), 55 (original emphasis). (The interview was conducted by Pascal Bonitzer and Jean Narboni in 1983.)

A person employing the judgment heuristic of "anchoring and adjustment" relies on a starting point to make (anchor) an inference, such as trying to estimate a quantity by thinking of why it might be larger or smaller than some given, initial value, or assessing his or her own abilities by anchoring on others' opinions. Typically, people adjust too little from a starting point. One may speculate that the plot of a film, too, may offer a "framing," or starting point, that acts to unduly restrict the range of our inferential activity. See, e.g., *The MIT Encyclopedia of the Cognitive Sciences*, 423–25, and Kunda, *Social Cognition*, 104.

69. I discuss a holistic and "horizontal" form of analysis in the third section of chapter 1, as well as the pertinence of a spectator's movements of "attention" to the analysis of camera movements in the conclusion of chapter 2.

70. William Johnson, "Coming to Terms with Color," in *The Movies as Medium*, ed. Lewis Jacobs (New York: Farrar, Straus & Giroux, 1970), 233 n. 21.

71. The perception of "transparency" comes from midlevel visual processing in the brain and is closely related to perceptions of both shadow and opaque occlusion. See generally *The MIT Encyclopedia of the Cognitive Sciences*, "Transparency," 845–47; and Arnheim, *Art and Visual Perception*, 253–258, 309–310. Wittgenstein explores the 'nonembodied' aspects of the logic, or grammar, of the word "transparency" in *Remarks on Colour*. He imagines a fictitious, transparent white glass that removes the colors from a movie, making the movie appear on the screen in black and white. See Part I, § 25 and Part III, § 184. Wittgenstein's approach suggests that it might be worth-

while to think about the 'hidden grammar' of a word by seeking to reveal the word's 'hidden analogies.' These embedded analogies (or radial extensions) might themselves be conceived on the analogy of an invisibly 'tinted' glass (a kind of 'folk theory') through which we may see the word. I will discuss this issue in the next chapter in terms of a *relativity* of 'description.'

If the above picture holds, then what would be analogous to a 'darker' word, or description, subject to invisible 'toning'? Would it be an embodied and entrenched word like "hand" in a proposition, as when G. E. Moore raises his hand and says, "Here is one hand, and here is another"? Note that if Moore simply raised his hand without speaking, he would not be making a statement. See Moore's "Proof of an External World" (1933) and also "A Defense of Common Sense" (1925) in *Philosophical Papers* (London: George Allen & Unwin, 1959).

72. The fanciful names given to Eastman Kodak's tinted Sonochrome film stocks in 1929 suggest how tinted color was perceived to be entirely "arbitrary": peach-blow, inferno, rose dorée, candle flame, sunshine, firelight, purple haze, fleur de lis, azure, nocturne, verdante, aqua green, argent, and caprice.

73. Toning makes it appear that a hue is embodied *in* an object, while tinting creates the impression that a hue has been overlaid *on* an object. Some situations seem to contradict this perceptual judgment, but the contradiction is only apparent. Consider, for example, a character who is wearing a white shirt. Tinting would give the shirt (and other light objects and areas) a new hue, and that hue would be seen to be "in" the image because it is "on" the character who is "in" the image. Still, the character's "original" shirt remains white in our mind because we ascribe the change in hue to the action of light itself (which normally is not seen as colored). Tinting the image, then, simply makes the normal white light look colored, as if a gel had been used on a light source or as if we were looking at the scene through a tinted windowpane. We continue to believe that the shirt is actually white; it just appears in a different hue because the light in the diegesis has been given a new color by extra-diegetic fiat, much as nondiegetic music might have been added to the scene as authorial commentary. The characters in the diegesis will see the shirt as white, too, and will continue to act accordingly. Thus, the spectator will see the hue of the character's shirt onscreen as having been tinted and overlaid, not as embodied. On the other hand, toning the shirt in a new hue would preserve the object-ness of the shirt because the gray scale would be preserved for all the objects and persons in the image (thus suggesting volume through a chiaroscuro effect). Toning would maintain the whiteness of the shirt while making it appear that darker objects in the image have a new embodied hue being reflected to us by normal light. We perceive these objects as having been changed even if the characters do not.

74. For example, tinting and toning are alike in that both may be accomplished in postproduction; both produce hues; both are composed of "colored" light from the theater screen; and both are processed by the same brain mechanisms. Although a toned hue, like color generally, appears to be possessed by, and embodied in, an object, what we actually see is the light that has *not* been absorbed by the object but, rather, *filtered* through it (in the case of toning) or *reflected* away from it (in the case of real-world objects). In tinting, the situation is similar: Light is passed through a glass filter before illuminating an object, or else normal light is reflected from an object but passes through a glass filter before reaching our eyes.

75. Implicit in my text is the idea that color as a device need not function in film or be theorized in a strictly embodied, basic-level way. I believe that color has startling new roles to play at subordinate and superordinate levels of description. These new roles will significantly change the relationship of color to other filmic elements and to qualities of the world being represented on film. Color need not appear only as an added Tint to an object; it may also become a Tone. Probing these relationships, however, must be deferred to another occasion.

76. See, e.g., Deleuze, *Cinema 2*, chap. 8, "Cinema, Body and Brain, Thought," 189–224.

77. Roland Barthes, *The Pleasure of the Text*, trans. Richard Miller (New York: Hill and Wang, 1975), 55–57 (my emphases of "movements," "never leaves the frame," and "nothing leaps out of the frame"); cf. 6–8. See especially Martin Lefebvre's analysis of a "figural experience" while watching a film, "On Memory and Imagination in the Cinema," *New Literary History* 30, 2 (Spring 1999), 481–98.

78. Robert Lapsley and Michael Westlake, *Film Theory: An Introduction* (New York: St. Martin's Press, 1988), 86.

79. Jean-Pierre Oudart, "Cinema and Suture" [orig. 1969], *Screen* 18, 4 (Winter 1977/78), 41. The translation appearing in *Screen* is reprinted in *Cahiers du Cinéma 1969–1972: The Politics of Representation* [vol. 3], ed. Nick Browne (Cambridge, Mass.: Harvard University Press, 1990), 45–57. For a summary of the major ideas underlying "suture," see Susan Hayward, *Cinema Studies: The Key Concepts* (New York: Routledge, 2nd ed. 2000), 378–85. Note that my analysis of theories of suture in this section is primarily a "vertical," dissective analysis; see the third section of chapter 1 above, "How Should Analysis Proceed?"

80. Oudart, "Cinema and Suture," 41.

81. Oudart's description of the shot (quoted in the text above) is inaccurate in an important respect. He says that after the Confederate soldiers suddenly rise

up through the bottom of the frame, the spectator takes a moment to realize that the soldiers have occupied "a rise above the river, which was hidden by the position of the camera." In fact, the shot is composed in a conventional manner employing the rule of 'one-thirds.' The far ridgeline, down which the Union troops have come, provides a 'horizon line' that is located one third down from the top of the image. The far bank of Rock River is located one third up from the bottom of the image. The "rise above the river" is perfectly visible at the bottom of the image and is not "hidden by the position of the camera." I believe that the spectator's surprise at seeing the Confederates appear is due to three factors: First, a new center of interest has suddenly been created that opens an entirely new plane of action in an area much nearer the camera than the Union troops; second, there was no indication in two immediately preceding shots from the identical camera position that it would be possible for a center of interest to appear in the bottom third of the image (the area in the bottom third was simply empty and seemed of no significance); third, the new center of interest has appeared in an unexpected way because actions that cross the top and bottom frame lines are rare (though even more rare is an action that moves behind the camera to appear from the 'wrong' direction). These three factors cause us to suddenly notice that we have *not* noticed the bottom third of the frame.

I believe there are additional psychological principles at work in "suture" related to a spectator's working memory and attention. Working memory is serial, highly selective, slow, limited to 5–9 bits of information, and highly responsive to sensory characteristics (as opposed to long-term memory, which tends to encode information in terms of its meaning or gist). Working memory holds only 1 or 2 ideas at a time, coordinates other forms of memory, and evaluates the degree of "progress" being made on a task. (You may test the capacity of working memory for yourself by trying to hold 1 or 2 *images* in mind while scanning the visible details of a scene.) Stephen Heath, drawing on Freud, recognizes the importance of working memory for a theory of suture. See Heath, *Questions of Cinema*, "On Suture," 108–09, and text accompanying note 101 below.

On overlooking certain important details that are clearly present (e.g., the "rise above the river" on which the Confederates suddenly appear in Oudart's illustration of "suture"), cf. Daniel T. Levin, "Change Blindness Blindness as Visual Metacognition," *Journal of Consciousness Studies* 9, nn. 5–6 (2002): 111–30. Consider also the theoretical implications of the well-known filmic device of the "cheat cut"; Branigan, *Narrative Comprehension and Film*, sect. "Forgetting and Revising," 83–85; sect. "Separation of Material and Structure," 140–42; and see 45–47, 182. A fine example of change blindness may be found in the opening of Buster Keaton's *Cops* (1922). Does the opposite phenomenon exist, that is, something that does not change yet is perceived as change? One thinks of the subtle and anodyne graphic matches of Yasujiro Ozu, which suggest stasis or repose yet tend to go unnoticed. See also the discussion of "sustaining" causality in the next chapter.

82. For Oudart, perceiving an image is a meshwork of different activities.

> It is of course a simplification to say that the spectator perceives an image, framed and delimited, since he does not perceive simultaneously the framing, the space, and the filmed object. Perception of the framing always eclipses vision of the object at the same time as it puts an end to the spectator's *jouissance* in the space.

"Cinema and Suture," 42. By "*jouissance* in the space," Oudart is referring to what I take to be stage 3 of his theory of a spectator's changing awareness of an image. Oudart seems to have constructed a vertical hierarchy among "the framing, the space, and the filmed object." Cf. Wittgenstein's 'horizontal' approach in note 115 below.

Oudart's use of the idea that the perception of one thing "eclipses vision" of another suggests that he is thinking of framing and suture as a form of perceptual 'masking.' The psychological effect of masking occurs in a variety of situations in several forms (including simultaneous, forward, and backward masking) and is an aspect of 'attention.' Suture theorists tend to emphasize the negative connotations of the idea of 'masking,' namely, that masking must be concealing something important. Daniel Dayan, for example, applies the notion of "masking" to the concealing of ideology in film. (See text accompanying note 92 below.) There are, however, notable survival advantages to masking (e.g., overriding old information with new). Also related to processes of masking and attention is a spectator's important effort toward building an internal map, or model, of the acoustic and spatial environment of an event. The point here is that one should be careful to discriminate among the numerous effects of a psychological process, if one wishes to make psychological claims.

83. In the same spirit as Oudart, here is Victor Burgin's account of looking at a still photograph:

> To look at a photograph beyond a certain period of time is to court a frustration; the image which on first looking gave pleasure has by degrees become a veil behind which we now desire to see. . . .To remain long with a single image is to risk the loss of our imaginary command of the look, to relinquish it to that absent other to whom it belongs by right — the camera. . . .The lens arranges all information according to laws of projec-

tion which place the subject as geometric point of origin of the scene in an imaginary relationship with real space, but facts intrude to deconstruct the initial response: the eye/(I) cannot move within the depicted space (which offers itself precisely to such movement), it can only move across it to the points where it encounters the frame. The subject's inevitable recognition of the *rule* of the frame may, however, be postponed by a variety of strategies which include "compositional" devices for moving the eye from the framing edge. "Good composition" may therefore be no more or less than a set of devices for prolonging our imaginary command of the point-of-view, our *self*-assertion, a device for retarding recognition of the autonomy of the frame, and the authority of the *other* it signifies. "Composition" (and indeed the interminable discourse about composition — formalist criticism) is therefore a means of prolonging the imaginary force, the real power to please, of the photograph, and it may be in this that it has survived so long, within a variety of rationalisations, as a criterion of value in visual art generally.

Victor Burgin, "Looking at Photographs" [orig. 1977], in *Thinking Photography*, ed. Victor Burgin (London: Macmillan, 1982), 152 (original emphases).

84. Although Oudart speaks in general of the 'suturing' shot as being a 'reverse field,' in the case of the initial shot he describes from *The General*, it is not possible to say how, or whether, the next shot is a reverse field. This shot shows a line of Confederate cannons. The foreground of the shot reveals no match or overlap with anything seen in the previous shot. That is, it is unclear how far away the cannons are and whether they are directly behind the Confederate soldiers who have been shown in the previous shot to have occupied the rise above the river. On Oudart's use of 'reverse field,' see "Cinema and Suture," 37, 39, 46. The device of shot/reverse shot is an example of a reverse field. For an approach to shot/reverse shot that is quite different from "suture," see Bordwell, "Convention, Construction, and Cinematic Vision," *Post–Theory: Reconstructing Film Studies*, 87–107. See also Bordwell's perceptive commentary on suture in *Narration in the Fiction Film*, 110–13.

85. Oudart, "Cinema and Suture," 37. On the exchange between the Absent One and a character, see also 36, 38, 39, 40, 42, 43, 45.

86. On Oudart's notion of a dual prospective and retrospective time, see "Cinema and Suture," 37.

87. Oudart contends that "The cinema is characterised by an antinomy of reading and *jouissance*. . . ." "Cinema and Suture," 42; see also 43, 44, 45.

88. Oudart, "Cinema and Suture," 35–36.

89. Oudart, "Cinema and Suture," 36.

90. Oudart, "Cinema and Suture," 42, 44.

91. Oudart, "Cinema and Suture," 40, 43.

92. See Daniel Dayan, "The Tutor-Code of Classical Cinema" [orig. 1974], in *Movies and Methods* [vol. I], 438–51. Two recent accounts of suture follow Dayan's interpretation of Oudart. See Jean-Pierre Geuens, *Film Production Theory* (Albany: State University of New York Press, 2000), chap. 7, "The Frame," 181–83; and Todd McGowan, "Looking for the Gaze: Lacanian Film Theory and Its Vicissitudes," *Cinema Journal* 42, n. 3 (Spring 2003), 39 and n. 34. This approach to suture bears similarities to V. I. Pudovkin's "invisible observer," which is used, in effect, to justify the continuity editing system. See Bordwell, *Narration in the Fiction Film*, chap. 1, "Mimetic Theories of Narration," sect. "The Invisible Observer," pp. 9–12.

93. See, e.g., the contrast Oudart draws between two Robert Bresson films, *The Trial of Joan of Arc* (1962) and *Au hasard, Balthazar* (1966), in which the latter fails for lack of suture; "Cinema and Suture," 44. A good test for a theory of suture would be to examine films that utilize strikingly different ways of framing "absence" and the "unseen," as in the following films: Bresson's *The Devil, Probably* (1977), Miklós Jancsó's *The Red and the White* (1967), Jean-Marie Straub and Danièle Huillet's *The Bridegroom, the Comedienne, and the Pimp* (1968), Andrei Tarkovsky's *Stalker* (1979), Béla Tarr and Ágnes Hranitzky's *Werckmeister Harmonies* (1997–2000), and Abbas Kiarostami's *The Wind Will Carry Us* (1999).

94. Dayan, "The Tutor-Code of Classical Cinema," 446. Dayan also uses much stronger language than "entrapment" to describe the injurious effects of suture. He says that the spectator "feels dispossessed of what he is prevented from seeing." Dayan refers to the Absent One as "[t]his ghost, who rules over the frame and robs the spectator of his pleasure." (448) In reference to the spectator's experience of time as simultaneously prospective and retrospective (stage 9 of my description of suture in the text), Dayan asserts that the "spectator is torn to pieces, pulled in opposite directions." He concludes that "Oudart insists on the brutality, on the tyranny" of suture. (450)

95. On Oudart's claim that the "exchange" between presence and absence occurs not between two shots but within a single shot, see "Cinema and Suture," 37, 39. Oudart uses the sonic metaphor "echo" fourteen times in his essay in order to focus, I believe, on this notion of absence in a single shot ("echo" suggests the intangible, invisible, and perhaps the imaginary). A similar metaphor, "flickering in eclipses" used nine times, is derived from Jacques-Alain Miller's general account of suture within Lacanian psychoanalysis (an eclipse produces a shadowlike 'echo' of light). Miller explores a further analogy: The

relation of zero (an 'absence') to the numbers is like the subject's relation to the signifying chain (discourse). See Miller's "Suture (elements of the logic of the signifier)" [orig. 1966], *Screen* 18, 4 (Winter 1977/78), 34. Oudart's notion of "absence" within a single shot is reminiscent of Bazin's idea of the *necessity* of something being continually "hidden from us" so that camera movement can function to maintain the spectator's faith in the reality of the film image through creation of an always-shifting "lateral depth of field." See discussion of "lateral depth of field" in the preceding chapter at note 34 and in note 30 above.

96. Silverman, *The Subject of Semiotics*, 195.

97. Silverman, *The Subject of Semiotics*, 204.

98. Silverman, *The Subject of Semiotics*, 205–06; see also 212–13.

99. Silverman, *The Subject of Semiotics*, 221; see also 206, 236, and 222–36.

100. See William Rothman, "Against 'The System of the Suture'" [orig. 1975], in *Movies and Methods* [vol. I], 451–59. In a similar vein, see Barry Salt, "The Last of the Suture?" (letter), *Film Quarterly* 31, 4 (Summer 1978), 64–65.

101. See Heath, *Questions of Cinema*, "Narrative Space" [orig. 1976], 19–75, and "On Suture" [orig. 1977], 76–112; and see the index entries on "suture" and "frame, framing." Heath also argues that the sound track must be considered as a suturing device; "On Suture," 99. For Heath, film *space* is narrativized into a *place* and each place, in turn, is replaced by a new one, forming a chain of places that culminates in the initial narrativized space being *re-placed* by a resolution. "Narrative Space," 62; "Film, System, Narrative" [orig. 1975], 136. Heath argues that "the work of classical continuity is not to hide or ignore offscreen space but, on the contrary, to contain it, to regularize its fluctuation in a constant movement of reappropriation." "Narrative Space," 45.

When the theory of suture is thus put within a *narrative* framework, then what Noël Carroll calls the "erotetic" model of narrative (which utilizes a question/answer model of narration) will bear some similarity to the way in which, in the theory of suture, the presence of a shot is able to raise a 'question' (an absence) that is 'answered' in the next shot. Cf. Carroll, "The Power of Movies," 89; Roland Barthes, *S/Z: An Essay*, trans. Richard Miller (New York: Hill and Wang, 1974), e.g., sect. 32, "Delay," 75–76; sect. 37, "The Hermeneutic Sentence," 84–86; sect. 62, "Equivocation I: Double Understanding," 144–45; and sect. 89, "Voice of Truth," 209–10. In a similar vein, see Barry Salt, "The Last of the Suture?" (letter) *Film Quarterly* 31,4 (Summer 1978), 64–65.

102. Slavoj Žižek, *The Fright of Real Tears: Krzysztof Kieślowski between Theory and Post-Theory* (London: British Film Institute, 2001), Part One, "The Universal: Suture Revisited," 31–33, 52–54, 55–56, 58, 65, 187 n. 47.

Katarzyna Marciniak extends Žižek's notion of a suture/desuture dialectic to propose a notion of "hypersuture" that leads to an "abjecting enclosure," an exhausting physical and conceptual quarantine for spectators. "Second Worldness and Transnational Feminist Practices: Agnieszka Holland's *A Woman Alone*" in *East European Cinemas*, ed. Anikó Imre (New York: Routledge, forthcoming 2005).

103. Žižek, *The Fright of Real Tears*, chap. 2, "Back to the Suture," 31–54.

104. Žižek, *The Fright of Real Tears*, 52–53 (original emphasis).

105. Žižek, *The Fright of Real Tears*, 39. Cf. Žižek's comments on the two "frames" of a painting — one visible, one invisible — and the "gap" between them; 5–6.

106. Žižek, *The Fright of Real Tears*, 58. Also "short-circuited" by the fact of suture in film and by the importance of the Gaze are, according to Žižek, such misguided theories as Post-Theory, cognitivism, and historicism. See chap. 3, "The Short-Circuit," 56, 58, 61, 65.

107. Žižek, *The Fright of Real Tears*, 68.

108. Žižek, *The Fright of Real Tears*, 58.

109. In general, what will count as a "shot" in a film theory is connected to what counts as a "frame." Different notions of a "frame" produce different notions of a "shot." See, e.g., note 38 above and the text accompanying note 63 above.

110. Oudart mentions jouissance on eight occasions. It can be translated as fascination, passion, erotic engagement, jubilation, or "vertiginous delight" (cf. stage 3 of my description of suture in the text). See Oudart, "Cinema and Suture," 38, 41, 42, 45, 47.

111. Pascal Bonitzer, "Deframings" [orig. 1978], in *Cahiers du Cinéma, Vol. 4, 1973–1978: History, Ideology, Cultural Struggle*, ed. David Wilson (New York: Routledge, 2000), 198–99. See generally, Lynne Kirby's review essay of Bonitzer's *Décadrages: Peinture et cinema* (1985), "Painting and Cinema: The Frames of Discourse," *Camera Obscura* 18 (Sept. 1988), 95–105. Another use of the concept of "deframing" may be found in Deleuze, *Cinema 2*, 214.

112. Bonitzer, "Deframings," 200 (footnote omitted). By contrast, Bonitzer says that in Godard's work "what is important is neither framing nor deframing, but what [the spectator sees that explicitly] shatters the frame. . . ." (201)

113. Bonitzer, "Deframings," 201; see also 200. Does the "sadism" of deframing lead to a masochistic aesthetic for the spectator? Cf. Gaylyn Studlar, "Masochism and the Perverse Pleasures of the Cinema," in *Movies and Methods*, Vol. II, 602–21. Notice that something human has been *drained away* in deframing, whereas in suture, according to Dayan, something has been *absorbed*. Although draining and absorbing are opposite processes, the underlying schematic image is that of a *container* for a liquid. Dayan contends:

The code, which *produces* an imaginary, ideological effect, is hidden by the message. Unable to see the workings of the code, the spectator is at its mercy. His imaginary is sealed into the film; the spectator thus absorbs an ideological effect without being aware of it. . . .

Dayan, "The Tutor-Code of Classical Cinema," 448–49 (original emphasis).

114. On kinds of causation, see esp. Lakoff and Johnson, *Philosophy in the Flesh*, chap. 11, "Events and Causes," 170–234. On methods of causal reasoning, see Branigan, *Narrative Comprehension and Film*, 39–40; on kinds of causation, 26–32; on the relation of causality and metaphor, 6, 49, 50, 203; and see index entry, "causality." The next chapter will consider some of the problems of theorizing causation.

In the course of a complex argument, Slavoj Žižek asserts that "what happens . . . is not that the object falls out of its frame, so that we get only the empty frame . . .; what happens, rather, is the exact opposite — the object is still there; . . . it is the frame that falls into what it frames . . . ." Here, clearly, another grammar (and causative language-game) for the word "frame" is in effect. *The Fragile Absolute or, Why Is the Christian Legacy Worth Fighting for?* (New York: Verso, 2000), 29.

115. Wittgenstein, *Philosophical Investigations* § 99 (original emphases); cf. §§ 71, 76–77, 98, 100–01. I am reminded of film viewing when Wittgenstein says,

I look at the landscape, my gaze ranges over it, I see all sorts of distinct and indistinct movement; *this* impresses itself sharply on me, *that* is quite hazy. After all, how completely ragged what we see can appear! And now look at all that can be meant by "description of what is seen." — But this just is what is called description of what is seen. There is not *one genuine* proper case of such description — the rest being just vague, something which awaits clarification, or which must just be swept aside as rubbish. [Part II, xi, 200 (original emphases).]

I believe that one aspect of what Wittgenstein is complaining about here is that in looking at the world we tend to privilege immediate conscious attention and what is sharply focused in the fovea centralis at the expense of peripheral vision and memory. The distribution of boxes in figure 4.1 is designed to suggest the permeable boundaries within a polysemous word. The lines of figure 4.1 could have been drawn in a blurred way to further suggest Wittgenstein's notion of the indistinct boundaries among a series of genuine descriptions of what is seen in a moment or meant by a word. For Wittgenstein, blurriness is not necessarily an imperfection (like an indistinct or unfinished sketch) but, instead, may be a step toward something new.

In *The Blue and Brown Books* Wittgenstein says, "Many words . . . don't have a strict meaning. But this is not a defect. To think it is would be like saying that the light of my reading lamp is no real light at all because it has no sharp boundary." (27) Wittgenstein asks, "Why should one be puzzled just by the lack of a definition of time, and not by the lack of a definition of 'chair'?" (26) He also argues that there is no sharp boundary that separates what is misleading in an analogy from its fruitful aspects. (28)

116. On fictions within a fiction, see Edward Branigan, "Nearly True: Forking Plots, Forking Interpretations — A Response to David Bordwell's 'Film Futures,'" *SubStance* 97, v. 31, n. 1 (2002), 105–14, and Branigan, *Narrative Comprehension and Film*, chap. 7, "Fiction," 192–217. What sort of word is "fiction"? When thought of as a subordinate category, it would seem to refer to a "suitable illusion" (because in the context of subordinate categorization what are real are the concrete, appropriate parts and details of a thing); as a basic-level concept, fiction would refer to an artistic genre; and as a superordinate concept, it would be a kind of metaphor, hypothesis, possibility, or counterfactual conditional.

117. The following are additional real and embodied situations that may be metaphorically linked to Wittgenstein's room with an open door (thereby creating new images for the activity of framing): a birdcage, an insect trap, and the "glass ceiling" encountered by women in the business and professional worlds. Furthermore, Wittgenstein's "open door" may be interpreted as a "convenient illusion," as in the case of a subjective contour (cf. definition 2 of the frame), or the "open door" may be turned inside out to create a "room" in the form of a Möbius strip (cf. definition 14, which invokes contradiction, ambivalence, and unconscious processes).

118. See comments by Wittgenstein in note 115 above and in the text accompanying note 56 above.

CHAPTER 5: WHEN IS A CAMERA?

An early sketch of a few of the ideas in the present chapter may be found in "*Quand y a-t-il caméra?*," *Champs Visuels: Revue interdisciplinaire de recherchessur l'image* 12–13 (Paris: L'Harmattan, Janvier 1999), 18–32 (special issue edited by Guillaume Soulez on "Penser, cadrer: le projet du cadre"). Work on the chapter was made possible by the Foreign Scholars Program at the University of Bergen, Norway, in February and March of 1999 and by a Research Grant in 1999 from the College of Letters and Science, University of California, Santa Barbara. I especially wish to thank Professor Peter Larsen in Bergen and Dean David Marshall in Santa Barbara for their unflagging support.

1. *The Collected Dialogues of Plato, Including the Letters,* ed. Edith Hamilton and Huntington Cairns (Princeton, N.J.: Princeton University Press, 1963), *Timaeus,* 19b–e.

2. Ludwig Wittgenstein, *Philosophical Investigations,* trans. G.E.M. Anscombe (Oxford: Blackwell, 3rd ed. 1967), § 90; cf. § 112. For a lucid example of how various analogies underlie our use of a concept, see Wittgenstein's analysis of some of the ways we talk about "time" using, for example, analogies with physical movement; *Wittgenstein's Lectures, Cambridge, 1932–1935: From the Notes of Alice Ambrose and Margaret Macdonald,* ed. Alice Ambrose (Amherst, New York: Prometheus Books, 2001), Part I, §§ 12–14, 22. Wittgenstein also offers a wonderfully inventive argument that the grammar of the phrase "in the same way" is intimately connected to (hidden, contradictory) analogies; Part II, § 18. I am aware that this phrase (or one similar . . .) appears in a number of my arguments.

   Later in this section I will discuss nine analogies with physical movement that are relied upon by Socrates in the epigraph. How we understand the "movement" of a camera is partly dependent on a conception of time. On analogies that underlie various conceptions of time, see, e.g., George Lakoff and Mark Turner, *More than Cool Reason: A Field Guide to Poetic Metaphor* (Chicago: University of Chicago Press, 1989), 34–49, and esp. George Lakoff and Mark Johnson, *Philosophy in the Flesh: The Embodied Mind and Its Challenge to Western Thought* (New York: Basic Books, 1999), chap. 10, "Time," 137–69.

   I draw on many of Wittgenstein's ideas in this chapter. Regrettably, his work has had almost no impact on film theory. What follows are most of the works in film studies that directly make use of Wittgenstein: *Wittgenstein, Theory and the Arts,* ed. Richard Allen and Malcolm Turvey (London: Routledge, 2001), Bryan Vescio, "Reading in the Dark: Cognitivism, Film Theory, and Radical Interpretation," *Style* 35, 4 (Winter 2001), 572–91; Manuel De Landa, "Wittgenstein at the Movies," in *Cinema Histories, Cinema Practices,* ed. Patricia Mellencamp and Philip Rosen [The American Film Institute Monograph Series, vol. 4] (Frederick, Md.: University Publications of America, 1984), 108–19. See also Malcolm Turvey, *The Enchanted Camera: Modernist Skepticism and Visual Redemption in Classical Film Theory* (New York University: Ph.D. diss., May 2002). In addition, Wittgenstein has been used to analyze the work of Jean Epstein, Jean-Luc Godard, and Neil Jordan, and to elucidate the dynamics of conversations between lovers: Malcolm Turvey, "Jean Epstein's Cinema of Immanence: The Rehabilitation of the Corporeal Eye," *October* 83 (Winter 1998), 25–50; Robert MacLean, "Opening the Private Eye: Wittgenstein and Godard's *Alphaville,*" *Sight and Sound* 47, 1 (Winter 1977–78), 46–49;

Richard Gull, "The Anti-Metaphysics Game: A Wittgensteinian Reading of *The Crying Game*," in *Film and Knowledge: Essays on the Integration of Images and Ideas*, ed. Kevin L. Stoehr (Jefferson, N.C.: McFarland, 2002), 81–94; Kay Young, *Ordinary Pleasures: Couples, Conversation, and Comedy* (Columbus: Ohio State University Press, 2001). Several other essays in *Film and Knowledge* also touch upon Wittgenstein's ideas, as do Stanley Cavell's essays on film.

3. In this book I adopt a tripartite division for describing motility: *Motion* is the subjective experience, *movement* is the objective act (i.e., an object in action), and *mobility* is the quality. *Move, moving, movable* denote the general case and make no commitment as to the three kinds. For example, a causal theory of perception might claim that a percept of motion has been created by the movement of an object that materializes mobility, and, more generally, the act of perception might be characterized as a "movement" of sense-data. Note that a similar tripartite division describes an abstract form of moving: *inference* is the mental process, *implication* is the objective act (of a speaker who indirectly expresses something), and *implicitness* is the quality. For example, a causal theory of communication might claim that what a perceiver infers has been implied by a speaker and is an implicit quality of the message. More controversial, perhaps, would be a tripartite division of narrative: plot (subjective), story (objective), and screen (quality). I will be concerned throughout this chapter with the similarities between literal and abstract forms of moving. We will discover that abstract forms of moving are often metaphorical projections designed to capture some aspect of an event as it is experienced within a social frame (e.g., the act of communication being characterized as a "movement" of ideas).

The distinction between motion and movement has a neurological parallel. A certain kind of brain injury leads to a person being unable to experience the motion associated with an object's continuous change in position, though the person sees that a movement has occurred — that an object has changed position — after the fact: Steam looks like a solid, and a cup does not fill gradually but is seen to be empty and then full. R. H. Hess, C. L. Baker, Jr., and J. Zihl, "The 'Motion-Blind' Patient: Low-Level Spatial and Temporal Filters," *The Journal of Neuroscience* 9, 5 (May 1989), 1628–1640. There may be an anlogue to this condition in film. Consider how the jump cuts of Jean-Luc Godard's *À bout de souffle* (*Breathless*, 1960) suppress motion while forcing a spectator to try to reconstitute it after the fact through the evident movements of things. A more subtle representation of the passage of time through the suppression of motion may be found in the "incremental variations" of Ozu films. See Edward Branigan, "The Space of *Equinox Flower*," in *Close Viewings: An Anthology of New Film Criticism*, ed. Peter

Lehman (Tallahassee: Florida State University Press, 1990), esp. 82–87, 98–103.

There is also a kind of neurological impairment in which a person can properly perceive an object *only* when it is moving, not stationary. The very technology of cinema mimics this condition, because without the movement of film through a projector there would be no picture in motion on the screen. In addition, consider how camera movement or editing may be used to clarify an ambiguous image or to reveal that an initial impression was mistaken.

4. I am thinking of the author as a narrative "argument" in several senses of argument, specifically, the author as: that which seeks to be *persuasive* in a discourse; as the *effect* of a felt persuasion; as that which we take to be a *summary* of the importance of some part of a work; as the *sum* of the relations that we imagine between assumptions, premises, and conclusions of a work; as an *analogy* to the substantive required by a predicate in grammar (e.g., the grammar we may employ in talking about a work); as an *independent variable* upon whose value a function depends; as the *particular value* assigned to a variable in a logical proposition. See generally, Edward Branigan, "Diegesis and Authorship in Film," *Iris* 7, v. 4, n. 2 (1986), 37–54. On the author as a "narrative" form of argument, see Branigan, *Narrative Comprehension and Film* (New York and London: Routledge, 1992).

5. Wittgenstein, *Philosophical Investigations*, §§ 455–57; cf. § 1.

6. Plato, op. cit., *Timaeus*, 20b.

7. Arguments by Socrates against artist-imitators may be found in Books 2, 3, and 10 of Plato's *Republic*.

8. What might count as camera "movement" (including cases in which there is no motion on the screen) was first raised as an issue in the final three sections of chapter 2.

9. The density of implications that emerge from the word "projection" already suggests a range of issues that will need to be addressed in order to understand some of the possibilities for deploying the term "camera." Consider the implications for film of these common projective activities: displaying, screening, perceiving, mapping, screening out, filling in, extrapolating, transforming, attributing, and scheming. In what ways might a literal or figurative experience of "motion" be connected to a projection of "movement"? See also Stephen Mamber, "Narrative Mapping," in *New Media: Theories and Practices of Digitextuality*, ed. Anna Everett and John T. Caldwell (New York: Routledge, 2003), 145–58. In another realm (that of the description of space and time in theories of quantum gravity), consider the revolutionary idea of the "holographic principle," whereby any "thing" may be completely described through its "projection" on a "screen." See, e.g., Lee Smolin, *Three*

Roads to Quantum Gravity (New York: Basic Books, 2001), chap. 12, "The Holographic Principle," 169–78.

10. See, e.g., Joseph D. Anderson, *The Reality of Illusion: An Ecological Approach to Cognitive Film Theory* (Carbondale: Southern Illinois University Press, 1996), 54–65, 90–110; Alain Berthoz, *The Brain's Sense of Movement*, trans. Giselle Weiss (Cambridge, Mass.: Harvard University Press, 2000); Richard L. Gregory, *Eye and Brain: The Psychology of Seeing* (Princeton, N.J.: Princeton University Press, 5th ed. 1997), 98–120; and a more technical book, Maurice Hershenson, *Visual Space Perception: A Primer* (Cambridge, Mass.: MIT Press, 1999). Far more than five senses exist (consider, for example, the vestibular senses; proprioceptors of the muscles and joints; and senses of space, balance, color, effort, and self); movement is sometimes considered the sixth sense. Movement and motion are often the focal points for a discussion of the nature of time in cinema and sometimes for claims about the nature of cinema. See, e.g., Arthur C. Danto, "Moving Pictures," in *Philosophizing Art: Selected Essays* (Berkeley and Los Angeles: University of California Press, 1999), 205–32; Mary Ann Doane, "Temporality, Storage, Legibility: Freud, Marey, and the Cinema," *Critical Inquiry* 22, 2 (Winter 1996), 313–43; but cf. David Bordwell, *Narration in the Fiction Film* (Madison: University of Wisconsin Press, 1985), chap. 6, "Narration and Time," 74–98. Note also that digital recording and playback systems for sound are based, like the hyper-photography of film, on principles of sampling and mental reconstruction.

11. Incidentally, Einstein's special theory of relativity prohibits only objects with finite mass (energy) from movements exceeding the speed of light. Other kinds of motion in the world may occur at velocities greater than the speed of light, for example, the rapid expansion of *space* in the early inflationary universe, the recession velocity of distant galaxies due to an ongoing expansion of space, and the point of intersection of wave fronts from two supernova. Perhaps the most profound and mysterious example of all is the instantaneous collapse of *probability* waves associated with the quantum mechanical properties of spatially distant entangled particles.

12. Jean Mitry, *The Aesthetics and Psychology of the Cinema*, trans. Christopher King (Bloomington, Ind.: Indiana University Press, 1997), 185 (original emphasis) from Part IV, "Rhythm and Moving Shots," 168–275.

13. Mitry, *The Aesthetics and Psychology of the Cinema*, 189 (original emphasis).

14. Further details on the psychophysics of continuity editing may be found in Anderson, *The Reality of Illusion*, chap. 6, "Continuity," 90–110. Putting two different movements together in a "match on action" is a special case. In general, a wide range of new effects (emergent motions) can be achieved by juxtaposing shots containing motions that have different speeds and

directions occurring at different distances and places in the image as well as in different perspectives by using, for example, lenses of different focal lengths. See, e.g., Rudolf Arnheim, *Film as Art* (Berkeley and Los Angeles: University of California Press, 1957), "Motion" [orig. 1934], 181–87.

15. Gilles Deleuze, *Cinema 1: The Movement-Image*, trans. Hugh Tomlinson and Barbara Habberjam (Minneapolis: University of Minnesota Press, 1986) and *Cinema 2: The Time-Image*, trans. Hugh Tomlinson and Robert Galeta (Minneapolis: University of Minnesota Press, 1989).

16. Since schemata will be mentioned several times in this chapter, I will briefly describe this concept from cognitive psychology. A person's knowledge does not consist of a list of unconnected facts but, rather, *coheres* in specifiable ways. A schema is one type of mental structure that makes knowledge cohere. A schema may be thought of as a graded set of expectations about experience in a given domain based on interpretations of past experience. It is not a "copy" of reality nor a collection of memories of sounds and images, but a set of expectations and skills based on a cluster of categories along with relevant constraints. This arrangement of knowledge is used to recognize, fill in, simplify, modify, recombine, order, classify, and predict new sensory data. Its effects are due *not to semiotic* codes (nor differential position, negative contrasts, arbitrary rules, or induction alone) but, rather, to *inferences* (as well as abduction, modeling, projection, hypotheses, exemplification, prototypes, metaphor, templates, trial and error, positive comparisons, judging probability, and other reasoning strategies). A schema does not determine the nature of events or objects through necessary and sufficient conditions. Instead, it is like an explanatory heuristic designed to quickly solve problems and to regulate attention and behavior in everyday situations. Knowledge is arranged in a hierarchy, from tentative and contingent conclusions about data (including "default" specifications) at one extreme to increasingly more probable, general, and invariant specifications governing a class or classes of data at the other extreme. A schema tests and refines sensory data at the same time that the data is testing the adequacy of the (implicit) criteria embodied in the schema. There are an enormous number of schemata of various types (e.g., template, prototype, procedural, and self-schemata), including ones that guide social behavior and put ideology into action. A schema is arranged in a (tangled) hierarchy with other super- and subframes of knowledge. I will discuss some of these frames of knowledge in the section of the text below entitled "When." See, e.g., Ulric Neisser, *Cognition and Reality: Principles and Implications of Cognitive Psychology* (San Francisco: W.H. Freeman, 1976); Ziva Kunda, *Social Cognition: Making Sense of People* (Cambridge, Mass.: MIT Press, 1999); Susan T. Fiske and Shelley E. Taylor, *Social*

Cognition (New York: McGraw-Hill, 2nd ed. 1991); Mark Johnson, *The Body in the Mind: The Bodily Basis of Meaning, Imagination, and Reason* (Chicago: University of Chicago Press, 1987); Mary Crawford and Roger Chaffin, "The Reader's Construction of Meaning: Cognitive Research on Gender and Comprehension," in *Gender and Reading: Essays on Readers, Texts, and Contexts*, ed. Elizabeth A. Flynn and Patrocinio Schweickart (Baltimore: Johns Hopkins University Press, 1986), 3–30.

17. Notice that the mental images of the "cameras" described in the text are not accompanied by sound. If these are the sorts of images of a camera that prevail, then we will be led toward the idea that the medium of film is essentially visual. I do not believe that a *medium* is defined only by its mechanical elements; that is, representation cannot be reduced to causal mechanics. Cf. James Lastra, "Reading, Writing, and Representing Sound," in *Sound Theory/Sound Practice*, ed. Rick Altman (New York: Routledge, 1992), 65–86.

18. Adam Abrams adds to the difficulties of speaking with James Bond in person:

> To extend Edward Branigan's analogy from "*When* Is a Camera?" if we could, like Buster Keaton in *Sherlock, Jr.* pass from our perspective in the audience into the fictional world of the film *Dr. No*, we might be able to meet and talk to James Bond. Bond, however, would be unaware of himself in many of the ways we might think of him — as, say, a symbol of Great Britain, a male fantasy-figure, an icon of patriarchy, etc. He might be perfectly willing to let us drive his Aston Martin, but he wouldn't recognize himself in the way we do — he'd only be aware of those roles which exist in his own (fictional) life — spy, Agent 007, lothario, etc.

"Rules of *This* Game: *Chinese Roulette* and the Spectator Experience" (University of California, Santa Barbara: unpub. ms., 2000), 9.

19. The examples that I discuss from *The Threepenny Opera* and *The Great Train Robbery* were suggested in 1999 by an anonymous reviewer of this chapter as counterexamples to my argument. However, for reasons stated in the text, I believe that the examples support the argument.

20. If I were to extend the line of reasoning employed at the end of chapter 2 and throughout chapter 4, then I would say that the goal is not to eliminate the gap between a spotlight and moonlight nor to reduce one to the other but, rather, to provide a series of intermediate conceptual links that preserve the causal efficacy of both the spotlight and the moonlight.

21. Here is another way of stating the argument that the causation of fictions cannot be reduced to the physical causation producing a fiction. If interpreting fictionally is analogous to ascribing the subjunctive mood to a sentence (a counterfactual conditional), then my claim would be that no list of indicative statements (about, say, spotlights, costumes, and actors) will add up to the subjunctive mood even though, for example, both the subjunctive and the indicative are expressed by "words" and both involve "reasons" for occurrences of interest.

The rationale for speaking of "adjacent" causatives is that the spotlight/moonlight problem seems to represent a "boundary" between causal realms. One almost wants to say that the spotlight and moonlight "cause each other" — to say that the need for moonlight causes a spotlight to be used, which is the reason that the moon gives light onstage. This violates the logic of the traditional concept of causation, however; that is, the effect of a cause cannot also be a cause of the cause, because then the effect would be a cause of itself, a cause *prior to* itself that has worked backward in time to create itself as a future effect. One might also be tempted to think of the spotlight as "sustaining" the moonlight much as table legs sustain and hold steady a tabletop that, in turn, sustains the legs in an upright fashion. The difficulty with employing sustaining causation in this case is that one still has no explanation for how electricity in the spotlight can truly interact with, and sustain, the light of the moon unless one reduces moonlight to a spotlight; but in this reductive case, of course, the fiction has been erased. (Sustaining causes will be discussed in more detail later in the chapter.) Another possibility would be to argue that our notion of a spotlight belongs to our model of the "concrete" world, while the moonlight belongs to another, superordinate model of the world. This is a more promising line of thought. I will consider a number of these "world models" in the section of the text below entitled "When." For the moment, it is enough to say that a given causative expression must be used *relative* to the appropriate world model. As one learns more about a given world, new models are created for new problems and projects.

22. "Supervenience" is a relation whereby elements of one type depend on — are supervenient on — elements of a different type. The types of elements involved in the relation might be properties, qualities, facts (including social, historical, and evolutionary facts), discourse, conceptual ranges, mental processes, or physical processes. The dependence relation is such that whenever there is a change in the elements of the supervening type, there must also be a change in the elements of the other, subvenient type, though there could be a change in the subvenient elements with no change in the supervenient elements. No causal or logical relation holds between the two groups of elements, nor is one group reducible or identical to the other. This means that any new group of subvenient ele-

ments that is found to be identical to the original set of subvenient elements will itself be in a relation of supervenience with a group of elements identical to those paired with the original set. For example, if something is judged to be "good" in one set of (subvenient) circumstances, then something new must also be "good" when the new circumstances are identical in all pertinent respects to the old circumstances. A thing is characterized as "good" (as supervening) only in *consequence* of possessing some other set of subvenient characteristics known as the "supervenience base." Another example: It may be argued that mental properties (including at least intentional states if not sensory experiences) are supervenient on neurobiological properties and/or physical-chemical properties. "Beauty" may also be a supervenient property. Supervenience is used to model a thing in terms of a *hierarchy* of connected levels. It should perhaps be contrasted to the notion of a "heterarchy" discussed in the previous chapter as a model for "radial meaning."

23. Cf. the spotlight-mentioned-as-moonlight with Nelson Goodman's concept of "expression" as "metaphorical exemplification." See *Languages of Art: An Approach to a Theory of Symbols* (Indianapolis: Hackett Publishing, 2nd ed., 1976), "Expression," 85–95.

24. Noël Carroll, *The Philosophy of Horror, or Paradoxes of the Heart* (New York: Routledge, 1990), 95–96 (my emphases). See also Branigan, *Narrative Comprehension and Film*, chap. 7, "Fiction," 192–217; Murray Smith, "Film Spectatorship and the Institution of Fiction," *The Journal of Aesthetics and Art Criticism* 53, 2 (Spring 1995), 113–27.

25. Although emotions felt by an audience member cannot be identical in all respects to those of a character, it would be wrong to assume that therefore *all* emotions a spectator feels must be completely detached and distant from a character on the model of a spectator who feels pity or laughs at a character's suffering rather than feeling the suffering. Reactions by an audience to a character's situation may be closely related to a character's emotions in a multitude of ways. See, e.g., *Passionate Views: Film, Cognition, and Emotion*, ed. Carl Plantinga and Greg M. Smith (Baltimore, Md.: Johns Hopkins University Press, 1999); Torben Grodal, *Moving Pictures: A New Theory of Film Genres, Feelings, and Cognition* (New York: Oxford University Press, 1997); Ed S. Tan, *Emotion and the Structure of Narrative Film: Film as an Emotion Machine*, trans. Barbara Fasting (Mahwah, N.J.: Lawrence Erlbaum, 1996); Murray Smith, *Engaging Characters: Fiction, Emotion, and the Cinema* (New York: Oxford University Press, 1995); Per Persson, *Understanding Cinema: A Psychological Theory of Moving Imagery* (Cambridge: Cambridge University Press, 2003), esp. chap. 4, "Character Psychology and Mental Attribution," 143–246; Greg M. Smith, *Film Structure and the Emotion System* (Cambridge: Cambridge University Press, 2003); Torben Grodal,

"Film, Character Simulation, and Emotion," in *Nicht allein das Laufbild auf der Leinwand . . . Strukturen des Films als Erlebnispotentiale*, ed. Jörg Friess, Britta Hartmann, and Eggo Müller (Berlin: Vistas Verlag, 2001), 115–27; Norbert Wiley, "Emotion and Film Theory," *Studies in Symbolic Interaction* 26 (New York: JAI, Elsevier Science, 2003), 169–87. See also Patrick Colm Hogan, *Cognitive Science, Literature, and the Arts: A Guide for Humanists* (New York: Routledge, 2003), chaps. 6 and 7, 140–90.

26. The human visual system works to construct what David Marr calls an "object-centered description" of space and depth, which is *independent* of our position, distance, and angle of view; that is, what we see is not an image like the one on the retina. See, e.g., Marr, *Vision: A Computational Investigation into the Human Representation and Processing of Visual Information* (San Francisco: W.H. Freeman, 1982); and *Visual Cognition*, ed. Steven Pinker (Cambridge, Mass.: MIT Press, 1984). There is a connection here between the idea of a spectator who is not literally confined to the lens of the camera and the idea of a type of film narration based on "invisible observation" in which there is no invisible observer to literally possess each view. Cf. note 41 in chapter 4 above.

27. According to Julian Hochberg and Virginia Brooks, "The fact is that we must parse most of the motion patterns we encounter [in watching film and in visual cognition generally] in terms of *purposeful* acts, not in terms of physically specifiable trajectories." Hochberg and Brooks explain that perception relies on schemata:

> [V]ery shortly after it has occurred [on the order of 1,200 milliseconds], the representation of an event, or of a part of an event, is *different* from the perception obtained during the event itself. Some specific physical information about space and time is lost with time. We assume that such losses occur as well after each change in direction or speed, or after each cutaway or change in scene. That is, unless the viewer has available some mental structure or schematic event into which the segments take their place, *and from which they can be regenerated when needed*, the continual movement in space becomes indeterminate in memory. . . . [Thus] most moving pictures are not assemblies of simple physical trajectories [or based on simple physical laws].

Hochberg and Brooks add, "It certainly does not take some ninety minutes to review in our minds the average movie's representation." "Movies in the Mind's Eye," in *Post-Theory: Reconstructing Film Studies*, ed. David Bordwell and Noël Carroll (Madison, Wis.: University of Wisconsin Press, 1996), 374,

379 (my emphasis of "purposeful" and "different"); see also 373. See also Anderson, *The Reality of Illusion*, chap. 6, "Continuity," 90–110.

A fundamental consideration in understanding the mind is the fact that, because of limited resources, the mind must manage energy. The nature of "mental representation" is in part a response to this problem of energy management. For example, the mind creates only a 2½-dimensional sketch of space, not a full 3-dimensional representation (which would quickly become unmanageable). The brain makes use of special schemata and procedures to access certain features of a spatial layout only when, and if, needed. That is, the brain lets the world itself store certain kinds of spatial information (the final ½-dimension). Moreover, this suggests that there is not a sharp divide between mind and world — an idea that I sought to illustrate from a different perspective in chapter 4 by analyzing the relation between language and world. See Marr, *Vision*; and Steven Pinker, *How the Mind Works* (New York: W.W.Norton & Co., 1997), sect. "Seeing in Two and a Half Dimensions," 256–61, and 137–38, 141. See also Peggy La Cerra and Roger Bingham, *The Origin of Minds: Evolution, Uniqueness, and the New Science of the Self* (New York: Harmony Books, 2002).

Here is another, more prosaic example of energy management. A squirrel does not memorize all of the locations where it has buried nuts but, instead, *knows how* to search for where they might have been buried (i.e., knows a routine, possesses a repertoire of actions). Perhaps some of the analytical terms discussed in chapter 2 have a *procedural* component so that part of their "meaning" is distributed in the film itself; that is, the meaning is partly unspecified and dependent on the interaction with a particular film. This approach is in line with my attempt to rework the question of meaning in the first section of chapter 3 and in chapter 4. Note that this approach to thinking puts much greater weight on procedures, practices, acting, heuristics, schematizing, and attending to transient assessments of information than it does on the construction of detailed mental models that are meant to accompany a thick stream of internal (semiotic) representations and/or inner expressions. Thus, a "pattern" is not defined simply by its existence in the physical world. See discussion of Daniel Dennett's "mild realism" in the text accompanying note 45 in chapter 4 above.

28. See Branigan, *Narrative Comprehension and Film*, sect. "How Many Cameras Are in a Film?," 157–60, and also 144–45. On narration and its levels (in which each level produces a distinct "camera"), see 63–124. Instead of describing levels of narration as "superimposed," one might say "supervenient." See note 22 above. In *Narrative Comprehension and Film* and in the text above, I refer to levels of narration as being "higher" according to their greater communicative "power"; in the language of supervenience, however, a higher-level narration

(e.g., an implied authorial narration) would act as the supervenience base for a lower-level (supervening) narration (e.g., a point-of-view shot).

29. Christian Metz, "The Imaginary Signifier," in *The Imaginary Signifier: Psychoanalysis and the Cinema*, trans. Celia Britton, Annwyl Williams, Ben Brewster, and Alfred Guzzetti (Bloomington: Indiana University Press, 1982), 51.

30. Compare, for instance, the neo-Bazinian account of photography in Stanley Cavell's *The World Viewed: Reflections on the Ontology of Film* (Cambridge, Mass.: Harvard University Press, enlarged edition 1979) with Christian Metz's fundamental rethinking of the relationship of photography to film (i.e., the effect on us of a "camera" when one watches a film) in "*Trucage* and the Film" [orig. 1972], *Critical Inquiry* 3, 4 (Summer 1977), 657–75 and "Photography and Fetish," *October* 34 (Fall 1985), 85 (". . . film is less a succession of photographs than, to a large extent, a destruction of the photograph. . . ."). In the spirit of Metz's argument, one may ask how many cameras are seen in a split screen? In a special effect in which the effects of the camera(s) are not seen? Some of André Bazin's important essays may be found in *What Is Cinema?*, vols. I and II, trans. Hugh Gray (Berkeley and Los Angeles: University of California Press, 1967 and 1971).

Metz's work illustrates a general shift in film theory away from questions of ontology, aesthetics, and realism toward epistemology, ideology, and history. In this chapter I will treat the notion of "identity" (an ontological question) as an interlocked set of *relatively* entrenched "descriptions" in a given world. In the language of supervenience, the search for a reductive ontology of film (the essence of the medium) has been replaced by so-called "wide-content" epistemological properties of film (descriptions) supervening on a base that extends beyond the current intrinsic physical characteristics that instantiate the supervening properties. See generally, *The MIT Encyclopedia of the Cognitive Sciences*, ed. Robert A. Wilson and Frank C. Keil (Cambridge, Mass.: MIT Press, 1999), "Supervenience," 812–14; Nelson Goodman and Catherine Z. Elgin, *Reconceptions in Philosophy and Other Arts and Sciences* (Indianapolis, Ind.: Hackett Publishing, 1988); W.J.T. Mitchell, *Picture Theory: Essays on Verbal and Visual Representation* (Chicago: University of Chicago Press, 1994); W.J.T. Mitchell, *Iconology: Image, Text, Ideology* (Chicago: University of Chicago Press, 1986).

If our comprehension of a film is not essentially photographic, one may argue that for the same reasons our comprehension of a photograph is not, or need not be, essentially photographic. Even though this may be true, I maintain that our comprehension of the "photographic" is different in the two media. When we know that we're looking at still photos, we calibrate our expectations to fit the medium at hand so that, for example, "objectivity" will be something a bit different in a photograph than in a film because objectivity must contrast with another possibility for "subjectivity" in a photograph than in a film, and "movement" will be seen to exist in photography in a less literal kind of way because immobility in photography is not the same as immobility in film. (In still photography, movement is depicted through the use of various pictorial techniques such as blurring together with special kinds of compositions, subject matter, and conventions, as in Étienne-Jules Marey's fixed-plate geometric chronophotography.) On the other hand, a freeze frame in film is not equivalent to a still photo because in the film we've *already* seen that it can move and, moreover, we've already *heard* it move. (Sound is generated by a movement in the world that disturbs the medium of air.) In general, our reaction to an image is primed to work within a frame of reference, and changing the medium (the conditions of viewing) changes the frame. My use of the word "medium" here is not meant to presuppose an ontology but merely refers to an ordinary, social judgment made at a particular time about how some properties of some materials, processes, and uses may be taken to form a group (a context, a medium). The elements of the group, as well as our judgments of the nature of the group, may change. For a complementary view, see Kevin Fisher, "Tracing the Tesseract: A Conceptual Prehistory of the Morph," in *Meta-Morphing: Visual Transformation and the Culture of Quick-Change*, ed. Vivian Sobchack (Minneapolis: University of Minnesota Press, 2000), 103–29 ("Unlike still photography, moving images actualize the intentional space of the image, implying a thickness to things, transforming the human face from Barthes's death mask into Balázs's living *microphysiognomy*"; 118, original emphasis, footnotes omitted.)

Noël Carroll argues that one always expects motion from still images in a film because of our prior knowledge about the nature of the film apparatus — the nature of the medium — but only during a first viewing of the film. For Carroll, our expectations change decisively on a second viewing. I believe that this depends on what one means by "viewing" a film, however. We may continue to feel suspense, horror, and other effects of a film even though we have previously seen the film. Similarly, an absolute rationality concerning whether something moves or not on a first viewing may not so easily usurp all imaginative re-viewings. It seems to me that some cognitive film theories are too limited by their emphasis on a first viewing, on immediate cues on the screen, on the determining shape of style, and on the irreversible time of plot presentation. I do not believe that these factors mechanically generate all of the important effects of a film in the way that a projector unwinds a reel of film. Moreover, these sorts of factors make the object seem far too precise and relegate "vagueness" to spectators who are generating "interpretations." See Noël Carroll, "Defining the Moving Image," in *Theorizing the Moving Image* (Cambridge: Cambridge University Press, 1996), 65. Cf. note 60 in chapter 2 above.

31. What sort of 'fact' may be depicted in a picture or photograph? Suppose that we are looking at a picture and we see the angled corners of a geometrical figure, but other parts of the picture are 'hazy' so that we cannot determine the exact number of sides of the figure or figures. We might conclude that the picture depicts an indeterminable figure and perhaps more than one, or, alternatively, we might conclude that the picture depicts something indeterminate, a set of figures, not all of which are present — say, those figures with three, four, or five sides within a certain range of sizes and ratios of sides. (That is, we believe that a number of figures *may* be made out of the angled corners in a variety of ways.) If the picture were a photograph, we might be inclined toward the first interpretation — that is, that there was once a determinate figure or figures in front of the camera but that now we are unable to determine the precise number of their sides. But is this the only conclusion that we may reach about a photograph? Is it always true that the manner in which a picture was made determines (or is even relevant to) what it refers to or means? I believe that at least for some photographs that are 'narrative' (i.e., that exemplify covering laws) and/or 'fictional,' what may be depicted is 'more' than what was once visible in front of the camera lens. These photographs are indeterminate (fuzzy, out of focus) in the second sense above: They may depict a sample or class of things, or a possible subset of such a class, without showing each and every member of the class or relevant subset. Thus, these photographs are figuratively blurry and sometimes, in addition, literally blurry. It may even be the case that a photograph is meant to represent a particular thing that was once in front of the lens (a singular occurrence) as well as the fact that the thing is *typical*. In short, it may be a fact that a photograph is blurry but the meaning of the blurriness may not be clear.

To put it differently, our thinking tends to slide too often from the fact of an object's *being*-in-front-of a camera to the object's having a *being*-in-common with the other objects that were in front of the camera (i.e., a realism). I do not claim that the photographic (being photographic) is in all cases not necessary to the meaning of a photograph. I am trying here to follow some of the strategies Wittgenstein employed in his later works: to avoid overgeneralizing, to look for or else to invent *intermediate* cases, and to say, 'in *some* cases, there is a difference.' For Wittgenstein, the 'looseness' or 'flexibility' of *resemblance* as a relation (as opposed to, say, 'necessity' or 'stipulation') is an advantage in clarifying how language (and engineering?) works. 'Resemblance' leads to 'gradations' of a category (as in radial meaning) rather than bright lines. In addition, the relation of 'resemblance' may be more responsive to a particular *way of looking* in a particular situation ('I see an intermediate case or a similarity with . . . and a connection to. . . .'). Wittgenstein is, thus, an embarrassment to reductive forms of analytic philosophy that seek the ultimate constituents of a thing and its logical structure — an analytic philosophy that strives to fashion a language in which things are either sharply focused/ resolved or dissolved/absent. See Wittgenstein, *Philosophical Investigations*, §§ 11–14, 122; and pp. 185, 198; cf. § 352.

Something about a photograph may indeed always be 'factual,' but it need not be because the photograph is photographic. Cf. René Descartes's assertion that neither a painting nor an image in the mind can be entirely false and fantastic in the "First Meditation: What can be called into doubt" of *Meditations on First Philosophy*, in *The Philosophical Writings of Descartes, Vol. II*, ed. John Cottingham, Robert Stoothoff, and Dugald Murdoch (Cambridge: Cambridge University Press, 1984), sixth and seventh paragraphs, 13–14. Note that instead of selecting 'angled corners' for my example of what may be in a picture or photograph, I could have 'focused' on other perceptible, and relative, properties of an object (e.g., color, location, orientation, texture, speed, melody). A range of important issues involving the relationship of photography to film may be found in Garrett Stewart, *Between Film and Screen: Modernism's Photo Synthesis* (Chicago: University of Chicago Press, 1999); and in Annette Michelson, Douglas Gomery, and Patrick Loughney, *The Art of Moving Shadows* (Washington, D.C.: National Gallery of Art, 1989). The issue of definiteness and indefiniteness was also discussed in notes 32 and 60 in chapter 2 above and in the text accompanying note 3 in chapter 3 above.

32. Cf. Wittgenstein, *Philosophical Investigations*, §§ 71, 76–77, 99.

33. See, e.g., Douwe Draaisma, *Metaphors of Memory: A History of Ideas about the Mind*, trans. Paul Vincent (Cambridge, U.K.: Cambridge University Press, 2000).

34. André Bazin's ontology, epistemology, and aesthetics of film may be limited in various ways. An extreme step, often taken, would be to reduce Bazin's theory to a simple claim about the spectator's strong "interest" in photographic "realism." This not only distorts the claims and subtleties of Bazin's theory but also leaves unexamined the enormously complicated issue of realism, many elements of which are *not visible* on the screen. This is not the place to survey the problem of realism; suffice it to say that for many (Anglo-American) spectators, Hitchcock's fictional narrative film *The Man Who Knew Too Much* (1956) is probably more realistic than Vertov's non-psychological though self-conscious, nonfictional and nonnarrative film *Man with a Movie Camera* (1929). Realism is not determined by how something comes to be, and looks to be, on the screen.

35. Throughout this chapter I will be emphasizing the importance of "ordinary language" in my discussions of such topics as causality, the ideas of Wittgenstein, abstract concepts as extensions of concrete models of the world (e.g., in the section below, "When"), as well as the nature of the ordinary discourse used by critics and spectators in speaking about a "camera." The importance of

ordinary language also means that *narrative* rhetoric — which is pervasive in our thinking about the world — should be of interest to philosophy. Narrative schemata constitute primary modes for knowledge representation and embody familiar forms of causation and causal efficacy. Accordingly, I make several references to narrative theory. I also mention some of the older, technical names for specific types of causation in the belief that this tradition captures at least a notion of "folk causality."

The historian Michel de Certeau summarizes three reasons that some twentieth-century philosophers have concentrated on the study of "ordinary language" in attempting to solve philosophical puzzles:

1. the usual ways of speaking do not have *any equivalent* in philosophical discourse and they cannot be translated into it because they are richer and more varied than it is; 2. [the usual ways of speaking] constitute a *reserve* of "distinctions" and "connections" accumulated by historical experience and stored up in everyday speech; 3. as linguistic *practices*, [the usual ways of speaking] manifest *logical complexities* unnoticed by scientific formalizations.

The Practice of Everyday Life, trans. Steven Rendall (Berkeley and Los Angeles: University of California Press, 1984), 12 (de Certeau's emphases; footnotes omitted).

36. On the problem of forms of causation that are too local and too strong, see Branigan, *Narrative Comprehension and Film*, sect. "Causality and Schema," 26–32.

37. Photographs are neither necessary nor sufficient for the truth of a documentary film. Furthermore, most documentaries make claims that are based on the fact that something being shown is in some way *typical*. But being a photograph does not guarantee being typical. See generally Trevor Ponech, "What is Non-fiction Cinema?" and Noël Carroll, "Fiction, Non-fiction, and the Film of Presumptive Assertion: A Conceptual Analysis," in *Film Theory and Philosophy*, ed. Richard Allen and Murray Smith (New York: Oxford University Press, 1997), 173–220; Carl R. Plantinga, *Rhetoric and Representation in Nonfiction Film* (Cambridge: Cambridge University Press, 1997); Branigan, *Narrative Comprehension and Film*, sect. "Nonfictional Pictures," 202–07.

38. Although normally one does not speak of a "negative" cause, I am here treating active forbearance as an act (to which, incidentally, legal liability may attach because in the proper circumstances forbearance will be deemed the "cause" of an event).

39. Apparently, not every physical change is caused; two examples are radio-active decay and energy fluctuations of the vacuum (as in the Casimir "effect"). It is a matter of debate whether there exist voluntary acts of agents that are uncaused.

40. Note that causes and actions have degrees of abstractness. For example, an action may be described in a relatively concrete way as "John sang 'happy birthday' to Chuck," but more abstractly as "John usually sings at parties," "John is musical," "John makes noises." Similarly, an "object" has degrees of literalness. For example, a specific object may be described as wooden, a table, a dining room table, a makeshift desk, a sort of shelf, or furniture. Causes at the appropriate level must be fit to the appropriate kind of object. I will return to the problem of "abstract" causes and "abstract" objects in the section below entitled "When." What degrees of abstractness can be attributed to the object camera? What actions are appropriate to it?

41. *Wittgenstein's Lectures*, Part I, § 15 (Wittgenstein's emphases).

42. John Searle's Chinese Room puzzle, introduced in 1980, would seem to have emerged from remarks by Wittgenstein in *Philosophical Investigations*; see, e.g., §§ 159, 162, 173, 344, and p. 176. Searle's puzzle remains a matter of current controversy. See, e.g., Robert I. Damper, "The Chinese Room Argument — Dead but Not Yet Buried," *Journal of Consciousness Studies* 11, nn. 5–6 (2004), 159–69.

43. *Philosophical Investigations*, § 621; see also §§ 611–13; on the danger of "assimilating descriptions," § 10. Cf. also *Wittgenstein's Lectures*, Part II (The Yellow Book), § 8. My interpretation in the text above of Wittgenstein's question (from § 621) should be compared with Arthur Danto's interpretation when he considers the distinction between "Works of Art and Mere Real Things," in chapter 1 of *The Transfiguration of the Commonplace: A Philosophy of Art* (Cambridge, Mass.: Harvard University Press, 1981), 4–6. See also Ludwig Wittgenstein, *Philosophical Occasions, 1912–1951*, ed. James C. Klagge and Alfred Nordmann (Indianapolis: Hackett, 1993), Appendix A, "Immediately Aware of the Cause" [notes taken by Rush Rhees, 1938], 410.

44. *Wittgenstein's Lectures*, ed. Ambrose, Part III, Michaelmas Term, Lecture V, p. 83.

45. On the perplexities of defining parts and objects (over which "causation" works), and on the relationships of parts and objects to ways of speaking, see, e.g., Wittgenstein, *Philosophical Investigations*, §§ 47–48, 59–64; cf. § 136; but cf. § 139(b). These perplexities extend equally to the problem of what counts as a word (a part) as opposed to a proposition (a whole); this distinction is not antecedently clear but depends on a situation, § 49. In addition,

a prominent concept in cognitive psychology (as well as in narratology) is a causal form of "expectation." Wittgenstein's analysis of expectation and similar words (§ 445) concludes with "It is in language that an expectation and its fulfillment make contact." See §§ 437–65; cf. §§ 487, 493, 495, 507. On the relationship of causal reasoning to metaphor and schemata, see, e.g., Branigan, *Narrative Comprehension and Film*, 20, 26–32, 33–34, 36, 39–40, 44–50, 116, 202–03. The relativity of parts and objects to a chosen frame (e.g., an expectation of a spectator in a narrative frame) suggests that the varieties of metonymy and synecdoche are truly unlimited and not susceptible to formal inventory.

Like Wittgenstein, Steven Pinker argues that language is intimately connected to both causation and thought:

> Space and force pervade language. Many cognitive scientists (including me) have concluded from their research on language that a handful of concepts about places, paths, motions, agency, and causation underlie the literal or figurative meanings of tens of thousands of words and constructions, not only in English but in every other language that has been studied. . . . These concepts and relations appear to be the vocabulary and syntax of mentalese, the language of thought. . . . And the discovery that the elements of mentalese are based on places and projectiles has implications for both where the language of thought came from and how we put it to use in modern times.

How the Mind Works, 355. See generally George Lakoff, *Women, Fire, and Dangerous Things: What Categories Reveal about the Mind* (Chicago: University of Chicago Press, 1987).

46. Wittgenstein's notion that an analogy may cause a misunderstanding should be compared with the Scholastics' idea of a *causa cognoscendi*, the reason or ground for — i.e., the cause of — a *truth*, which was distinguished from a *causa fiendi*, the cause of the existence of something. Cf. "casuistry." Note that one need not think of an "analogy" as a purely mental or conceptual relationship that causes either misunderstanding or understanding. Wittgenstein would probably argue that "analogies" might be found at least partially in the concrete ways that language is employed in our *behavior*. Cf. Wittgenstein, *Philosophical Investigations*, §§ 325, 475, 480, 630, 682. One would also need to think about how and when (i.e., under what circumstances) the word "mental" is used to mark something as being different from the "physical" and, hence, as requiring a different theory of causation in explaining a new sort of 'action-game' or "language-game"; see §§ 328, 360, 421, 608, 630, and pp. 179–80, 196; see also §§ 611–13, 621.

47. Stanley Cavell, *Cities of Words: Pedagogical Letters on a Register of the Moral Life* (Cambridge, Mass.: Harvard University Press, 2004), 33–34.

48. Wittgenstein, *Philosophical Occasions*, 397.

49. *Philosophical Investigations*, § 14 (Wittgenstein's emphasis). See also §§ 7, 10–13, 19; on "negation," §§ 547–51, 554–57; on "communication," §§ 3, 304, 356, 363, cf. §§ 491–92; on whether all games have a common nature, §§ 66–71, 75, 100; on a "form of life," §§ 19, 23, 241; on 'sustaining causes,' cf. § 421; on "assimilation," cf. § 607; on "language-games," §§ 7, 65.

    I use the term 'action-game' simply to emphasize one aspect of a "language-game." Wittgenstein characterizes the overall process of using words as follows: "I shall also call the whole, consisting of language and the *actions* into which it is woven, the 'language-game.'" (§ 7, my emphasis; see also §§ 37, 65) He says, "Here the term 'language-*game*' is meant to bring into prominence the fact that the *speaking* of language is part of an activity, or of a form of life." (§ 23, original emphasis) "And to imagine a language means to imagine a form of life." (§ 19) In Wittgenstein's example of a "language more primitive than ours" (a "complete primitive language"), one person "needs" a certain kind of stone in *building* a wall, calls out its name, and another person "brings" the stone (§ 2). In addition, finding "a new way of speaking" may lead to "a new sensation" and "a new way of looking at things": "As if you had invented a new way of painting; or, again, a new metre, or a new kind of song." (§§ 400–01) For Wittgenstein, a "form of life" is a particular intertwining of a culture, worldview, communal activities (goals, values, canons of rationality), and language. See Hans-Johann Glock, *A Wittgenstein Dictionary* (Oxford: Blackwell, 1996), "form of life," 124–29.

50. Performances, including, for example, knowing how to write and use language, play a musical instrument, and ride a bicycle, would perhaps today be referred to as "procedural" knowledge and ascribed to procedural schemata.

51. See *Wittgenstein's Lectures*, Part II (The Yellow Book), §§ 4, 6.

52. This example of a nearly vacuous causal formula about film is derived from André Bazin's description of "lateral depth of field," quoted in note 34 of chapter 3 above.

53. In my text I have borrowed and adapted some words and phrasing of Wittgenstein from *Philosophical Investigations*, §§ 173, 175, 177, 178. It would seem that one could watch a film in all of the ways that Wittgenstein lists in § 172 as examples of the experience of "being guided" and, doubtless, in other ways as well; also suggestive about 'watching' a film are his comments on "reading" in §§ 156–71.

54. *Philosophical Investigations*, §§ 23 (addendum), 73–74, cf. 420; p. 193; §§ 536–37, 539, pp. 209–10, cf. p. 199; pp. 206, 210; pp. 202, 206, 209.

See also p. 200. Seeing a thing's aspect as being particular or general would also seem to be related to seeing fictionally because Wittgenstein refers to a fiction as a "genre-picture"; §§ 518, 522, 525; cf. § 499. Cf. also § 99 ("indefinite sense") with Branigan, *Narrative Comprehension and Film*, chap. 7, "Fiction," 192–217 (fiction as "nonspecific" or "partially determined reference").

55. On the close kinship of aspects and word meanings, see *Philosophical Investigations*, pp. 210, 214.

56. I would argue that when a chess piece is used in a new context, such as to plug a hole, its *shape* appears under a new "aspect" (in the sense Wittgenstein uses the word "aspect"). In relation to the hole, its shape will be seen differently: Parts that were previously unimportant may now become salient, whereas other parts that were previously important go unnoticed. The shape of the chess piece is remodeled by our perception according to the way it may be seen to interact with the shape of the hole. One might contend that the properties of the chess piece appearing in the new circumstances were, in fact, already present when it was on the chessboard. But, if so, then how many properties are present within a chess piece (i.e., how many kinds of new circumstances might be imagined that may exist in the future in relation to the chess piece)? Similar remarks apply to the changing aspect of the *movement* of a chess piece when transferred from a chessboard to, say, a pendulum of a clock (i.e., when transferred from being part of a chess game to being part of a clock, or to being part of some other imaginable 'action-game').

Here's another example of this way of thinking. Some writers have said that the categories of classical, modern, and postmodern do not apply to the medium of film because film has *always possessed* a latent postmodernism (e.g., fluidity of space and time). If this is true, then exactly how many properties are present in the medium of film? As with the chess piece, this line of thinking allows one to find (to reinvent) whatever properties one wishes in a thing by reading backward in time. See *Reinventing Film Studies*, ed. Christine Gledhill and Linda Williams (New York: Oxford University Press, 2000).

57. Wittgenstein, *Philosophical Occasions*, 191.

58. The notion of a "camera" is tied up with our thinking about how we think when making sense of a narrative in film and equally about how a visible narrative acquires its meaning and circulates through society in a *verbal, synoptic* form. See esp. works by David A. Black, *Law in Film: Resonance and Representation* (Urbana: University of Illinois Press, 1999), chaps. 1, 2, and 5, 13–33, 34–51, and 99–108; "*Homo Confabulans*: A Study in Film, Narrative, and Compensation," *Literature and Psychology* 47, 3 (2001), 25–37; and, "Synopsis: A Theory of Symbolic Representation," *The Yale*

Journal of Criticism 10, 2 (Fall 1997), 423–36 (for corrected illustration, see v. 11, n. 1, Spring 1998, 313). Cf. Bryan Vescio's notion that film is a series of visual and aural metaphors endlessly paraphrasable; "Reading in the Dark: Cognitivism, Film Theory, and Radical Interpretation," *Style* 35, 4 (Winter 2001), 577–79. See also Robert Stam, *Subversive Pleasures: Bakhtin, Cultural Criticism, and Film* (Baltimore: Johns Hopkins University Press, 1989), chap. 2, "Language, Difference, and Power," 57–84; Henry Jenkins, *Textual Poachers: Television Fans and Participatory Culture* (New York: Routledge, 1992). For David Black:

> The cumulative verbal response to a film need not take the form of spoken words or even an inwardly audible running commentary. It may take such forms; but more fundamentally, and more exactly, it consists of the readiness to speak, the authority to recount the film. (*Law in Film*, 30; see also 26–27.)

59. David Bordwell claims that a camera is a vivid, "heuristic construct" made by critics to fit certain of their purposes within an institution and tradition of craft practices. He invites critics to scrutinize their presuppositions: "What is the basis for taking the image displayed on-screen to be the trace of 'the camera,' for assuming that camera to have a 'look,' for assigning that look to a filmmaker or narrator or enunciator or viewer?" (251) One might continue in this vein by asking whether the printed words in a novel are the trace of (what exactly?) the "pen" and whether we normally hear music as the trace of *objects* being plucked or blown into, or the trace of persons so doing. We *could imagine* such tracings, of course, and the savoring of a vibrato for its human touch, but this is not what we ordinarily do when we read or listen to music. See Bordwell's quite remarkable *Making Meaning: Inference and Rhetoric in the Interpretation of Cinema* (Cambridge, Mass.: Harvard University Press, 1989), esp. chaps. 5–9, 105–223, and on a camera, 162–64, 175–77, 251. See also his *Narration in the Fiction Film* (Madison: University of Wisconsin Press, 1985), 119–20.

For Jean-Louis Comolli, a camera serves dominant political and economic institutions rather than institutions of criticism. He argues that a camera is the result of an ideological demand for a certain kind of (bourgeois) realism in the image based on movement, depth, and canons of verisimilitude. See "Machines of the Visible," in *The Cinematic Apparatus*, ed. Teresa de Lauretis and Stephen Heath (New York: St. Martin's Press, 1980), 130 ("Contrary to what the technicians seem to believe, the restoration of movement and depth are not effects of the camera; it is the camera which is the effect, the solution to the problem of that restoration."). See also Comolli, "Mechanical Bodies, Ever More Heavenly," *October* 83 (Winter 1998), 20–21, but cf. 23 n. 5;

Jonathan L. Beller, "Capital/Cinema," in *Deleuze & Guattari: New Mappings in Politics, Philosophy, and Culture,* ed. Eleanor Kaufman and Kevin Jon Heller (Minneapolis: University of Minnesota Press, 1998), 77 ("[C]inematic movement is an extension of capital circulation: the cinematic image develops out of the commodity-form. . . .").

Another top-down conception of a camera is the approach of Kaja Silverman, who draws heavily on 1970s film theory and such writers as Jacques Lacan, Jean-Louis Baudry, Stephen Heath, and Jean-Louis Comolli. She finds that a camera is best defined by combining ideological and psychoanalytic terms because these terms are able to capture such crucial camera effects as the following: identification, mastery, suture, masking, disavowal, misrecognition (*méconnaissance*), mortification, trauma, the castration of the eye from the gaze, the look, memory, and a potential resistance to material practices. Some of these effects are exploited only in some films; that is, only some cameras are subversive and progressive. See "What Is a Camera?, or: History in the Field of Vision," *Discourse* 15, 3 (Spring 1993), 3–56. Silverman asserts:

> In fact, the only truly productive gaze in the cinema is that of the camera; that gaze produces the images with which the viewer identifies, and which he or she loves. In short, the camera "looks" the viewer as subject [sic]. However, just as a shot of a character within the fiction engaged in the activity of seeing functions to cover over the camera's coercive gaze, so the representation of the male subject [male viewer] in terms of vision has the effect of attributing to him qualities which in fact belong to that same apparatus [the camera] — qualities of potency and authority.

Kaja Silverman, *The Subject of Semiotics* (New York: Oxford University Press, 1983), 223.

For a very different approach to the ideological ground of film and its devices, see, e.g., *Post-Theory: Reconstructing Film Studies,* ed. David Bordwell and Noël Carroll, (Madison: University of Wisconsin Press, 1996) and Melinda Szaloky, who analyzes the representation of women within patriarchy by using feminist linguistics, social cognition, and Pierre Bourdieu's notion of the *habitus* in "Silence Fiction: Rethinking (Under)Representations of the 'Feminine' Through Social Cognition," *CiNéMAS* 12, 2 (Winter 2002), 89–115 (special issue on "Cinema and Cognition"); and in Szaloky, *Silence Fiction: Women's Voice and Film* (University of Oslo: M.A. Thesis in Media Science, 1999).

60. John Kreidl, *Jean-Luc Godard* (Boston: Twayne Publishers, 1980), 135–36 (original emphasis).

61. Jean-Louis Baudry, "Ideological Effects of the Basic Cinematographic Apparatus," in *Narrative, Apparatus, Ideology: A Film Theory Reader*, ed. Philip Rosen (New York: Columbia University Press, 1986), 292; Jean Mitry, *Esthétique et psychologie du cinéma* (Paris: Presses Universitaires de France, 1965), 179 (Mitry's emphasis).

62. *Hugo Münsterberg on Film: The Photoplay — A Psychological Study and Other Writings*, ed. Allan Langdale (New York: Routledge, 2002), 91; Münsterberg, *The Film — A Psychological Study: The Silent Photoplay in 1916* (New York: Dover Publications, 1970, o.p.; orig. 1916), 41.

63. Jean Epstein, "The Cinema Continues" [orig. 1930], in *French Film Theory and Criticism: A History/Anthology, 1907–1939 (Vol. II: 1929–1939)*, ed. Richard Abel (Princeton, N.J.: Princeton University Press, 1988), 64.

64. Jean Epstein, "On Certain Characteristics of *Photogénie*" [orig. 1923], in "Bonjour Cinéma and Other Writings," *Afterimage* 10 (Autumn 1981), 21.

65. Some of the ideas of Kracauer and Benjamin are discussed in chapter 4.

66. Jean Epstein, "*Photogénie* and the Imponderable" [orig. 1935], in *French Film Theory and Criticism*, 189. Malcolm Turvey connects Epstein's ideas to Wittgenstein's notion of "aspect-dawning" in "Jean Epstein's Cinema of Immanence: The Rehabilitation of the Corporeal Eye," *October* 83 (Winter 1998), 25–50.

67. Deleuze, *Cinema 2: The Time-Image* [orig. 1985], 23 (original ellipsis points). For another approach to what Deleuze refers to as a "camera-consciousness" that moves "in accordance with the functions of thought," see Bruce F. Kawin, *Mindscreen: Bergman, Godard, and First-Person Film* (Princeton, N.J.: Princeton University Press, 1978); and Kawin, "An Outline of Film Voices," *Film Quarterly* 38, 2 (Winter 1984–85), 38–46.

What follows is an extensive comment on the nature of a camera offered by Deleuze during an interview:

As for the camera, with all its propositional functions, it's a sort of third eye, the mind's eye. You [the two interviewers] cite Hitchcock: he does, it's true, bring the viewer into the film, as Truffaut and Douchet have shown. But that's nothing to do with the look. It's rather because he frames the action in a whole network of relations. Say the action's a crime. Then these relations are another dimension that allows the criminal to "give" his crime to someone else, to transfer or pass it on to someone else. Rohmer and Chabrol saw this really well. The relations aren't actions but symbolic acts that have a purely mental existence (gift, exchange, and so on). And they're what the camera reveals: framing and camera movement display mental relations. If Hitchcock's so English, it's because what interests him is the problem and the paradoxes of relation. The frame for him is like a tapestry frame: it holds within it the network of relations, while the action is just a thread moving in and out of the network. What Hitchcock thus brings into cinema is, then, the mental image. It's not a matter of the look, and if the camera's an eye, it's the mind's eye. So Hitchcock has a special place in cinema: he goes beyond the action-image to something deeper, mental relations, a kind of vision. Only, instead of seeing this as a breaking-down of the action image, and of the movement-image in general, he makes it a consummation, saturation, of that image. So you might equally well say he's the last of the classic directors, or the first of the moderns.

Gilles Deleuze, "On *The Movement-Image,*" in *Negotiations, 1972–1990,* trans. Martin Joughin (New York: Columbia University Press, 1995), 54–55; cf. 52. (The interview was conducted by Pascal Bonitzer and Jean Narboni in 1983.)

68. Gerald Mast, "On Framing," *Critical Inquiry* 11, 1 (September 1984), 102, including film stills (my emphases and square brackets).

69. G. E. Moore, "Wittgenstein's Lectures in 1930–33" (Part III), *Mind* 64, 253 (Jan. 1955): 18–19 (original emphases; my selection from Moore spans three paragraphs and comes from a lecture given by Wittgenstein in 1933); reprinted in Wittgenstein's *Philosophical Occasions, 1912–1951,* ed. James C. Klagge and Alfred Nordmann (Indianapolis: Hackett, 1993), 105–06.

For Wittgenstein, aesthetic "reasons" given in answer to the question "Why do you like it?" are "of the nature of further descriptions," and further descriptions are connected to what is judged to be "right" as defined by prototypes and ideals (what the thing is *like*). An "ideal," says Wittgenstein, arises from "a certain very complicated role it [plays] in the life of people." The purpose of aesthetic descriptions is to draw attention to specific features (in the exact way that Wittgenstein's "aspects" dawn, flash, or change) rather than to explain the features. By contrast, the question "Do you like it?" is not an aesthetic question for Wittgenstein. It is tied to science and psychology (e.g., whether the thing produced a pleasant feeling or is otherwise agreeable, or *likeable*); to answer this second question, one must examine symptoms (e.g., 'the film last night gave me a headache'), test empirical attributes of the artwork, form hypotheses, and verify the truth by finding "causes" and explanations. Aesthetic descriptions for Wittgenstein are not based on the science of psychology, which deals with causes, but derive instead from language-games, which deal with (the statement of) reasons and ideals. He says,

> The word "beauty" is used for a thousand different things. Beauty of face is different from that of flowers and animals. That one is playing utterly different [language-] games is evident from the difference that emerges in the discussion of each. We can only ascertain the meaning of the word "beauty" by seeing how we use it. (*Wittgenstein's Lectures*, ed. Ambrose, Part I, § 32; see §§ 31–35)

Basically, my response to Wittgenstein's distinction between "reasons" and "causes" is to transfer (dissolve?) the distinction into a greatly expanded notion of "cause." This has been one of my aims throughout the present chapter, such as in the sections "Camera Fiction" and "Sustaining and Other Causes" and the present section "When." I believe that my approach is consistent with both Wittgenstein's ideas and a second-generation cognitive science and, for that matter, consistent with many works of first-generation cognitive film theory, including the work of David Bordwell because he has been exemplary in locating a cognitive psychology of film viewing within historical settings and tasks, as Wittgenstein demands, for there is a crucial historical component to 'prototypes and ideals.' (Prototypes and ideals function somewhat like 'grammatical rules' in that they provide a standard or measure for assessing 'use' and offering 'reasons.') Wittgenstein's approach to aesthetic judgment focuses on top-down effects (intentional and internal effects on our judgment) rather than on external cues and causes from the artwork (bottom-up). The specific kinds of things that may be seen in an image will depend on what the rules of our interpretation allow us to say. Cognitive film theories, at least to an important degree, seek to address how these top-down judgments come to pass and how we construct reasons. One of the aims of many cognitive film theories is to investigate the (top-down) models of thought found in, for example, schemata, radial meanings, and prototypes — from which, in turn, spring 'reasons' and 'descriptions.' This is why cognitive film theory is partly misnamed: It is not so much a theory about film like the others but a way of thinking about the possibility of film theory — how one may make a theoretical claim through the use of a particular language and set of metaphors. Wittgenstein may be anti-Theory, but not antitheory. On expanding the notion of causation, see note 72 below. On some rules of interpretation, see, e.g., Bordwell, *Making Meaning*, and Thomas Elsaesser and Warren Buckland, *Studying Contemporary American Film: A Guide to Movie Analysis* (London: Arnold, 2002).

70. Other objects that do not qualify for our model of the concrete world are those that suddenly become soft, pass through one another, jump to a new

location, become their mirror image, be their mirror image simultaneously, disappear temporarily, are masked, or are composed of an instruction set (e.g., a grocery list or computer program). A number of the foregoing "fantastic" objects, however, may be useful in certain other descriptions of the world, such as in quantum physics.

Richard Scarry's children's books well dramatize our conception of push-pull causality by depicting a vast array of occurrences that splash, fall, spring up, ricochet, drip, fly out, or are motor driven. On our basic-level model of the concrete world and its causality, see, e.g., Robin Horton, "Tradition and Modernity Revisited," in *Rationality and Relativism*, ed. Martin Hollis and Steven Lukes (Cambridge: MIT Press, 1982), 201–60. Film scholars have drawn on this model to address such issues as the nature of character, the device of shot/reverse shot, and the art film. See Murray Smith, *Engaging Characters: Fiction, Emotion, and the Cinema* (Oxford: Oxford University Press, 1995), "The Person Schema and Primary Theory," 20–24; David Bordwell, "Convention, Construction, and Cinematic Vision," in *Post-Theory: Reconstructing Film Studies*, ed. David Bordwell and Noël Carroll (Madison: University of Wisconsin Press, 1996), 87–107; and Torben Kragh Grodal, "Art Film, the Transient Body, and the Permanent Soul," *Aura* 6, 3 (2000), 33–53.

71. "Basic-level" categories along with subordinate and superordinate categories were discussed in chapter 4. Basic-level concepts are one of the central discoveries of a second-generation cognitive science that deals with embodied processes of mind. See Lakoff and Johnson, *Philosophy in the Flesh*, 75–78, 90. On projections from basic-level concepts and on "folk-generic" knowledge (i.e., projections from what I have been calling the concrete, "living room" model of the world), see 26–30, 90–91. On language and 'basic-level causation,' see note 45 above.

72. Lakoff and Johnson, *Philosophy in the Flesh*, 30. In addition, Lakoff and Johnson argue that causality is understood in terms of a set of basic-level prototypes with "radial" extensions toward less central literal cases and then further outward toward various metaphorical descriptions of (real) causation. See chap. 11, "Events and Causes," 170–234. Wittgenstein was well aware of the complicated grammar of the word "cause" and its relevance to aesthetic issues. He analyzes the "cause-effect language-game" in terms of a person's intuitive sense — immediate awareness — of a prototypical situation (p. 373). This, I believe, makes the basic meaning of causation nonconscious, embodied, and radial. Wittgenstein, "Cause and Effect: Intuitive Awareness," from *Philosophical Occasions*, 368–426. See also *L. Wittgenstein: Lectures & Conversations on Aesthetics, Psychology and Religious Belief, Compiled from Notes taken by Yorick Smythies, Rush Rhees and James Taylor*, ed. Cyril

Barrett (Berkeley and Los Angeles: University of California Press, 1992), "Lectures on Aesthetics," Part II, 11–18. See also Glock, *A Wittgenstein Dictionary*, "causation," 72–76.

73. Ordinary containers are often used to conceptualize such abstractions as time, space, gestalt structure, mind, self, category, predication, and logical relationships. On container metaphors and the container schema, see, e.g., Lakoff and Johnson, *Philosophy in the Flesh*, 31–32, 117, 153, 156–51, 275, 338, 380–82, 544–45. Wittgenstein, like Lakoff and Johnson, questions the objectivity of such notions as category, proposition, logic, and language by, in effect, probing the limits of thinking in terms of containers; see, e.g., *Philosophical Investigations*, § 99 and §§ 88–122.

Notice that when the container schema is used to visualize a "camera" as a receptacle holding a film emulsion — such as Plato's wax tablet stored in the mind — one is forced by the nature of this "picture" of the camera to confront as a major issue the relationship between what is held inside (on the emulsion) and what remains outside. How was something outside removed or "taken" to the inside? What kinds of thing may be brought inside? Was the thing damaged or "distorted" in the process? What is the purpose of such a transfer and in what manner can the things brought inside be returned to the world? In preserving objects inside, is the camera like a "drawer" or more like a "tabletop" (considering the flatness of the film emulsion and the flatness of the screen on which film is projected)? The answers to these questions (which are addressed in various film theories) will begin to point toward a particular aesthetics — how a camera may be used efficiently and effectively as a container and the appropriate manner in which the container may be penetrated or broken. Note that when the camera is conceived as a container, it operates by actual *touch* — that is, it grasps certain structural aspects of an object, transforming a thing into a "figure" by wrenching it from an external "ground." There are, of course, alternatives to imagining the camera as a container. For example, the camera might function as part of a "language" or, as discussed earlier, the camera might be a "guide." Because there seem to be many metaphors and projections governing the camera, not one, there would seem to be many cameras, not one.

74. On the relationship of narrative to the source-path-goal schema, see, e.g., Mark Johnson, *Moral Imagination: Implications of Cognitive Science for Ethics* (Chicago: University of Chicago Press, 1993), chap. 7, "The Narrative Context of Self and Action," 150–84; Lakoff and Johnson, *Philosophy in the Flesh*, 32–34, 36, 42–44.

75. On everyday reasoning, see generally Lakoff and Johnson, *Philosophy in the Flesh*; on preserving inferential structure, see 3–7, 21–22, 91, 527–28. See also Kunda, *Social Cognition*, chaps. 3, 4, and 5 on judgment heuristics,

explanatory principles, and the operation of memory, 53–209. On the use of everyday reasoning by film writers, see, e.g., Bordwell, *Making Meaning*.

76. Jacques Aumont argues that the term "camera movement" is "a term of convenience, too imprecise for a theoretical vocabulary." He worries that some movements and motions in/of the image are undecidable by merely looking at them. But why should our perception of "camera movement" be reduced to, or hampered by, technical questions about physical cameras? Is a 'theory' about film and its spectators simply an effort to reconstitute production circumstances? Despite Aumont's uneasiness about "camera movement," however, he quite confidently discusses the materiality of a camera apparatus that produces shots that happen *not* to be 'in movement' or, rather, *seem not* to be 'in movement' though possibly moving (as discussed in the text above, section "Motion Picture"). Is it only the appearance of some obvious "movement" (Aumont) on the screen that makes the camera indistinct, vague, figurative, or self-referential ("too imprecise for a theoretical vocabulary"), whereas otherwise the immobile-appearing camera is literal and certain? For Aumont, the essence of film seems to be photographicity and, thus, the unmoving image is already proof of the presence of a camera that becomes the *definite* camera, *the* source from which springs the film and all of its effects. See Aumont, The Image, trans. Claire Pajackowska (London: British Film Institute, 1997), 168.

77. See, e.g., Branigan, *Narrative Comprehension and Film*, chap. 4, "Levels of Narration," 86–124, esp. subsection "Text under a Description," 111–14; and 125–42.

78. On some models for the emotions, see, e.g., notes 25 and 59 above.

79. Vivian Sobchack, "Toward Inhabited Space: The Semiotic Structure of Camera Movement in the Cinema," *Semiotica* 41, 1/4 (1982), 319–20 (Sobchack's emphases, footnote omitted); cf. 330–31 and nn. 5, 9, 18. Sobchack continues to think about camera movement in "The Active Eye: A Phenomenology of Cinematic Vision," *Quarterly Review of Film and Video* 12, 3 (1990), 21–36.

Here's another illustration of the usual tripartite description of the camera (mechanical, concrete, and cognitive/emotive):

In Godard's *La Chinoise* [1967], some youthful Maoists are shown in their communal apartment engaging in an ideological dispute. One group sits at one end of the room, the other at the opposite end [concrete]. Instead of cutting from one group to the other with their dialogue, Godard dollys back and forth for the duration of the scene, a conspicuous and apparently clumsy technique [mechanical]. . . . The pendular movements of the camera convey metaphorically the monotonous [emotive?] but necessary refinement of ideas of the dialectical process. . . . [E]ach swing of the camera represents a thesis or antithesis [cognitive].

Louis D. Giannetti, "The Aesthetic of the Mobile Camera," in *Godard and Others: Essays on Film Form* (Rutherford, N.J.: Fairleigh Dickinson University Press, 1975), 74.

80. Sobchack, "Toward Inhabited Space," 317–18 (my emphasis). The reference to Maurice Merleau-Ponty is from his *Phenomenology of Perception*, trans. Colin Smith (London: Routledge & Kegan Paul, 1962), 137.

81. On "when" something is, cf. Nelson Goodman, *Ways of Worldmaking* (Indianapolis: Hackett Publishing Co., 1978), chap. 4, "When Is Art?," 57–70. See also the special issue devoted to "More Ways of Worldmaking" of *The Journal of Aesthetic Education* 25, 1 (Spring 1991). Goodman's definition of "use" may be a bit too narrow; e.g., 70. "Use" includes the possibility of multiple — and possibly competing, implicit, and/or entrenched — descriptions of an object. The problem with an ontological question, with asking what something "is" in order to trim away the "inessential" properties, is that one too easily loses sight of the purpose (the context) for asking the question and, further, one is too often committed to those properties made salient by present, local circumstances. Note that, for Wittgenstein, a "use" begins not with the naming of something but with a "description" of it. See *Philosophical Investigations*, §§ 26, 49; cf. § 663.

Film is often said to be, or to involve, "performance" or "performances of actions" or "presentations of events." This is still too general a formulation. Many sorts of time (performance) may be depicted, embodied, suggested, repressed, or imagined in watching a film. I cannot here undertake an analysis of time in the cinema, except to note that the proper question to ask is "when is time?"

82. A fine example of historicizing the metaphor that a camera "can see" can be found in Malcolm Turvey, "Can the Camera See? Mimesis in *Man with a Movie Camera*," *October* 89 (Summer 1999), 25–50. Turvey examines specific social, political, and scientific ideas of the late nineteenth century and early twentieth century in the Soviet Union in order to situate the theory and practice of Dziga Vertov. The films of Stan Brakhage are then said to take Vertov's metaphor "to its logical extreme" and the films of Andy Warhol and Michael Snow "to turn this tradition on its head" (49). Nevertheless, Turvey seems hostile to any attempt to historicize *other* metaphors for camera sight, for example, metaphors based on psychoanalysis (30–31, 34). Again, I believe that there is no single camera — no single theory, no single metaphor, no single use — there are, as it were, only 'genres.' This is not a claim that a camera is neutral but, rather, that, like a word, a camera is destined to

acquire a meaning only when it is the instrument of a critic's or spectator's (perceived) interests and projects, when it becomes one of the metaphors we live by. Needless to say, humans live, and have lived, by many metaphors.

For an example of a quite different interpretation of the camera movements of Snow's *La Région centrale* (1971) than offered by Turvey, see Sobchack, "Toward Inhabited Space," 331–32. For Turvey, Snow's film is "machinic narcissism" reflecting "the period of advanced capitalism — when the absolute *indifference* of capital to human life enters advanced art with a vengeance" (49–50; Turvey's emphasis). By contrast, Sobchack argues that "although [camera] movement may be all [in *La Région centrale*], it is yet embodied and intentional and inhabits space in human terms — even as the filmmaker hides behind a hill [while the camera is in movement]. (We might ask from whom he is hiding: the camera? the viewer? himself?)" Sobchack adds generally, "Even in its most mechanical presence and at its supposed farthest remove from human intentionality, the camera still moves intentionally and means to mean in its movement." To understand the difference between the claims of Turvey and Sobchack, one would need to historicize their metaphors for thinking about the camera. Is the proof to be found only by looking at *La Région centrale*? I think not.

83. Richard Rorty, "Inquiry as Recontextualization: An Anti-Dualist Account of Interpretation," in *Objectivity, Relativism, and Truth: Philosophical Papers, Vol. I* (Cambridge: Cambridge University Press, 1991), 99–100 (original emphasis). A sophisticated and nuanced account of the philosophical issues involving the relation of mental states to the world may be found in Daniel C. Dennett, "Real Patterns," *The Journal of Philosophy* 88, 1 (Jan. 1991), 27–51.

84. Rorty, "Texts and Lumps," in *Objectivity, Relativism, and Truth*, 81 (original emphasis). Rorty's comment explains why Plato's theory of human memory as a wax tablet that receives impressions is wrong. Long-term memory has been shown to be neither a copy of the world nor static, but to be an (ongoing, changing) interpretation of the world according to various ways of looking — that is, of assembling facts under (ongoing, changing) descriptions.

85. For Wittgenstein, naming an object (e.g., 'camera') is not yet a "move" according to the rules of a "language-game." A "move" amounts to placing a fact under a description sanctioned by the rules of a game. Wittgenstein asserts, "[N]aming and describing do not stand on the same level: naming is a preparation for description. Naming is so far not a move in the language-game — any more than putting a piece in its place on the board is a move in chess. We may say: *nothing* has so far been done, when a thing has been named. It has not even got a name except in the language-game." Thus, I would assert, we cannot know what the word "camera" means on a given

occasion without knowing how it is being used within descriptions of the occasion. The important moves of a camera are those it makes in a language-game. Wittgenstein, *Philosophical Investigations*, § 49 (original emphases).

86. Wittgenstein, *Philosophical Investigations*, § 439.

87. Nelson Goodman and Catherine Z. Elgin, *Reconceptions in Philosophy and Other Arts and Sciences* (Indianapolis, Ind.: Hackett Publishing, 1988), 158 (original emphases). On "rightness," see sects. "Rightness of Categories" and "Symbol by Sample," 14–23, and sect. "The World," 49–53; see also index entry, "rightness." See generally Jerome Bruner, *Actual Minds, Possible Worlds* (Cambridge, Mass.: Harvard University Press, 1986).

88. Goodman and Elgin, *Reconceptions in Philosophy*, 155–56, 157 (original emphasis).

89. I have borrowed the idea of a "schedule of descriptions" from Arthur Danto, "Moving Pictures," 213. We may take the idea one step further. If each common type of 'camera' is defined by a 'schedule of authorized descriptions,' then what is important in using the word 'camera' is to recognize the *partial overlap* of some of the descriptions between two given 'schedules' that provides a distinctive, "continuous transition" between those two uses of the word 'camera.' (Cf. Wittgenstein's comment that appears as an epigraph for chapter 4.) There will be different transitions between different pairs of uses of the word 'camera.' In this approach one does not search for what each camera may have in common with all of the others (even if there is something in common) nor does one concede that each camera is simply 'another or different *kind*' or that there is a discrete group of functions performed by a camera, separate from all the others. Instead, what is important is the grammar of the *transition* between two uses of the word 'camera,' two schedules of descriptions. Figure 4.1 may be taken to represent these many cameras. I have at least partially outlined 'schedules of descriptions' for the words 'movement' (chapters 2 and 5), 'point of view' (chapter 2), 'camera' (chapters 3 and 5), and 'frame' (chapter 4). In addition, this chapter seeks to raise questions about the use of the concept of 'causation,' which has produced such formulas as those listed in figure 5.1.

90. *The Collected Dialogues of Plato*, ed. Hamilton and Cairns, Theaetetus, 189e – 190a (my emphasis); see also 196a; and Sophist, 263e.

91. Wittgenstein, *Philosophical Investigations*, §§ 455–57.

92. See Branigan, *Narrative Comprehension and Film*, subsection "Text under a Description," 111–14. Language is central to thought even though the mind employs forms of representation other than words, some of which are conscious, such as images. Cf. Wittgenstein, *Philosophical Investigations*, §§ 649, 663. Note that a single mental image cannot stand for an entire category for any

classification higher than a basic-level category. For example, a person may summon a mental image of a chair but not a mental image of "furniture." Lakoff and Johnson, *Philosophy in the Flesh*, 27. Sergei Eisenstein, recognizing the limitations of imagery, notably insisted that film strive to be a language rather than mere pictures of basic-level things.

The relationship of language to film comprehension is too complex to discuss, but I offer five suggestive quotations:

> Language can say, even if sometimes only with approximation, what all the other codes can say, while the inverse is not true. . . . [L]anguage does much more than [translate] vision. . . . To speak of the image is in reality to speak the image; not essentially a [translation] but a comprehension, a resocialization. . . . Nomination completes the perception as much as it translates it; an insufficiently verbalizable perception is not fully a perception in the social sense of the word.

Christian Metz, "The Perceived and the Named," trans. Steven Feld and Shari Robertson, *Studies in Visual Communication* 6, 3 (Fall 1980), 62–63.

> [N]atural languages signify and refer to, but do not provide translations of non-linguistic realities. Rather, they provide *tools* for the *description and interpretation* of non-linguistic phenomena, including films, as well as for the expression of more abstract conceptualizations that have no perceptible counterparts in "reality," such as the cognitive relationships spectators entertain with events on the screen. Or, for that matter, in reality. What would something like a *desire* or a *memory* look like? What is a thing like "before" or "after"? Those prepositions express the way speakers conceptualize their relations with other entities in his or her spatial (or, by metaphor), temporal environment, but they do not "denote" some perceptible entities. Neither do they "translate" some objective relationship, which exists independently of its cognitive conceptualization.

Jan Simons, "'Enunciation': From Code to Interpretation," in *The Film Spectator: From Sign to Mind*, ed. Warren Buckland (Amsterdam: Amsterdam University Press, 1995), 193 and 193 n. 6 (my emphasis of the first four words).

> Here is a little demonstration to help focus again on the facts. Try to stop your inner speech for ten seconds. . . . I find it impossible to do for

more than five seconds or so. It is the simplest possible demonstration, but it shows how dependent we are on the flow of inner speech, which is one dimension of our working memory.

Bernard J. Baars, "In the Theatre of Consciousness: Global Workspace Theory, A Rigorous Scientific Theory of Consciousness," *Journal of Consciousness Studies* 4, 4 (1997), 302. On the nature of mental imagery and the possibility of an amodal "interlingua" or "mentalese," see Oliver Sacks, "A Neurologist's Notebook: The Mind's Eye — What the Blind See," *The New Yorker* (July 28, 2003), 48–59.

If there is one single aspect of human mental function that is more closely tied up with symbolic processes than any other, it is surely our use of language. Language is, indeed, the ultimate symbolic mental function, and it is virtually impossible to conceive of thought as we know it in its absence. For words, it is fair to say, function as the units of human thought, at least as we are aware of it. They are certainly the medium by which we explain our thoughts to one another and, as incomparably social creatures, seek to influence what is going on in one another's brains. Thus, if we are seeking a single cultural releasing factor that opened the way to symbolic cognition, the invention of language is the most obvious candidate. Indeed, it is perhaps the only plausible one that it has so far proved possible to identify.

Ian Tattersall, "How We Came to Be Human," *Scientific American* 285, 6 (Dec. 2001), 61. This article is an excerpt from Tattersall's book *The Monkey in the Mirror: Essays on the Science of What Makes Us Human* (New York: Harcourt, 2002). See also Peter J. Richerson and Robert Boyd, *Not by Genes Alone: How Culture Transformed Human Evolution* (Chicago: University of Chicago Press, 2005).

Computers were originally just supposed to be number-crunchers, but now their number-crunching has been harnessed in a thousand imaginative ways to create new virtual machines, such as video games and word processors, in which the underlying number-crunching is almost invisible, and in which the new powers seem quite magical. Our brains, similarly, weren't designed . . . for word processing, but now a large portion — perhaps even the lion's share — of the activity that takes place in adult human brains is involved in a sort of word processing: speech production and comprehension, and the serial rehearsal and rearrangement of linguistic items, or better, their neural surrogates. And these activities magnify and transform the underlying hardware powers in ways that seem (from the "outside") quite magical.

Daniel C. Dennett, *Consciousness Explained* (Boston: Little, Brown and Co., 1991), 225; on consciousness as a product of cultural evolution, quoted in the text, see 219 (my emphasis). Extending Dennett's computer analogy, one might say that the various cameras discerned by critics are *virtual* cameras made out of (a critic's, an institution's, a filmmaker's) rules and procedures rather than glass, metal, and wire. If film is an "illusion," then it is a "user illusion" based on a spectator's changing interaction with the film as a "virtual machine," an evolving *interface* utilizing "virtual cameras."

93. Tzvetan Todorov, *The Poetics of Prose*, trans. Richard Howard (Ithaca, N.Y.: Cornell University Press, 1977), 93–94.

Works Cited

I have divided the works cited into a set of loose categories so as to aid the reader in finding the relevant bibliography and better illustrate the structure of this book. Works that are especially noteworthy *in relation* to this book's concerns are marked with an asterisk. Here are the categories:

A. ART HISTORY

Baxandall, Michael. *Painting and Experience in Fifteenth-Century Italy*. Oxford, U.K.: Clarendon Press, 1972.

Derrida, Jacques. *The Truth in Painting*. Translated by Geoff Bennington and Ian McLeod. Chicago: University of Chicago Press, 1987.

Duro, Paul, ed. *The Rhetoric of the Frame: Essays on the Boundaries of the Artwork*. Cambridge, U.K.: Cambridge University Press, 1996.

Elkins, James. *On Pictures and the Words That Fail Them*. Cambridge, U.K.: Cambridge University Press, 1998.

———. *Our Beautiful, Dry, and Distant Texts: Art History as Writing*. New York: Routledge, 2000.

———. "Preface to the Book A Skeptical Introduction to Visual Culture." *Journal of Visual Culture 1* (April 2002), 93–99.

———. *Visual Studies: A Skeptical Introduction*. New York: Routledge, 2003.

Gombrich, E.H. "Illusion and Art." In *Illusion in Nature and Art*, edited by R. L. Gregory and E. H. Gombrich. New York: Charles Scribner's Sons, 1973.

Krauss, Rosalind E. *The Optical Unconscious*. Cambridge, Mass.: MIT Press, 1993.

B. COGNITIVE SCIENCE

Antony, Michael V. "Is 'Consciousness' Ambiguous?" *Journal of Consciousness Studies 8* (February 2001), 19–44.

Baars, Bernard J. "In the Theatre of Consciousness: Global Workspace Theory, A Rigorous Scientific Theory of Consciousness." *Journal of Consciousness Studies 4* (1997), 292–309.

Brockmeier, Jens. "Ineffable Experience." *Journal of Consciousness Studies 9* (Sept./Oct. 2002), 79–95.

Crawford, Mary, and Roger Chaffin. "The Reader's Construction of Meaning: Cognitive Research on Gender and Comprehension." In *Gender and Reading: Essays on Readers, Texts, and Contexts*, edited by Elizabeth A. Flynn and Patrocinio Schweickart. Baltimore: Johns Hopkins University Press, 1986.

Crick, Francis. *The Astonishing Hypothesis: The Scientific Search for the Soul*. London: Simon & Schuster, 1994.

Damasio, Antonio. *The Feeling of What Happens: Body and Emotion in the Making of Consciousness*. New York: Harcourt Brace, 1999.

Damper, Robert I. "The Chinese Room Argument — Dead but Not Yet Buried." *Journal of Consciousness Studies 11* (2004), 159–69.

*Dean, Jeffrey T. "The Nature of Concepts and the Definition of Art." *The Journal of Aesthetics and Art Criticism 61* (Winter 2003), 29–35.

Dennett, Daniel. "Cognitive Wheels: The Frame Problem of AI." In The *Robot's Dilemma: The Frame Problem in Artificial Intelligence*, edited by Zenon W. Pylyshyn. Norwood, N.J.: Ablex Publishing, 1987.

*———. *Consciousness Explained*. Boston: Little, Brown and Co., 1991.

Draaisma, Douwe. *Metaphors of Memory: A History of Ideas about the Mind*. Translated by Paul Vincent. Cambridge, U.K.: Cambridge University Press, 2000.

Fauconnier, Gilles, and Mark Turner. *The Way We Think: Conceptual Blending and the Mind's Hidden Complexities*. New York: Basic Books, 2002.

Fireman, Gary D., Ted E. McVay, Jr., and Owen J. Flanagan, eds. *Narrative and Consciousness: Literature, Psychology and the Brain*. Oxford, U.K.: Oxford University Press, 2003.

Fiske, Susan T., and Shelley E. Taylor. *Social Cognition*. New York: McGraw-Hill, 2nd ed. 1991.

Forceville, Charles. "The Conspiracy in the Comfort of Strangers: Narration in the Novel and the Film." *Language and Literature* 11 (2002), 119–35.

———. "Visual Representations of the Idealized Cognitive Model of Anger in the Asterix Album La Zizanie." *Journal of Pragmatics* 37 (2005), 69–88.

*Hart, F. Elizabeth. "The Epistemology of Cognitive Literary Studies." *Philosophy and Literature* 25 (October 2001), 314–34.

Harth, Erich. "Art and Reductionism." *Journal of Consciousness Studies* 11 (March/April 2004), 111–16.

Herman, David, ed. *Narrative Theory and the Cognitive Sciences*. Stanford, Calif.: Center for the Study of Language and Information, 2003.

Hernadi, Paul. "Why Is Literature: A Coevolutionary Perspective on Imaginative Worldmaking." *Poetics Today* 23 (Spring 2002), 21–42. Special issue on "Literature and the Cognitive Revolution."

Hogan, Patrick Colm. *The Mind and Its Stories: Narrative Universals and Human Emotions*. Cambridge, U.K.: Cambridge University Press, 2003.

———. *Cognitive Science, Literature, and the Arts: A Guide for Humanists*. New York: Routledge, 2003.

Holland, Norman N. "Where Is a Text? A Neurological View." *New Literary History* 33 (Winter 2002), 21–38.

Horton, Robin. "Tradition and Modernity Revisited." In *Rationality and Relativism*, edited by Martin Hollis and Steven Lukes. Cambridge, Mass.: MIT Press, 1982.

Johnson, David Martel. *How History Made the Mind: The Cultural Origins of Objective Thinking*. Chicago: Open Court, 2003.

*Johnson, Mark. *The Body in the Mind: The Bodily Basis of Meaning, Imagination, and Reason*. Chicago: University of Chicago Press, 1987.

———. *Moral Imagination: Implications of Cognitive Science for Ethics*. Chicago: University of Chicago Press, 1993.

Journal of Aesthetics and Art Criticism 62 (Spring 2004): special issue on "Art, Mind, and Cognitive Science."

Journal of Consciousness Studies 9 (2002): special issue on "Is the Visual World a Grand Illusion?"

Kunda, Ziva. *Social Cognition: Making Sense of People*. Cambridge, Mass.: MIT Press, 1999.

La Cerra, Peggy, and Roger Bingham. *The Origin of Minds: Evolution, Uniqueness, and the New Science of the Self*. New York: Harmony Books, 2002.

*Lakoff, George. *Women, Fire, and Dangerous Things: What Categories Reveal about the Mind*. Chicago: University of Chicago Press, 1987.

*Lakoff, George, and Mark Johnson. *Metaphors We Live By*. Chicago: University of Chicago Press, 1980.

*———. *Philosophy in the Flesh: The Embodied Mind and Its Challenge to Western Thought*. New York: Basic Books, 1999.

Lakoff, George, and Mark Turner. *More than Cool Reason: A Field Guide to Poetic Metaphor*. Chicago: University of Chicago Press, 1989.

Levin, Daniel T. "Change Blindness Blindness as Visual Metacognition." *Journal of Consciousness Studies* 9 (2002), 111–30.

*Minsky, Marvin. *The Society of Mind*. New York: Simon and Schuster, 1985.

Neisser, Ulric. "The Processes of Vision." In *Perception: Mechanisms and Models*, edited by Richard Held and Whitman Richards. San Francisco: W.H. Freeman, 1972. Reprinted from *Scientific American* 219 (Sept. 1968), 204–14.

*———. *Cognition and Reality: Principles and Implications of Cognitive Psychology*. San Francisco: W.H. Freeman, 1976.

*Pinker, Steven. *How the Mind Works*. New York: W.W. Norton & Co., 1997.

———. *The Blank Slate: The Modern Denial of Human Nature*. New York: Viking Penguin, 2002.

Port, Robert F., and Timothy van Gelder, eds. *Mind as Motion: Explorations in the Dynamics of Cognition*. Cambridge, Mass.: MIT Press, 1995.

Richards, Richard A. "A Fitness Model of Evaluation." *The Journal of Aesthetics and Art Criticism* 62 (Summer 2004), 263–75.

Richerson, Peter J., and Robert Boyd. *Not by Genes Alone: How Culture Transformed Human Evolution*. Chicago: University of Chicago Press, 2005.

Sacks, Oliver. "A Neurologist's Notebook: The Mind's Eye — What the Blind See." *The New Yorker* (July 28, 2003), 48–59.

Smyth, Mary M., and Steven E. Clark. "My Half-Sister Is a THOG: Strategic Processes in a Reasoning Task." *The British Journal of Psychology* 77 (May 1986), 275–87.

Sperber, Dan, and Deirdre Wilson. *Relevance: Communication and Cognition*. Oxford, U.K.: Blackwell, 2nd ed. 1995.

*Spolsky, Ellen. "Darwin and Derrida: Cognitive Literary Theory as a Species of Post-Structuralism." *Poetics Today* 23 (Spring 2002), 43–62.

Tattersall, Ian. "How We Came to Be Human." *Scientific American* 285 (Dec. 2001), 56–63.

———. *The Monkey in the Mirror: Essays on the Science of What Makes Us Human.* New York: Harcourt, 2002.

Tooby, John, Leda Cosmides, and Ellen Spolsky. "Dialogue." *SubStance* 94/95 (2001), 199–202. Special issue "On the Origin of Fictions: Interdisciplinary Perspectives."

Van der Heijden, A.H.C. "Attention." In *A Companion to Cognitive Science*, edited by William Bechtel and George Graham. Oxford, U.K.: Blackwell, 1998.

*Wilson, Robert A., and Frank C. Keil, eds. *The MIT Encyclopedia of the Cognitive Sciences.* Cambridge, Mass.: MIT Press, 1999.

C. FILM

C1. AESTHETICS AND CRITICISM

Abrams, Adam. "Rules of This Game: Chinese Roulette and the Spectator Experience." Unpub. ms., 2000.

Andrew, Dudley. "The Gravity of 'Sunrise.'" *Quarterly Review of Film Studies* 2 (August 1977), 356–87. Revised as "The Turn and Return of Sunrise" in *Film in the Aura of Art*. Princeton, N.J.: Princeton University Press, 1984.

———. "The Frame-Mobile and the Age of Cinema." In *Limina/le soglie del film — Film's Thresholds [X International Film Studies Conference]*, edited by Veronica Innocenti and Valentina Re. Italy: University of Udine, 2004.

Arijon, Daniel. *Grammar of the Film Language.* New York: Hastings House, 1976.

Armes, Roy. *The Ambiguous Image: Narrative Style in Modern European Cinema.* Bloomington: Indiana University Press, 1976.

Aumont, Jacques. *The Image.* Translated by Claire Pajackowska. London: British Film Institute, 1997.

Aumont, Jacques, Alain Bergala, Michel Marie, and Marc Vernet. *Aesthetics of Film.* Translated and revised by Richard Neupert. Austin: University of Texas Press, 1992.

Bordwell, David. "Imploded Space: Film Style in The Passion of Jeanne d'Arc." *Purdue Film Studies* [vol. 1]. Pleasantville, N.Y.: Redgrave, 1976.

———. "The Art Cinema as a Mode of Film Practice." *Film Criticism* 4 (Fall 1979): 56–64.

———. *The Films of Carl-Theodor Dreyer.* Berkeley and Los Angeles: University of California Press, 1981.

———. *On the History of Film Style.* Cambridge, Mass.: Harvard University Press, 1997.

———. "Intensified Continuity: Visual Style in Contemporary American Film." *Film Quarterly* 55 (Spring 2002), 16–28.

337

———. *Figures Traced in Light: On Cinematic Staging*. Berkeley and Los Angeles: University of California Press, 2005.

*Bordwell, David, and Kristin Thompson. *Film Art: An Introduction*. New York: McGraw-Hill, 7th ed. 2004.

Brakhage, Stan. "Metaphors on Vision." *Film Culture* 30 (1963).

Branigan, Edward. "The Space of Equinox Flower." In *Close Viewings: An Anthology of New Film Criticism*, edited by Peter Lehman. Tallahassee: Florida State University Press, 1990.

Burch, Noël. *To the Distant Observer: Form and Meaning in the Japanese Cinema*. Berkeley and Los Angeles: University of California Press, 1979.

Charney, Leo, and Vanessa R. Schwartz, eds. *Cinema and the Invention of Modern Life*. Berkeley and Los Angeles: University of California Press, 1995.

Cocteau, Jean. *Jean Cocteau: The Art of Cinema*. Edited by André Bernard and Claude Gauteur. Translated by Robin Buss. New York: Marion Boyars, 1992.

Durgnat, Raymond. *Films and Feelings*. Cambridge, Mass.: M.I.T. Press, 1967.

———. *A Long Hard Look at 'Psycho.'* London: British Film Institute, 2002.

Fieschi, Jean-André. "F. W. Murnau." In *Cinema — A Critical Dictionary: The Major Film-Makers* [vol. 2], edited by Richard Roud. New York: The Viking Press, 1980.

Fisher, Kevin. "Tracing the Tesseract: A Conceptual Prehistory of the Morph." In *Meta-Morphing: Visual Transformation and the Culture of Quick-Change*, edited by Vivian Sobchack. Minneapolis: University of Minnesota Press, 2000.

Gledhill, Christine, and Linda Williams, eds. *Reinventing Film Studies*. New York: Oxford University Press, 2000.

Gull, Richard. "The Anti-Metaphysics Game: A Wittgensteinian Reading of The Crying Game." In *Film and Knowledge: Essays on the Integration of Images and Ideas*, edited by Kevin L. Stoehr. Jefferson, N.C.: McFarland, 2002.

Hedges, Inez. *Breaking the Frame: Film Language and the Experience of Limits*. Bloomington, Ind.: Indiana University Press, 1991.

Jenkins, Henry. *Textual Poachers: Television Fans and Participatory Culture*. New York: Routledge, 1992.

Johnson, William. "Coming to Terms with Color." In *The Movies as Medium*, edited. by Lewis Jacobs. New York: Farrar, Straus & Giroux, 1970.

Kirby, Lynne. *Parallel Tracks: The Railroad and Silent Cinema*. Durham, N.C.: Duke University Press, 1996.

Kreidl, John. *Jean-Luc Godard*. Boston: Twayne Publishers, 1980.

Lehman, Peter, ed. *Close Viewings: An Anthology of New Film Criticism*. Tallahassee: Florida State University Press, 1990.

MacLean, Robert. "Opening the Private Eye: Wittgenstein and Godard's *Alphaville*." *Sight and Sound* 47 (Winter 1977–78), 46–49.

McLaughlin, James. "All in the Family: Alfred Hitchcock's 'Shadow of a Doubt.'" *Wide Angle* 4 (1980), 12–19.

Michelson, Annette, Douglas Gomery, and Patrick Loughney. *The Art of Moving Shadows*. Washington, D.C.: National Gallery of Art, 1989.

Neale, Steve. "Art Cinema as Institution." *Screen* 22 (1981), 11–39.

Perez, Gilberto. *The Material Ghost: Films and Their Medium*. Baltimore: Johns Hopkins University Press, 1998.

Perkins, V. F. "The Cinema of Nicholas Ray." In *Movie Reader*, edited by Ian Cameron. New York: Praeger, 1972.

———. *Film as Film: Understanding and Judging Movies*. Baltimore, Md.: Penguin, 1972.

Peterson, James. *Dreams of Chaos, Visions of Order: Understanding the American Avant-Garde Cinema*. Detroit: Wayne State University Press, 1994.

Petric, Vlada. "Tarkovsky's Dream Imagery." *Film Quarterly* 43 (Winter 1989–90), 28–34.

Polan, Dana. "Formalism and Its Discontents." *Jump Cut* 26 (1981).

Reisz, Karel, and Gavin Millar. *The Technique of Film Editing*. New York: Hastings House, 2nd ed. 1968.

Roberts, Kenneth, and Win Sharples. *A Primer for Filmmaking*. Indianapolis, Ind.: Pegasus, 1971.

Rothman, William. "Alfred Hitchcock's *Murder!*: Theater, Authorship and the Presence of the Camera." *Wide Angle* 4 (1980), 54–61.

———. *The "I" of the Camera: Essays in Film Criticism, History, and Aesthetics*. Cambridge, U.K.: Cambridge University Press, 2nd ed. 2004.

Sarris, Andrew. *The American Cinema: Directors and Directions, 1929–1968*. New York: E.P. Dutton, 1968.

Sesonske, Alexander. *Jean Renoir: The French Films, 1924–1939*. Cambridge, Mass.: Harvard University Press, 1980.

Silverman, Kaja, and Harun Farocki. *Speaking about Godard*. New York: New York University Press, 1998.

Stam, Robert. *Subversive Pleasures: Bakhtin, Cultural Criticism, and Film*. Baltimore: Johns Hopkins University Press, 1989.

———. *Reflexivity in Film and Literature: From Don Quixote to Jean-Luc Godard*. New York: Columbia University Press, 1992.

Thompson, Kristin. *Eisenstein's Ivan the Terrible: A Neoformalist Analysis*. Princeton, N.J.: Princeton University Press, 1981.

———. *Breaking the Glass Armor: Neoformalist Film Analysis*. Princeton, N.J.: Princeton University Press, 1988.

Truffaut, François. *Hitchcock*. New York: Simon and Schuster, rev. ed. 1984.

Tybjerg, Casper. "The Sense of The Word." In *Film Style and Story: A Tribute to Torben Grodal*, edited by Lennard Højbjerg and Peter Schepelern. University of Copenhagen: Museum Tusculanum Press, 2003.

Wees, William. "The Cinematic Image as a Visualization of Sight." *Wide Angle* 4 (1980), 28–37.

Weinbren, Grahame, and Christine Brinckmann. "Selective Transparencies: Pat O'Neill's Recent Films." *Millennium Film Journal* 6 (Spring 1980), 50–72.

Williams, Forest. "The Mastery of Movement: An Appreciation of Max Ophuls." *Film Comment* 5 (Winter 1969), 70–74.

Wollen, Peter. "Rope: Three Hypotheses." In *Alfred Hitchcock: Centenary Essays*, edited by Richard Allen and S. Ishii-Gonzalès. London: British Film Institute, 1999.

Wood, Robin. *Sexual Politics and Narrative Film: Hollywood and Beyond*. New York: Columbia University Press, 1998.

Wuss, Peter. "The Documentary Style of Fiction Film in Eastern Europe: Narration and Visual Style." In *Film Style and Story: A Tribute to Torben Grodal*, edited by Lennard Højbjerg and Peter Schepelern. University of Copenhagen: Museum Tusculanum Press, 2003.

C2. CAMERA

Anderson, Joseph D. "Moving through the Diegetic World of the Motion Picture." In *Film Style and Story: A Tribute to Torben Grodal*, edited by Lennard Højbjerg and Peter Schepelern. University of Copenhagen: Museum Tusculanum Press, 2003.

Astruc, Alexandre. "The Birth of a New Avant-garde: La Caméra-stylo." In *The New Wave*, edited by Peter Graham. New York: Doubleday, 1968.

Bacher, Lutz. *The Mobile Mise en Scene: A Critical Analysis of the Theory and Practice of Long-Take Camera Movement in the Narrative Film*. New York: Arno Press, 1978.

*Bordwell, David. "Camera Movement, the Coming of Sound, and the Classical Hollywood Style." In *Film: Historical-Theoretical Speculations [The 1977 Film Studies Annual: Part Two]*. Pleasantville, N.Y.: Redgrave, 1977.

*———. "Camera Movement and Cinematic Space." In *Explorations in Film Theory: Selected Essays* from Ciné-Tracts, edited by Ron Burnett. Bloomington: Indiana University Press, 1991.

Boultenhouse, Charles. "The Camera as a God." In *Film Culture Reader*, edited by P. Adams Sitney. New York: Cooper Square Press, 2000.

Branigan, Edward. "The Spectator and Film Space — Two Theories." *Screen* 22 (1981), 55–78.

———. "What Is a Camera?" In *Cinema Histories, Cinema Practices*, edited by Patricia Mellencamp and Philip Rosen [The American Film Institute Monograph Series, vol. 4]. Frederick, Md.: University Publications of America, 1984.

———. "Quand y a-t-il caméra?" ["When Is a Camera?"] *Champs Visuels: Revue interdisciplinaire de recherchessur l'image* 12–13 (Janvier 1999) [Paris: L'Harmattan], 18–32. Special issue on "Penser, cadrer: le project du cadre."

————. "How Frame Lines (and Film Theory) Figure." In *Film Style and Story: A Tribute to Torben Grodal*, edited by Lennard Højbjerg and Peter Schepelern. University of Copenhagen: Museum Tusculanum Press, 2003.

*Comolli, Jean-Louis. "Machines of the Visible." In *The Cinematic Apparatus*, ed. by Teresa de Lauretis and Stephen Heath. New York: St. Martin's Press, 1980.

*Danto, Arthur C. "Moving Pictures." In *Philosophizing Art: Selected Essays*. Berkeley and Los Angeles: University of California Press, 1999.

Durgnat, Raymond. "The Restless Camera." *Films and Filming* 15 (Dec. 1968), 14–18.

Geuens, Jean-Pierre. "Visuality and Power: The Work of the Steadicam." *Film Quarterly* 47 (Winter 1993–94), 8–17.

Giannetti, Louis D. "The Aesthetic of the Mobile Camera." In *Godard and Others: Essays on Film Form*. Rutherford, N.J.: Fairleigh Dickinson University Press, 1975.

*Johnson, Kenneth. "The Point of View of the Wandering Camera." *Cinema Journal* 32 (Winter 1993), 49–56.

Lightman, Herb A. "The Fluid Camera." *American Cinematographer* 27 (March 1946), 82, 102–03.

MacDougall, David. "When Less Is Less: The Long Take in Documentary." *Film Quarterly* 46 (Winter 1992–93), 36–46. Reprinted in *Film Quarterly: Forty Years — A Selection*, edited by Brian Henderson and Ann Martin with Lee Amazonas. Berkeley and Los Angeles: University of California Press, 1999.

Mast, Gerald. "On Framing." *Critical* Inquiry 11 (September 1984), 82–109.

*Metz, Christian. "Trucage and the Film." *Critical Inquiry* 3 (Summer 1977), 657–75.

Moore, Rachel O. *Savage Theory: Cinema as Modern Magic*. Durham, N.C.: Duke University Press, 2000.

*Nizhny, Vladimir. *Lessons with Eisenstein*. Translated by Jay Leyda. New York: Hill and Wang, 1962.

*O'Leary, Brian. "Camera Movements in Hollywood's Westering Genre: A Functional Semiotic Approach." *Criticism* 45 (Spring 2003), 197–222.

*————. "Hollywood Camera Movements and the Films of Howard Hawks: A Functional Semiotic Approach." *New Review of Film and Television Studies* 1 (November 2003), 7–30.

Pichel, Irving. "Seeing with the Camera." *The Hollywood Quarterly of Film, Radio and Television* 1 (Winter 1946), 138–45. Reprinted in *Hollywood Directors 1941–1976*, edited by Richard Koszarski. New York: Oxford University Press, 1977. Also reprinted as "Change of Camera Viewpoint." In *The Movies as Medium*, edited by Lewis Jacobs. New York: Farrar, Straus & Giroux, 1970.

Salt, Barry. "A Note on 'Hollywood Camera Movements and the Films of Howard Hawks: A Functional Semiotic Approach' by Brian O'Leary." *New Review of Film and Television Studies* 3 (May 2005), 101–103.

*Silverman, Kaja. "What Is a Camera?, or: History in the Field of Vision." *Discourse* 15 (Spring 1993), 3–56.

*Sobchack, Vivian. "Toward Inhabited Space: The Semiotic Structure of Camera Movement in the Cinema." *Semiotica* 41 (1982), 317–35.

———. "The Active Eye: A Phenomenology of Cinematic Vision." *Quarterly Review of Film and Video* 12 (1990), 21–36.

*Turvey, Malcolm. "Can the Camera See? Mimesis in *Man with a Movie Camera*." *October* 89 (Summer 1999), 25–50.

Vernet, Marc. "The Look at the Camera." *Cinema Journal* 28 (Winter 1989), 48–63.

Vineyard, Jeremy. *Setting Up Your Shots: Great Camera Moves Every Filmmaker Should Know*. Studio City, Calif.: Michael Wiese Productions, 1999.

C3. CLASSICAL THEORY

Andrew, Dudley. "Realism and Reality in Cinema: The Film Theory of André Bazin and Its Source in Recent French Thought." Ph.D. diss., University of Iowa, 1972.

———. *Concepts in Film Theory*. Oxford, U.K.: Oxford University Press, 1984.

———. *André Bazin*. New York: Columbia University Press, new preface, 1990.

Arnheim, Rudolph. *Film als Kunst*. Berlin: Ernst Rowohlt Verlag, 1932.

———. *Film*. Translated by L. M. Sieveking and Ian F. D. Morrow. London: Faber & Faber, 1933.

———. *Film as Art*. Berkeley and Los Angeles: University of California Press, 1957.

Balázs, Béla. *Theory of the Film: Character and Growth of a New Art*. Translated by Edith Bone. New York: Dover, 1970.

Bazin, André. *Qu'est-ce que le cinéma?*, vols. I–IV. Paris: Éditions du Cerf, 1958.

———. *What Is Cinema?* [vol. I]. Translated by Hugh Gray. Berkeley and Los Angeles: University of California Press, 1967.

———. *What Is Cinema?* [vol. II]. Translated by Hugh Gray. Berkeley and Los Angeles: University of California Press, 1971.

*———. *Jean Renoir*. Translated by W. W. Halsey II and William H. Simon. New York: Simon & Schuster, 1973.

———. *Orson Welles: A Critical View*. Translated by Jonathan Rosenbaum. New York: Harper & Row, 1978.

———. *The Cinema of Cruelty: From Buñuel to Hitchcock*. Edited by François Truffaut. Translated by Sabine d'Estrée. New York: Seaver, 1982.

Bordwell, David. "The Musical Analogy." *Yale French Studies* 60 (1980), 141–56.

Branigan, Edward. "To Zero and Beyond: Noël Burch's Theory of Film Practice." In *Defining Cinema*, edited by Peter Lehman. New Brunswick, N.J.: Rutgers University Press, 1997.

Buckle, Gerard. *The Mind and the Film*. New York: Arno, 1970.

Burch, Noël. *Theory of Film Practice*. Translated by Helen R. Lane. New York: Praeger, 1973. Reprinted in part by Princeton University Press, Princeton, N.J., 1981.

———. "Porter, or Ambivalence." *Screen* 19 (1978/9), 91–105.

Burch, Noël, and Jorge Dana. "Propositions." *Afterimage* 5 (Spring 1974), 40–67.

Carroll, Noël. "Kracauer's Theory of Film." In *Defining Cinema*, edited by Peter Lehman. New Brunswick, N.J.: Rutgers University Press, 1997.

Comolli, Jean-Louis. "Film/Politics (2): L'Aveu: 15 Propositions." In *Cahiers du Cinéma 1969–1972: The Politics of Representation*, edited by Nick Browne. Cambridge, Mass.: Harvard University Press, 1990.

Eisenstein, Sergei. *The Film Sense*. Edited and translated by Jay Leyda. New York: Harcourt, Brace & World, 1942.

———. *Film Form: Essays in Film Theory*. Translated by Jay Leyda. New York: Harcourt, Brace & World, 1949.

———. "Colour Film." In *Movies and Methods: An Anthology* [vol. I], edited by Bill Nichols. Berkeley and Los Angeles: University of California Press, 1976.

———. *S. M. Eisenstein: Selected Works, Vol. I Writings, 1922–34*. Edited and translated by Richard Taylor. Bloomington and Indianapolis: Indiana University Press, 1988.

———. *S. M. Eisenstein: Selected Works, Vol. II, Towards a Theory of Montage*. Edited and translated by Michael Glenny and Richard Taylor. London: British Film Institute, 1991.

Epstein, Jean. "On Certain Characteristics of Photogénie" from "Bonjour Cinéma and Other Writings." *Afterimage* 10 (Autumn 1981), 8–39.

———. "The Cinema Continues" and "Photogénie and the Imponderable." In *French Film Theory and Criticism: A History/Anthology, 1907–1939 (Vol. II: 1929–1939)*, edited by Richard Abel. Princeton, N.J.: Princeton University Press, 1988.

Henderson, Brian. *A Critique of Film Theory*. New York: E. P. Dutton, 1980.

Koch, Gertrud. *Siegfried Kracauer: An Introduction*. Translated by Jeremy Gaines. Princeton, N.J.: Princeton University Press, 2000.

Kracauer, Siegfried. *Theory of Film: The Redemption of Physical Reality*. Princeton, N.J.: Princeton University Press, 1997.

Lindgren, Ernest. *The Art of the Film*. New York: Collier Books, 1963.

Mast, Gerald. "Kracauer's Two Tendencies and the Early History of Film Narrative." *Critical Inquiry* 6 (Spring 1980), 455–76.

Metz, Christian. "Current Problems of Film Theory: Christian Metz on Jean Mitry's *L'Esthétique et Psychologie du Cinéma, Vol II*." *Screen* 14 (Spring/Summer 1973), 40–87.

Mitry, Jean. *Esthétique et Psychologie du Cinéma*. Paris: Presses Universitaires de France, 1965.

———. *The Aesthetics and Psychology of the Cinema*. Translated by Christopher King. Bloomington: Indiana University Press, 1997.

*Münsterberg, Hugo. *The Film — A Psychological Study: The Silent Photoplay in 1916*. New York: Dover Publications, 1970. Reprinted and expanded as *Hugo Münsterberg on Film: The Photoplay — A Psychological Study and Other Writings*, edited by Allan Langdale. New York: Routledge, 2002.

New German Critique 54 (Fall 1991), special issue on Siegfried Kracauer.

Pudovkin, V. I. *Film Technique and Film Acting*. Translated by Ivor Montagu. New York: Grove Press, revised and enlarged ed., 1970.

Turvey, Malcolm. "Jean Epstein's Cinema of Immanence: The Rehabilitation of the Corporeal Eye." *October* 83 (Winter 1998), 25–50.

———. *The Enchanted Camera: Modernist Skepticism and Visual Redemption in Classical Film Theory*. Ph.D. diss., New York University, 2002.

C4. COGNITIVE THEORY

*Anderson, Joseph D. *The Reality of Illusion: An Ecological Approach to Cognitive Film Theory*. Carbondale: Southern Illinois University Press, 1996.

*Bordwell, David. *Making Meaning: Inference and Rhetoric in the Interpretation of Cinema*. Cambridge, Mass.: Harvard University Press, 1989.

*———. "A Case for Cognitivism." *Iris* 9 (Spring 1989), 11–40.

*———. "A Case for Cognitivism: Further Reflections." *Iris* 11 (Summer 1990), 107–12.

———. "Cognition and Comprehension: Viewing and Forgetting in Mildred Pierce." *Journal of Dramatic Theory and Criticism* 6 (Spring 1992), 183–98.

———. "Contemporary Film Studies and the Vicissitudes of Grand Theory." In *Post-Theory: Reconstructing Film Studies*, edited by David Bordwell and Noël Carroll. Madison: University of Wisconsin Press, 1996.

*———. "Convention, Construction, and Cinematic Vision." In *Post-Theory: Reconstructing Film Studies*, edited by David Bordwell and Noël Carroll. Madison: University of Wisconsin Press, 1996.

*Bordwell, David, and Noël Carroll, eds. *Post-Theory: Reconstructing Film Studies*. Madison: University of Wisconsin Press, 1996.

Branigan, Edward. "Sound, Epistemology, Film." In *Film Theory and Philosophy*, edited by Richard Allen and Murray Smith. New York: Oxford University Press, 1997.

*Buckland, Warren, ed. *The Film Spectator: From Sign to Mind*. Amsterdam: Amsterdam University Press, 1995.

*———. *The Cognitive Semiotics of Film*. Cambridge, U.K.: Cambridge University Press, 2000.

———. "Orientation in Film Space: A Cognitive Semiotic Approach." *Recherches en communication* 19 (2003), 87–102. Special issue on "Cognitive Semiotics."

Carroll, Noël. "Prospects for Film Theory: A Personal Assessment." In *Post-Theory: Reconstructing Film Studies*, edited by David Bordwell and Noël Carroll. Madison: University of Wisconsin Press, 1996.

———. "Fiction, Non-fiction, and the Film of Presumptive Assertion: A Conceptual Analysis." In *Film Theory and Philosophy*, edited by Richard Allen and Murray Smith. New York: Oxford University Press, 1997.

CiNéMAS 12 (Winter 2002), special issue on "cinema and cognition."

Currie, Gregory. *Image and Mind: Film, Philosophy and Cognitive Science*. Cambridge, U.K.: Cambridge University Press, 1995.

*Grodal, Torben. *Moving Pictures: A New Theory of Film Genres, Feelings, and Cognition*. Oxford, U.K.: Oxford University Press, 1997.

*———. "Art Film, the Transient Body, and the Permanent Soul." *Aura* 6 (2000), 33–53.

———. "Film, Character Simulation, and Emotion." In *Nicht allein das Laufbild auf der Leinwand . . . Strukturen des Films als Erlebnispotentiale*, edited by Jörg Friess, Britta Hartmann, and Eggo Müller. Berlin: Vistas Verlag, 2001.

———. "The Experience of Realism in Audiovisual Representation." In *Realism and "Reality" in Film and Media [Northern Lights Film and Media Studies Yearbook 2002]*, edited by Anne Jerslev. University of Copenhagen: Museum Tusculanum Press, 2002.

Grodal, Torben, Bente Larsen, and Iben Thorving Laursen, eds. *Visual Authorship: Creativity and Intentionality in Media [Northern Lights Film and Media Studies Yearbook 2004]*. University of Copenhagen: Museum Tusculanum Press, 2005.

*Hochberg, Julian, and Virginia Brooks. "Movies in the Mind's Eye." In *Post-Theory: Reconstructing Film Studies*, edited by David Bordwell and Noël Carroll. Madison: University of Wisconsin Press, 1996.

Iris 9 (Spring 1989), special issue on "Cinema and Cognitive Psychology."

Jullier, Laurent. *Cinéma et cognition*. Paris: L'Harmattan, 2002.

Larsen, Peter. "Urban Legends: Notes on a Theme in Early Film Theory." In *City Flicks: Indian Cinema and the Urban Experience*, edited by Preben Kaarsholm. Calcutta: Seagull Books, 2004.

Lefebvre, Martin. "On Memory and Imagination in the Cinema." *New Literary History* 30 (Spring 1999), 481–98.

*Persson, Per. *Understanding Cinema: A Psychological Theory of Moving Imagery*. Cambridge, U.K.: Cambridge University Press, 2003.

Plantinga, Carl R. *Rhetoric and Representation in Nonfiction Film*. Cambridge, U.K.: Cambridge University Press, 1997.

*———. "Cognitive Film Theory: An Insider's Appraisal." *CiNéMAS* 12 (Winter 2002), 15–37.

Plantinga, Carl, and Greg M. Smith, eds. *Passionate Views: Film, Cognition, and Emotion*. Baltimore: Johns Hopkins University Press, 1999.

Ponech, Trevor. "What Is Non-fiction Cinema?" In *Film Theory and Philosophy*, edited by Richard Allen and Murray Smith. New York: Oxford University Press, 1997.

*Simons, Jan. "'Enunciation': From Code to Interpretation." In *The Film Spectator: From Sign to Mind*, edited by Warren Buckland. Amsterdam: Amsterdam University Press, 1995.

*———. "Film, Language, and Conceptual Structures: Thinking Film in the Age of Cognitivism." Ph.D. diss., University of Amsterdam, 1995.

Smith, Greg M. *Film Structure and the Emotion System*. Cambridge, U.K.: Cambridge University Press, 2003.

*Smith, Murray. *Engaging Characters: Fiction, Emotion, and the Cinema*. Oxford, U.K.: Oxford University Press, 1995.

———. "Film Spectatorship and the Institution of Fiction." *The Journal of Aesthetics and Art Criticism* 53 (Spring 1995), 113–27.

Szaloky, Melinda. "Silence Fiction: Women's Voice and Film." M.A. thesis, University of Oslo, 1999.

———. "Silence Fiction: Rethinking (Under)Representations of the 'Feminine' Through Social Cognition." *CiNéMAS* 12 (Winter 2002), 89–115.

Tan, Ed S. *Emotion and the Structure of Narrative Film: Film as an Emotion Machine*. Translated by Barbara Fasting. Mahwah, N.J.: Lawrence Erlbaum, 1996.

*Vescio, Bryan. "Reading in the Dark: Cognitivism, Film Theory, and Radical Interpretation." *Style* 35 (Winter 2001), 572–91.

Wiley, Norbert. "Emotion and Film Theory." *Studies in Symbolic Interaction* 26 (New York: JAI, Elsevier Science, 2003), 169–87.

C5. NARRATOLOGY/NARRATIVE ANALYSIS

Aumont, Jacques. "The Point of View." *Quarterly Review of Film and Video* 11 (1989), 1–22.

Black, David A[lan]. "Genette and Film: Narrative Level in the Fiction Cinema." *Wide Angle* 8 (1986), 19–26.

*———. "Synopsis: A Theory of Symbolic Representation." *The Yale Journal of Criticism* 10 (Fall 1997), 423–36. Corrected illustration is in vol. 11 (Spring 1998), 313.

*———. *Law in Film: Resonance and Representation*. Urbana: University of Illinois Press, 1999.

*———. "Homo Confabulans: A Study in Film, Narrative, and Compensation." *Literature and Psychology* 47 (2001), 25–37.

*Bordwell, David. *Narration in the Fiction Film*. Madison: University of Wisconsin Press, 1985.

Branigan, Edward. *Point of View in the Cinema: A Theory of Narration and Subjectivity in Classical Film*. Berlin and New York: Mouton, 1984.

———. "Diegesis and Authorship in Film." *Iris* 7 (1986), 37–54.

———. "'Here Is a Picture of No Revolver!': The Negation of Images and Methods for Analyzing the Structure of Pictorial Statements." *Wide Angle* 8 (1986), 8–17.

*———. *Narrative Comprehension and Film*. New York and London: Routledge, 1992.

———. "Nearly True: Forking Plots, Forking Interpretations — A Response to David Bordwell's 'Film Futures.'" *SubStance* 97 (2002), 105–14.

Brewster, Ben. "A Bunch of Violets." Unpub. ms., 1995.

Browne, Nick. "The Spectator-in-the-Text: The Rhetoric of Stagecoach." *Film Quarterly* 29 (Winter 1975–76), 26–38. Reprinted in *Narrative, Apparatus, Ideology: A Film Theory Reader*, edited by Philip Rosen. New York: Columbia University Press, 1986.

———. "Narration as Interpretation: The Rhetoric of *Au Hasard, Balthazar*." In *The Rhetoric of Filmic Narration*. Ann Arbor, Mich.: UMI Research Press, 1976. Revised as "Narrative Point of View: The Rhetoric of *Au Hasard, Balthazar*." *Film Quarterly* 31 (Fall 1977), 19–31.

———. "Film Form/Voice-Over: Bresson's *The Diary of a Country Priest*." *Yale French Studies* 60 (1980), 233–40.

Buckland, Warren. "Narration and Focalisation in *Wings of Desire*." *CineAction* 56 (Sept. 2001), 26–33.

Casetti, Francesco. "The Communicative Pact." In *Towards a Pragmatics of the Audiovisual: Theory and History, Vol. 1*, edited by Jürgen E. Müller. Munich: Nodus Publikationen, 1994.

———. *Inside the Gaze: The Fiction Film and Its Spectator*. Translated by Nell Andrew with Charles O'Brien. Bloomington: Indiana University Press, 1998.

Chatman, Seymour. *Story and Discourse: Narrative Structure in Fiction and Film*. Ithaca, N.Y.: Cornell University Press, 1978.

———. "Characters and Narrators: Filter, Center, Slant, and Interest-Focus." *Poetics Today* 7 (1986), 189–204.

———. *Coming to Terms: The Rhetoric of Narrative in Fiction and Film*. Ithaca, N.Y.: Cornell University Press, 1990.

*Elsaesser, Thomas, and Warren Buckland. *Studying Contemporary American Film: A Guide to Movie Analysis*. London: Arnold, 2002.

Gaudreault, André, and François Jost. "Enunciation and Narration." In *A Companion to Film Theory*, edited by Toby Miller and Robert Stam. Oxford: Blackwell, 1999.

Gunning, Tom. "The Work of Film Analysis: Systems, Fragments, Alternation." *Semiotica* 144 (2003), 343–57.

Henderson, Brian. "Tense, Mood, and Voice in Film (Notes After Genette)." *Film Quarterly* 36 (Summer 1983), 4–17. Reprinted in *Film Quarterly: Forty Years — A Selection*, edited by Brian Henderson and Ann Martin with Lee Amazonas. Berkeley and Los Angeles: University of California Press, 1999.

Kania, Andrew. "Against the Ubiquity of Fictional Narrators." *The Journal of Aesthetics and Art Criticism* 63 (Winter 2005), 47–54.

Kawin, Bruce F. *Mindscreen: Bergman, Godard, and First-Person Film.* Princeton, N.J.: Princeton University Press, 1978.

———. "An Outline of Film Voices." *Film Quarterly* 38 (Winter 1984–85), 38–46.

Kinder, Marsha. "The Subversive Potential of the Pseudo-Iterative." *Film Quarterly* 43 (Winter 1989–90), 3–16. Reprinted in *Film Quarterly: Forty Years — A Selection*, edited by Brian Henderson and Ann Martin with Lee Amazonas. Berkeley and Los Angeles: University of California Press, 1999.

Mamber, Stephen. "Narrative Mapping." In *New Media: Theories and Practices of Digitextuality*, edited by Anna Everett and John T. Caldwell. New York: Routledge, 2003.

Metz, Christian. *L'Énonciation impersonnelle, ou le site du film.* Paris: Méridiens Klincksieck, 1991.

———. "The Impersonal Enunciation, or the Site of Film (In the margin of recent works on enunciation in cinema)." *New Literary History* 22 (Summer 1991), 747–72.

Pipolo, Tony. "The Aptness of Terminology: Point of View, Consciousness and *Letter from an Unknown Woman*." *Film Reader* 4 (1979), 166–79.

Pye, Douglas. "Movies and Point of View." *Movie* 36 (2000), 2–34.

Rush, Jeffrey S. "'Lyric Oneness': The Free Syntactical Indirect and the Boundary Between Narrative and Narration." *Wide Angle* 8 (1986), 27–33.

Thompson, Kristin. "The Concept of Cinematic Excess." In *Narrative, Apparatus, Ideology: A Film Theory Reader*, edited by Philip Rosen. New York: Columbia University Press, 1986.

———. *Storytelling in the New Hollywood: Understanding Classical Narrative Technique.* Cambridge, Mass.: Harvard University Press, 1999.

Tomasulo, Frank P. "Narrate and Describe? Point of View and Narrative Voice in *Citizen Kane's* Thatcher Sequence." *Wide Angle* 8 (1986), 45–52.

*Wilson, George M. *Narration in Light: Studies in Cinematic Point of View.* Baltimore: Johns Hopkins University Press, 1986.

———. "Le Grand Imagier Steps Out: The Primitive Basis of Film Narration." *Philosophical Topics* 25 (Spring 1997), 295–318.

C6. PHILOSOPHICAL FILM AESTHETICS

Allen, Richard. *Projecting Illusion: Film Spectatorship and the Impression of Reality.* Cambridge, U.K.: Cambridge University Press, 1995.

———. "Looking at Motion Pictures." In *Film Theory and Philosophy*, edited by Richard Allen and Murray Smith. New York: Oxford University Press, 1997.

Andrew, Dudley. "The Unauthorized Auteur Today." In *Film and Theory: An Anthology*, edited by Robert Stam and Toby Miller. Oxford, U.K.: Blackwell, 2000.

Barthes, Roland. *Camera Lucida: Reflections on Photography.* Translated by Richard Howard. New York: Hill and Wang, 1981.

Beller, Jonathan L. "Capital/Cinema." In *Deleuze & Guattari: New Mappings in Politics, Philosophy, and Culture,* edited by Eleanor Kaufman and Kevin Jon Heller. Minneapolis: University of Minnesota Press, 1998.

Bruno, Giuliana. "Collection and Recollection: On Film Itineraries and Museum Walks." In *Camera Obscura, Camera Lucida: Essays in Honor of Annette Michelson,* edited by Richard Allen and Malcolm Turvey. Amsterdam: Amsterdam University Press, 2003.

Burgin, Victor. "Looking at Photographs." In *Thinking Photography,* edited by Victor Burgin. London: Macmillan, 1982.

Carroll, Noël. "Language and Cinema: Preliminary Notes for a Theory of Verbal Images." *Millennium Film Journal* 7/8/9 (Fall/Winter 1980–1981), 186–217.

———. *Mystifying Movies: Fads & Fallacies in Contemporary Film Theory.* New York: Columbia University Press, 1988.

———. *The Philosophy of Horror, or Paradoxes of the Heart.* New York: Routledge, 1990.

———. *Theorizing the Moving Image.* Cambridge, U.K.: Cambridge University Press, 1996.

Cavell, Stanley. *The World Viewed: Reflections on the Ontology of Film.* Cambridge, Mass.: Harvard University Press, enlarged edition 1979.

——— *Cities of Words: Pedagogical Letters on a Register of the Moral Life.* Cambridge, Mass.: Harvard University Press, 2004.

Comolli, Jean-Louis. "Mechanical Bodies, Ever More Heavenly." *October* 83 (Winter 1998), 19–24.

Deleuze, Gilles. *Cinema 1: The Movement—Image.* Translated by Hugh Tomlinson and Barbara Habberjam. Minneapolis: University of Minnesota Press, 1986.

———. *Cinema 2: The Time-Image.* Translated by Hugh Tomlinson and Robert Galeta. Minneapolis: University of Minnesota Press, 1989.

———. *Negotiations, 1972–1990.* Translated by Martin Joughin. New York: Columbia University Press, 1995.

Gaut, Berys. "Cinematic Art." *The Journal of Aesthetics and Art Criticism* 60 (Fall 2002), 299–312.

Gerstner, David A., and Janet Staiger, eds. *Authorship and Film.* New York: Routledge, 2003.

Irwin, William, ed. *The Death and Resurrection of the Author?* Westport, Conn.: Greenwood Press, 2002.

Kirby, Lynne. "Painting and Cinema: The Frames of Discourse." *Camera Obscura* 18 (Sept. 1988), 95–105.

*Lastra, James. "Reading, Writing, and Representing Sound." In *Sound Theory/Sound Practice,* edited by Rick Altman. New York: Routledge, 1992.

Ponech, Trevor. "Visual Perception and Motion Picture Spectatorship." *Cinema Journal* 37 (Fall 1997), 85–100.

Rosen, Philip. *Change Mummified: Cinema, Historicity, Theory*. Minneapolis: University of Minnesota Press, 2001.

Sobchack, Vivian. *The Address of the Eye: A Phenomenology of Film Experience*. Princeton, N.J.: Princeton University Press, 1992.

Stewart, Garrett. *Between Film and Screen: Modernism's Photo Synthesis*. Chicago: University of Chicago Press, 1999.

*Szaloky, Melinda. "Sounding Images in Silent Film: Visual Acoustics in Murnau's Sunrise." *Cinema Journal* 41 (Winter 2002), 109–31.

*———. "Making New Sense of Film Theory Through Kant: A Novel Teaching Approach." *New Review of Film and Television Studies* 3 (May 2005), 33–58. Special issue on "Film and Television Studies Pedagogy."

Turim, Maureen. "Postmodern Metaphors and the Images of Thought." *Polygraph* 13 (2001), 112–19.

C7. PSYCHOANALYSIS

Baudry, Jean-Luis. "Ideological Effects of the Basic Cinematographic Apparatus." In *Narrative, Apparatus, Ideology: A Film Theory Reader*, edited by Philip Rosen. New York: Columbia University Press, 1986.

———. "The Apparatus: Metapsychological Approaches to the Impression of Reality in the Cinema." In *Narrative, Apparatus, Ideology: A Film Theory Reader*, edited by Philip Rosen. New York: Columbia University Press, 1986.

Bergstrom, Janet, ed. *Endless Night: Cinema and Psychoanalysis, Parallel Histories*. Berkeley and Los Angeles: University of California Press, 1999.

Burch, Noël. *Life to Those Shadows*. Translated by Ben Brewster. Berkeley and Los Angeles: University of California Press, 1990.

Casebier, Janet Jenks, and Allan Casebier. "Selective Bibliography on Dream and Film." *Dreamworks* 1 (Spring 1980), 88–93.

Doane, Mary Ann. *Femmes Fatales: Feminism, Film Theory, Psychoanalysis*. New York: Routledge, 1991.

———. "Temporality, Storage, Legibility: Freud, Marey, and the Cinema." *Critical Inquiry* 22 (Winter 1996), 313–43.

Eberwein, Robert T. *Film & The Dream Screen: A Sleep and a Forgetting*. Princeton, N.J.: Princeton University Press, 1984.

*Elsaesser, Thomas. "Tales of Sound and Fury: Observations on the Family Melodrama." In *Movies and Methods: An Anthology, Vol. II*, edited by Bill Nichols. Berkeley and Los Angeles: University of California Press, 1985.

Lapsley, Robert, and Michael Westlake. *Film Theory: An Introduction*. New York: St. Martin's Press, 1988.

*Metz, Christian. *The Imaginary Signifier: Psychoanalysis and the Cinema*. Translated by Celia Britton, Annwyl Williams, Ben Brewster, and Alfred Guzzetti. Bloomington: Indiana University Press, 1982.

———. "Photography and Fetish." *October* 34 (Fall 1985), 81–90.

Mulvey, Laura. *Visual and Other Pleasures*. Bloomington: Indiana University Press, 1989.

Penley, Constance. *The Future of an Illusion: Film, Feminism, and Psychoanalysis*. Minneapolis: University of Minnesota Press, 1989.

Rodowick, D. N. *The Crisis of Political Modernism: Criticism and Ideology in Contemporary Film Theory*. Urbana: University of Illinois Press, 1988.

Studlar, Gaylyn. "Masochism and the Perverse Pleasures of the Cinema." In *Movies and Methods: An Anthology, Vol. II*, edited by Bill Nichols. Berkeley and Los Angeles: University of California Press, 1985.

Willemen, Paul. "The Fugitive Subject." In *Raoul Walsh*, edited by Phil Hardy. Edinburgh: Edinburgh Film Festival, 1974.

———. "Reflections on Eikhenbaum's Concept of Internal Speech in the Cinema." *Screen* 15 (Winter 1974/75), 59–70.

———. "The Ophuls Text: A Thesis." In *Ophuls*, edited by Paul Willemen. London: British Film Institute, 1978.

———. *Looks and Frictions: Essays in Cultural Studies and Film Theory*. Bloomington: Indiana University Press, 1994.

Žižek, Slavoj. "'In His Bold Gaze My Ruin Is Writ Large.'" In *Everything You Always Wanted to Know about Lacan (But Were Afraid to Ask Hitchcock)*, edited by Slavoj Žižek. New York: Verso, 1992.

———. "The Hitchcockian Blot." In *Alfred Hitchcock: Centenary Essays*, edited by Richard Allen and S. Ishii-Gonzalès. London: British Film Institute, 1999.

———. *The Fragile Absolute or, Why Is the Christian Legacy Worth Fighting for?* New York: Verso, 2000.

C8. SEMIOTICS

Buckland, Warren. "Film Semiotics." In *A Companion to Film Theory*, edited by Toby Miller and Robert Stam. Oxford: Blackwell, 1999.

*Eco, Umberto. *A Theory of Semiotics*. Bloomington: Indiana University Press, 1976.

Iris 10 (April 1990), special issue on "Christian Metz & Film Theory."

Kinneavy, James. *A Theory of Discourse: The Aims of Discourse*. New York: W.W. Norton, 1971.

Metz, Christian. *Film Language: A Semiotics of the Cinema*. Translated by Michael Taylor. New York: Oxford University Press, 1974.

———. *Language and Cinema*. Translated by Donna Jean Umiker-Sebeok. The Hague: Mouton, 1974.

———. "The Perceived and the Named." Translated by Steven Feld and Shari Robertson. *Studies in Visual Communication* 6 (Fall 1980), 56–68.

Stam, Robert. *Film Theory: An Introduction*. Oxford: Blackwell, 2000.

Stam, Robert, Robert Burgoyne, and Sandy Flitterman-Lewis. *New Vocabularies in Film Semiotics: Structuralism, Post-Structuralism and Beyond*. New York: Routledge, 1992.

Projecting a Camera

C9. SUTURE

Bonitzer, Pascal. "Deframings." In *Cahiers du Cinéma, Vol. 4, 1973–1978: History, Ideology, Cultural Struggle*, edited by David Wilson. New York: Routledge, 2000.

Dayan, Daniel. "The Tutor-Code of Classical Cinema." In *Movies and Methods: An Anthology* [vol. I], edited by Bill Nichols. Berkeley and Los Angeles: University of California Press, 1976.

Geuens, Jean-Pierre. *Film Production Theory*. Albany: State University of New York Press, 2000.

Hayward, Susan. *Cinema Studies: The Key Concepts*. New York: Routledge, 2nd ed. 2000.

*Heath, Stephen. *Questions of Cinema*. New York: Macmillan, 1981.

Marciniak, Katarzyna. "Second Worldness and Transnational Feminist Practices: Agnieszka Holland's *A Woman Alone*." In *East European Cinemas*, edited by Anikó Imre. New York: Routledge, forthcoming 2005.

McGowan, Todd. "Looking for the Gaze: Lacanian Film Theory and Its Vicissitudes." *Cinema Journal* 42 (Spring 2003), 27–47.

Miller, Jacques-Alain. "Suture (Elements of the Logic of the Signifier)." *Screen* 18 (Winter 1977/78), 24–34.

Oudart, Jean-Pierre. "Cinema and Suture." *Screen* 18 (Winter 1977/78), 35–47. Reprinted in *Cahiers du Cinéma 1969–1972: The Politics of Representation* [vol. 3], edited by Nick Browne. Cambridge, Mass.: Harvard University Press, 1990.

Rothman, William. "Against 'The System of the Suture.'" In *Movies and Methods: An Anthology* [vol. I], edited by Bill Nichols. Berkeley and Los Angeles: University of California Press, 1976.

Salt, Barry. "The Last of the Suture?" *Film Quarterly* 31 (Summer 1978), 64–65.

Silverman, Kaja. *The Subject of Semiotics*. New York: Oxford University Press, 1983.

Žižek, Slavoj. *The Fright of Real Tears: Krzysztof Kieślowski between Theory and Post-Theory*. London: British Film Institute, 2001.

D. LITERATURE

D1. NARRATOLOGY/NARRATIVE ANALYSIS

Bal, Mieke. *Narratology: Introduction to the Theory of Narrative*. Toronto: University of Toronto Press, 2nd ed. 1997.

*Barthes, Roland. *S/Z*. Translated by Richard Miller. New York: Hill and Wang, 1974.

Booth, Wayne C. "Distance and Point-of-View: An Essay in Classification." *Essays in Criticism* 11 (Jan. 1961), 60–79.

———. *The Rhetoric of Fiction*. Chicago: University of Chicago Press, 2nd ed. 1983.

Chatman, Seymour. *Reading Narrative Fiction*. New York: Macmillan, 1993.

Friedman, Norman. "Point of View in Fiction: The Development of a Critical Concept." *PMLA* 70 (Dec. 1955), 1160–1184.

Genette, Gérard. *Narrative Discourse: An Essay in Method.* Translated by Jane E. Lewin. Ithaca, N.Y.: Cornell University Press, 1980.

———. *Narrative Discourse Revisited.* Translated by Jane E. Lewin. Ithaca, N.Y.: Cornell University Press, 1988.

Herman, David. *Universal Grammar and Narrative Form.* Durham, N.C.: Duke University Press, 1995.

Lanser, Susan Sniader. *The Narrative Act: Point of View in Prose Fiction.* Princeton, N.J.: Princeton University Press, 1981.

Morson, Gary Saul. *Narrative and Freedom: The Shadows of Time.* New Haven: Yale University Press, 1994.

New Literary History 32 (Summer 2001): special issue on "Voice and Human Experience."

*Prince, Gerald. *A Dictionary of Narratology.* Lincoln: University of Nebraska Press, 1987.

Rimmon-Kenan, Shlomith. *Narrative Fiction: Contemporary Poetics.* London: Methuen, 1983.

Schafer, Roy. "Action and Narration in Psychoanalysis." *New Literary History* 12 (Autumn 1980), 61–85.

Turner, Victor. "Social Dramas and Stories about Them." *Critical Inquiry* 7 (Autumn 1980), 141–68. Special issue "On Narrative" reprinted with additional essays as *On Narrative*, edited by W.J.T. Mitchell. Chicago: University of Chicago Press, 1981.

Uspensky, Boris. *A Poetics of Composition: The Structure of the Artistic Text and Typology of a Compositional Form.* Translated by Valentina Zavarin and Susan Wittig. Berkeley and Los Angeles: University of California Press, 1973.

Van Peer, Willie, and Seymour Chatman, eds. *New Perspectives on Narrative Perspective.* Albany: State University of New York Press, 2001.

White, Hayden. "The Value of Narrativity in the Representation of Reality." *Critical Inquiry* 7 (Autumn 1980), 5–27. Special issue "On Narrative" reprinted with additional essays as *On Narrative*, edited by W.J.T. Mitchell. Chicago: University of Chicago Press, 1981.

Young, Kay. *Ordinary Pleasures: Couples, Conversation, and Comedy.* Columbus: Ohio State University Press, 2001.

D2. THEORY

Barthes, Roland. *Critical Essays.* Translated by Richard Howard. Evanston, Ill.: Northwestern University Press, 1972.

———. *The Pleasure of the Text.* Translated by Richard Miller. New York: Hill and Wang, 1975.

*———. *Image, Music, Text.* Translated by Stephen Heath. New York: Hill and Wang, 1977.

Jakobson, Roman. "Linguistics and Poetics." In *The Structuralists: From Marx to Lévi-Strauss,* edited by Richard and Fernande de George. Garden City, N.Y.: Anchor Books, 1972.

Mitchell, W.J.T. *Iconology: Image, Text, Ideology.* Chicago: University of Chicago Press, 1986.

———. *Picture Theory: Essays on Verbal and Visual Representation.* Chicago: University of Chicago Press, 1994.

Robbe-Grillet, Alain. *For a New Novel: Essays on Fiction.* Translated by Richard Howard. New York: Grove, 1965.

Todorov, Tzvetan. *The Poetics of Prose.* Translated by Richard Howard. Ithaca, N.Y.: Cornell University Press, 1977.

———. *Theories of the Symbol.* Translated by Catherine Porter. Oxford: Basil Blackwell, 1982.

E. PHILOSOPHY

Adajian, Thomas. "On the Prototype Theory of Concepts and the Definition of Art." *The Journal of Aesthetics and Art Criticism* 63 (Summer 2005), 231–36.

Aldrich, Virgil. *Philosophy of Art.* Englewood Cliffs, N.J.: Prentice-Hall, 1963.

Allen, Richard, and Malcolm Turvey, eds. *Wittgenstein, Theory and the Arts.* London: Routledge, 2001.

Ayer, A. J. *Probability and Evidence.* New York: Macmillan, 1972.

Beardsley, Monroe C. *Aesthetics from Classical Greece to the Present: A Short History.* New York: Macmillan, 1966.

Benjamin, Walter. *Illuminations.* Edited by Hannah Arendt. Translated by Harry Zohn. New York: Schocken, 1969.

———. *The Arcades Project.* Translated by Howard Eiland and Kevin McLaughlin. Cambridge, Mass.: Harvard University Press, 1999.

Bouwsma, O. K. *Philosophical Essays.* Lincoln: University of Nebraska Press, 1965.

*———. *Toward a New Sensibility: Essays of O. K. Bouwsma,* edited by J. L. Craft and Ronald E. Hustwit. Lincoln and London: University of Nebraska Press, 1982.

———. *Wittgenstein: Conversations, 1949–1951,* edited by J.L. Craft and Ronald E. Hustwit. Indianapolis: Hackett, 1986.

Cohen, Ted. "The Philosophy of Taste: Thoughts on the Idea." In *The Blackwell Guide to Aesthetics,* edited by Peter Kivy. Oxford, U.K.: Blackwell Publishing, 2004.

Danto, Arthur. *The Transfiguration of the Commonplace: A Philosophy of Art.* Cambridge, Mass.: Harvard University Press, 1981.

De Certeau, Michel. *The Practice of Everyday Life.* Translated by Steven Rendall. Berkeley and Los Angeles: University of California Press, 1984.

De Landa, Manuel. "Wittgenstein at the Movies." In *Cinema Histories, Cinema Practices*, edited by Patricia Mellencamp and Philip Rosen [The American Film Institute Monograph Series, vol. 4]. Frederick, Md.: University Publications of America, 1984.

*Dennett, Daniel C. "Real Patterns." *The Journal of Philosophy* 88 (Jan. 1991), 27–51.

Descartes, René. *The Philosophical Writings of Descartes, Vols. I and II*, edited by John Cottingham, Robert Stoothoff, and Dugald Murdoch. Cambridge, U.K.: Cambridge University Press, 1984.

Ellis, John M. *Language, Thought, and Logic*. Evanston, Ill.: Northwestern University Press, 1993.

*Glock, Hans-Johann. *A Wittgenstein Dictionary*. Oxford: Blackwell, 1996.

Goodman, Nelson. *Languages of Art: An Approach to a Theory of Symbols*. Indianapolis, Ind.: Hackett, 2nd ed. 1976.

*———. *Ways of Worldmaking*. Indianapolis: Hackett Publishing Co., 1978.

———. *Fact, Fiction, and Forecast*. Cambridge, Mass.: Harvard University Press, 4th ed. 1983.

*Goodman, Nelson, and Catherine Z. Elgin. *Reconceptions in Philosophy and Other Arts and Sciences*. Indianapolis, Ind.: Hackett Publishing, 1988.

Grayling, A. C. *Wittgenstein: A Very Short Introduction*. New York: Oxford University Press, 2001.

Hernadi, Paul. *Cultural Transactions: Nature, Self, Society*. Ithaca, N.Y.: Cornell University Press, 1995.

Journal of Aesthetic Education 25 (Spring 1991), special issue on Nelson Goodman, "More Ways of Worldmaking."

Langer, Susanne K. *Feeling and Form: A Theory of Art*. New York: Charles Scribner's Sons, 1953.

Merleau-Ponty, Maurice. *Phenomenology of Perception*. Translated by Colin Smith. London: Routledge & Kegan Paul, 1962.

Moore, G[eorge] E[dward]. "Wittgenstein's Lectures in 1930–33" (Part III). *Mind* 64 (Jan. 1955), 1–27. Part I is in *Mind* 63 (Jan. 1954), 1–15; Part II is in *Mind* 63 (July 1954), 289–316. Reprinted in *Philosophical Occasions, 1912–1951*, edited by James C. Klagge and Alfred Nordmann. Indianapolis: Hackett, 1993.

———. *Philosophical Papers*. London: George Allen & Unwin, 1959.

Plato. *The Collected Dialogues of Plato, Including the Letters*, edited by Edith Hamilton and Huntington Cairns. Princeton, N.J.: Princeton University Press, 1963.

Plato: Complete Works, edited by John M. Cooper and D.S. Hutchinson. Indianapolis and Cambridge: Hackett Publishing, 1997.

Rajchman, John, and Cornel West, eds. *Post-Analytic Philosophy*. New York: Columbia University Press, 1985.

Rorty, Richard. *Contingency, Irony, and Solidarity*. Cambridge, U.K.: Cambridge University Press, 1989.

———. *Objectivity, Relativism, and Truth: Philosophical Papers, Vol. I*. Cambridge, U.K.: Cambridge University Press, 1991.

———. *Essays on Heidegger and Others: Philosophical Papers, Vol. 2*. Cambridge, U.K.: Cambridge University Press, 1991.

Savedoff, Barbara E. "Frames." *The Journal of Aesthetics and Art Criticism* 57 (Summer 1999), 345–56.

Scruton, Roger. "Photography and Representation." *Critical Inquiry* 7 (Spring 1981), 577–603.

Sparshott, F. E. "Goodman on Expression." *The Monist* 58 (April 1974), 187–202.

Stevenson, Charles L. "On the 'Analysis' of a Work of Art." In *Contemporary Studies in Aesthetics*, edited by Francis J. Coleman. New York: McGraw-Hill, 1968.

Strawson, P. F. *Analysis and Metaphysics: An Introduction to Philosophy*. Oxford, U.K.: Oxford University Press, 1992.

Thomasson, Amie L. "The Ontology of Art and Knowledge in Aesthetics." *The Journal of Aesthetics and Art Criticism* 63 (Summer 2005), 221–29.

Wittgenstein, Ludwig. *The Blue and Brown Books: Preliminary Studies for the "Philosophical Investigations."* New York: Harper & Row, 2nd ed. 1960.

*———. *Philosophical Investigations*. Translated by G.E.M. Anscombe. Oxford, U.K.: Blackwell, 3rd ed. 1967.

———. *Remarks on Colour*. Edited by G.E.M. Anscombe. Translated by Linda L. McAlister and Margarete Schättle. Berkeley and Los Angeles: University of California Press, 1977.

———. *L. Wittgenstein: Lectures & Conversations on Aesthetics, Psychology and Religious Belief, Compiled from Notes Taken by Yorick Smythies, Rush Rhees and James Taylor*. Edited by Cyril Barrett. Berkeley and Los Angeles: University of California Press, 1992.

———. *Philosophical Occasions, 1912–1951*. Edited by James C. Klagge and Alfred Nordmann. Indianapolis: Hackett, 1993.

———. *Wittgenstein's Lectures, Cambridge, 1932–1935: From the Notes of Alice Ambrose and Margaret Macdonald*. Edited by Alice Ambrose. Amherst, New York: Prometheus Books, 2001.

Wollheim, Richard. "Representation: The Philosophical Contribution to Psychology." *Critical Inquiry* 3 (Summer 1977), 709–23.

F. PICTORIAL COMPOSITION

Arnheim, Rudolf. *The Power of the Center: A Study of Composition in the Visual Arts — The New Version*. Berkeley and Los Angeles: University of California Press, 1988.

Dow, Arthur Wesley. *Composition; A Series of Exercises in Art Structure for the Use of Students and Teachers*. Berkeley and Los Angeles: University of California Press, 13th ed. 1997.

Freeburg, Victor Oscar. *Pictorial Beauty on the Screen*. New York: Arno Press, 1970.

Kepes, Gyorgy. *Language of Vision*. Chicago: Paul Theobald, 1944.

Nilsen, Vladimir. *The Cinema as a Graphic Art (On a Theory of Representation in the Cinema)*. Translated by Stephen Garry. New York: Hill and Wang, 1959. Reprinted by Garland Publishing, New York, 1985.

Turim, Maureen. "Symmetry/Asymmetry and Visual Fascination." *Wide Angle* 4 (1980), 38–47.

G. PSYCHOLOGY

Arnheim, Rudolf. *Toward a Psychology of Art*. Berkeley and Los Angeles: University of California Press, 1966.

———. *Art and Visual Perception: A Psychology of the Creative Eye [The New Version]*. Berkeley and Los Angeles: University of California Press, rev. ed. 1974.

———. *The Dynamics of Architectural Form*. Berkeley and Los Angeles: University of California Press, 1977.

Berthoz, Alain. *The Brain's Sense of Movement*. Translated by Giselle Weiss. Cambridge, Mass.: Harvard University Press, 2000.

Bruner, Jerome. *Actual Minds, Possible Worlds*. Cambridge, Mass.: Harvard University Press, 1986.

———. "Self-Making and World-Making." *The Journal of Aesthetic Education* 25 (Spring 1991), 67–78.

———. *Making Stories: Law, Literature, Life*. New York: Farrar, Straus and Giroux, 2002.

Freud, Sigmund. "The 'Uncanny.'" In *The Standard Edition of the Complete Psychological Works of Sigmund Freud, Vol. XVII (1917–1919)*, edited by James Strachey. London: The Hogarth Press, 1955.

———. *Beyond the Pleasure Principle*. Translated and edited by James Strachey. New York: W.W. Norton & Co., 1961.

———. *The Psychopathology of Everyday Life*. Translated by Alan Tyson. Edited by James Strachey. New York: W.W. Norton & Co., 1965.

Gombrich, E. H., Julian Hochberg, and Max Black. *Art, Perception, and Reality*. Baltimore: Johns Hopkins University Press, 1972.

Gregory, Richard L. *Eye and Brain: The Psychology of Seeing*. Princeton, N.J.: Princeton University Press, 5th ed. 1997.

Hershenson, Maurice. *Visual Space Perception: A Primer*. Cambridge, Mass.: MIT Press, 1999.

Hess, R. H., C. L. Baker, Jr., and J. Zihl. "The 'Motion-Blind' Patient: Low-Level Spatial and Temporal Filters." *The Journal of Neuroscience* 9 (May 1989), 1628–1640.

*Laplanche, J., and J.-B. Pontalis. *The Language of Psycho–Analysis.* Translated by Donald Nicholson-Smith. New York: W.W. Norton, 1973.

Marr, David. *Vision: A Computational Investigation into the Human Representation and Processing of Visual Information.* San Francisco: W.H. Freeman, 1982.

Pinker, Steven, ed. *Visual Cognition.* Cambridge, Mass.: MIT Press, 1984.

Rock, Irvin. "The Perception of Disoriented Figures." *Scientific American* 230 (July 1974), 78–85.

———. "Anorthoscopic Perception." *Scientific American* 244 (Sept. 1981), 145–53.

H. RESIDUUM

Brecht, Bertolt. The *Threepenny Opera.* Translated by Ralph Manheim and John Willett. New York: Arcade, 1994.

Carroll, Lewis. *The Annotated Alice: The Definitive Edition [Alice's Adventures in Wonderland & Through the Looking-Glass].* Introduction and notes by Martin Gardner. New York: W.W. Norton & Co., 2000.

Dahl, Roald. *James and the Giant Peach.* New York: Puffin Books, 1961.

Joyce, James. *Ulysses.* New York: Vintage Books, 1961.

Kafka, Franz. *The Complete Stories.* New York: Schocken, 1995.

McCarthy, Mary. "C.Y.E." In *Cast a Cold Eye.* New York: Harcourt Brace Jovanovich, 1950.

Scarry, Richard. *Bedtime Stories.* New York: Random House, 1989.

———. *A Day at the Fire Station.* New York: Golden Books, 2003.

Smolin, Lee. *Three Roads to Quantum Gravity.* New York: Basic Books, 2001.

Index

The Index includes the Preface, Notes, and Works Cited (in which authors are linked to a category, e.g., B, C5), but not the Acknowledgments. If one wishes to read this book through its index — by using the index as an outline of the book's arguments — one might begin with the chart that accompanies the entry, "frame, fifteen types of." Additional charts may be found under "camera," "framing," "meaning," and "metaphor, optical."

narrations 122; Grodal 109, 117, ch. 4 nn. 34, 54, ch. 5 n. 70;
heterarchy, not hierarchy 122; indefiniteness 146; nonanalytical
editing 122
as-if 223–24
as-is 223–24
aspect-dawning (Wittgenstein) 113, 198–200, 206, 223, ch. 5 nn. 54, 55, 56,
66, 69
Astruc, Alexandre ch. 3 n. 47, C2
attention 57–63:
and ambiguity 62; Bazin 77–78; attention to material form 75;
attention maps abstract spaces 62; of camera 36, 61–63; and
camera position 58, 63; and causation 190; and close-up ch. 4
n. 21; creates a camera 93; deep focus 55; dissective 13, ch. 1 n. 18;
filmic metaphors for 61–62; able to attend to only one or two
things at a time 62; Descartes ch. 2 n. 60; Durgnat 92; involuntary
62; Lindgren 78; maintain audience attention (Lightman) 35; may
shift ten-fifteen times/second 61; metaphor based on (opposed to
surface-depth metaphor) 126; Münsterberg ch. 2 n. 61; narration
prompts attention 30; narrativizing shot scale prompts attention
ch. 2 n. 10; perceptual masking ch. 4 n. 82; preconscious ch. 3
n. 72; and schemata ch. 5 n. 16; privileging of immediate attention
ch. 4 n. 115; during suture 135–37; synoptic 13, 16, ch. 1 n. 18;
unmotivated draws attention 26; while watching 18, 165; and
working memory 127, ch. 4 n. 81; *see also* camera movement,
perception of; unobtrusiveness principle
Au Hasard, Balthazar (Bresson, 1966) ch. 3 n. 53, ch. 4 n. 93
Aumont, Jacques:
camera ch. 5 n. 76; edge contrast ch. 4 n. 19; narrativization of
shot scale ch. 2 n. 10; theory of filmic point of view 49, ch. 2 n. 28;
works cited C1, C5
aura (Benjamin) 106, 132, ch. 4 n. 26; *see also* excess
Austin, J(ohn) L(angshaw) 191
authorship:
art cinema 98; auteur/Author 15, 18, ch. 1 nn. 11, 21, 23; authors
who imitate (Plato) ch. 3 n. 56; Barthes' view 2–7; birth of the
reader 3, 6; and communication 81, ch. 2 n. 31; death of 2–3, 7,
ch. 1 nn. 7, 23; definition ch. 5 n. 4; as description ch. 1 n. 21;
expression of Author 81; and fictiveness 168–69; film Author/Artist's
power ix; as first reader 5; as form of impersonation 7; forms of
address 84; and illusionism ch. 3 n. 56; impersonal 3; reader-author
7 fig. 1.1; and objectivity 3; Plato ch. 3 n. 56; in reductionism
and connectionism (two analytical methods) 15–16; as rhetoric
ch. 3 n. 56; Rothman ch. 3 n. 44; theories of ch. 4 n. 50; *see also*
impersonality; narration; point of view
Ayer, A.J. ch. 3 n. 36, E

Bechtel, William ch. 2 n. 59, B

Beggar's Opera, The (ballad opera by John Gay, 1728) 171

Beller, Jonathan L. ch. 5 n. 59, C6

Bellour, Raymond:
  dissective analysis ch. 1 n. 18

Belvaux, Rémy ch. 2 n. 56

Benjamin, Walter 107, 205, ch. 3 n. 14, ch. 4 nn. 22, 24, 26, ch. 5 n. 65, E

Benning, James 27

Bergala, Alain ch. 2 n. 10, C1

Bergman, Ingmar ch. 3 n. 53, ch. 4 nn. 32, 42, ch. 5 n. 67

Bergson, Henri ch. 4 n. 68

Bergstrom, Janet ch. 4 n. 42, C7

Bernard, André ch. 2 n. 1, C1

Berthoz, Alain ch. 5 n. 10, G

Bertolucci, Bernardo ch. 4 n. 32

Bingham, Roger ch. 4 n. 60, ch. 5 n. 27, B

Birds, The (Hitchcock, 1963) 50

Black, David Alan xix:
  on Genette ch. 2 n. 24; on narrative ch. 4 n. 4, ch. 5 n. 58; synopsis ch. 5 n. 58; works cited C5

Black, Max ch. 3 n. 45, G

blot, double framing of (Žižek) 42, 44, 47–50, 52, 112, ch. 4 n. 42; *see also* excess

Bond, James 167, 168–69, 170, 177, 189, ch. 5 n. 18

Bonitzer, Pascal ch. 4 n. 68, ch. 5 n. 67:
  deframing 142–43, 144, 145, ch. 2 n. 48; works cited C9

Bonzel, André ch. 2 n. 56

Booth, Wayne C.:
  theory of literary point of view 43, ch. 2 nn. 22, 31, ch. 3 n. 76; works cited D1

Bordwell, David xix, ch. 3 nn. 10, 13, 71, ch. 4 nn. 63, 65, 116, ch. 5 n. 27:
  analysis ch. 1 n. 18; art cinema 98, 109, ch. 3 n. 56, ch. 4 nn. 3, 33; camera ch. 5 n. 59; camera position and spectator attention 58, 63, ch. 2 n. 55; composition ch. 4 n. 20; critical rhetoric ch. 3 n. 68, ch. 4 n. 11, ch. 5 nn. 69, 75; on Genette ch. 2 n. 24; historical poetics ch. 1 n. 24; invisible observer ch. 4 n. 92; long take ch. 2 n. 10; middle-level research vs. piecemeal theorizing ch. 1 n. 24; moderate constructivism 19, 123, 147, ch. 2 n. 31, ch. 4 nn. 6, 61; narrative ch. 2 n. 6; shot/reverse shot ch. 4 n. 84, ch. 5 n. 70; *Sunrise* ch. 2 n. 57; theory of filmic point of view 48, ch. 2 nn. 11, 25, 31; time ch. 5 n. 10; types of cameras ch. 3 n. 2; unmotivated camera ch. 2 n. 3, ch. 4 n. 38; Wittgenstein ch. 5 n. 69; works cited C1, C2, C3, C4, C5

Borzage, Frank 91, ch. 3 n. 62

bottom-up perceptual processing:
  aesthetics (Wittgenstein) ch. 5 n. 69; Brakhage 114; color 129; cues and projector time 118; dawning of aspects 198–200; definition 117–18,

dissective attention (Stevenson) 13, 16, ch. 1 n. 18
distinct *see* "clear and distinct"
Doane, Mary Ann ch. 4 n. 42, ch. 5 n. 10, C7
documentary 219, ch. 5 n. 37; *see also* realism; typicality
Douchet, Jean ch. 5 n. 67
Dow, Arthur Wesley ch. 4 n. 20, F
Draaisma, Douwe ch. 5 n. 33, B
dream *see* camera, eight theoretical conceptions of
Dreyer, Carl-Theodor 27, 142, ch. 2 n. 3, ch. 3 n. 71, ch. 4 n. 34
Dr. No (Young, 1962) 168, 174, 177, ch. 5 n. 18
Dr. Strangelove (Kubrick, 1964) 148
Duras, Marguerite 142
Durgnat, Raymond:
      anthropomorphism 37, 38, ch. 2 n. 17, ch. 3 n. 54; camera 91–93, ch. 3
      n. 72; offscreen space ch. 4 n. 36; tendencies of camera movements
      ch. 2 n. 50; works cited C1, C2
Duro, Paul ch. 4 n. 13, A

eagle, examples of types of representation of 66–67, 68, 76, ch. 3 nn. 4, 74
Easy Street (Chaplin, 1917) 108, 207–208
Eberwein, Robert T. ch. 3 n. 60, ch. 4 n. 42, C7
Eclisse, L' (Antonioni, 1962) 30
ecological conventions (Grodal) 19, 99, 123, 147, ch. 2 n. 31, ch. 4 nn. 6, 61;
      see also middle-level approaches to film theory
Eco, Umberto ch. 3 n. 50, C8
Edison, Thomas 2, 74
editing:
      analytical 33–35; bottom-up and top-down forms of 118; camera
      movement as form of 78; cheat cut ch. 4 n. 81; continuity 163–66,
      176, ch. 5 n. 14; defined through set theory (Deleuze) ch. 4 n. 68;
      dislocated style ch. 2 n. 2; essence of cinema 78; grande syntagmatique
      of Metz ch. 2 n. 32; hierarchy vs. heterarchy 122; hyperdiegetic ch. 4
      n. 63; hysterical 52; as incomplete camera movements 162, ch. 2 n. 2;
      interior/latent (or internal/implicit) montage (plan-séquence) ch. 2
      nn. 10, 32; jump cut 203, ch. 4 n. 18, ch. 5 n. 3; local vs. distributed
      juxtapositions 122; match on action 163–65; Metz and fetishism ch. 4
      n. 42; nonanalytical 122; overlap with concept of "movement" between
      frames 11, 148, 160–166; overlap with concept of "movement"
      between shots 60, 61, 159, 162, 202, ch. 2 n. 2; overlap with concept
      of "postwandering" camera movement 60–61; overlap with definition
      of shot ch. 4 n. 38; perception of 176–78; problem of defining 19,
      61, 122, ch. 2 n. 32, ch. 4 nn. 38, 63, 109; Pudovkin ch. 2 n. 13;

Epstein, Jean 204–205, 206, ch. 3 n. 14, ch. 4 n. 26, ch. 5 nn. 2, 63–64, 66, C3
Equinox Flower (Ozu, 1958) ch. 5 n. 3
essence *see* a priori; ontology
Eustache, Jean 142
Everett, Anna ch. 5 n. 9, C5
everyday discourse/practice:
> camera linked to 15, 18; and the everyday body 119; Kracauer 106;
> about light xv–xvi, 128; in/out of ordinary time 109–10; sources of
> 211; as symbol system 1, 22; see also basic-level categories; "form
> of life"; frame, fifteen types of, no. 8 implicit everyday rationale;
> Kracauer; language, ordinary; talk
excess/surplus:
> Andrew ch. 4 n. 26; Barthes ch. 4 n. 26; as basic-level category ch. 4
> n. 26; and cinephilia ch. 4 n. 26; created through inspection 106;
> definition ch. 4 n. 26; deframing as anti-excess ch. 4 n. 113; as disframing
> ch. 4 n. 42; as downstream metaphor ch. 4 n. 26; and fiction 170; as
> metaphorical projection xv; Thompson ch. 4 n. 26; toning exceeds tinting
> 131; as upstream metaphor ch. 4 n. 26; *see also* aura; blot
expression:
> art cinema 98; Arnheim ch. 3 n. 46; in close-up shot (Balázs) 1; and
> empathy 80, 81; Romanticism 81, ch. 3 n. 44; theory of 80–81, ch. 3 n. 44;
> *see also* camera, eight theoretical conceptions of; meaning in film narrative

Falls, The (Greenaway, 1980) ch. 4 n. 48
family resemblance (Wittgenstein) 122 fig. 4.1, ch. 4 nn. 1, 61, ch. 5 n. 31 [cf. the
> notion of family resemblance with the "case law system" used to fashion
> legal principles]:
> "Art" ch. 4 n. 15; and aspect-dawning 198–200; "camera" 148, 216,
> ch. 5 n. 89 *see also* camera, eight theoretical conceptions of – camera,
> general conceptions of; "causation" xviii, ch. 5 n. 72; "chair" ch. 4 n. 115;
> "editing" 19, 61, ch. 4 nn. 38, 63, *see also* editing; "figure" 102; "frame"
> 6, 102–15, 121–22, 145, 147–48; "game" ch. 1 n. 15, ch. 5 n. 49; "good"
> 97, 102, 119, ch. 4 n. 1, ch. 5 n. 22; "guide/guiding" 195–97; "intention"
> 116; "language" ch. 1 n. 15; "look" 141; "movement" ch. 4 n. 62; nature
> of family resemblance ch. 4 n. 61; "on the screen" 148; "open" 102;
> "realism" 99–100; "resemblance" ch. 4 n. 61; "see" 77, 178, 211, ch. 5
> n. 82; "shot" ch. 4 nn. 18, 38, 109; other radial words 195, ch. 4 n. 1;
> "time" ch. 4 n. 115; "voice" *see* voice; what "misleads" in an analogy
> ch. 4 n. 115; "zero" ch. 4 n. 12; *see also* ambiguity; radial category
Farocki, Harun ch. 3 n. 55, C1
Fassbinder, Rainer Werner ix, ch. 4 nn. 20, 32, ch. 5 n. 18
Fauconnier, Gilles ch. 4 n. 35, B

not seeing through or in place of the camera 91, 92, 93, 105, 110, 167, 176–78, ch. 3 n. 75, ch. 4 n. 52, ch. 5 n. 26; and unobtrusiveness principle 84

projecting:

a camera xvi, 20, 36, 90–91, ch. 5 n. 73; camera knowledge 15; always in a direction 222; expression 1, 80–81; in family resemblance ch. 4 n. 61; Freud 124; from ordinary belief 176, 206; in horizontal intersection analysis 13; mental 5, 177; by metaphor 120, 121, 123; by using a grammar 218–20; an ontology xv–xvi; a life/our lives into a camera 15; projections to live by xvii; significance 93–94; spaces 93; meanings of word "projection" ch. 5 n. 9; *see also* metaphor; narrativize

Psycho (Hitchcock, 1960) 10, 91, ch. 2 n. 56, ch. 3 n. 72, ch. 4 nn. 36, 42

psychoanalysis *see* camera, eight theoretical conceptions of, no. 7 phantasy/dream; frame, fifteen types of, no. 14 psychic state; Freud; Lacan; suture; Žižek

Pudovkin, V.I. 35, 44, 52, ch. 2 n. 13, ch. 4 n. 92, C3

Pye, Douglas

theory of filmic point of view 52, ch. 2 n. 30; works cited C5

Pylyshyn, Zenon W. ch. 4 n. 43, B

Quine, W. V. xv

quotations:

texts comprised of 2, 3, 16, ch. 1 n. 8; *see also* description, under

radial category (dispersal of meaning):

ambiguity 6; analogy for ch. 4 n. 16; anchored by body 115; brief formula for 223–24; "camera" as 148, 216, ch. 5 n. 89; "causation" as xviii, ch. 5 n. 72; critique of radial (Adajian) ch. 4 n. 15; decentering ch. 1 n. 12; "frame" as 102–15, 121–22, 147–48, 200; graphic representation of 121–22, fig. 4.1; and heterarchy ch. 5 n. 22; homonymy and polysemy 101; and horizontal intersection 16; interlocking metaphors 20; Lakoff 101–102; and language-games 6, 219, ch. 1 n. 15; multiplicity of frames 6; preexisting analogies 102; of theoretical terms ch. 3 n. 4; schema of 122 fig. 4.1; Thomasson ch. 4 n. 15; *see also* ambiguity; family resemblance; figure 4.1, interpretations of; heterarchy; interpretation

Raff, Norman 74

Rainer, Yvonne ch. 4 n. 32

Rajchman, John ch. 2 n. 60, E

Ray, Nicholas 27, ch. 2 n. 2

Re, Valentina ch. 4 n. 26, C1

reader/readings:

author as first reader 5; reader-author 7; birth of reader 3, 6; inscribed quotations ch. 1 n. 8; multiple readings/interpretations 25, 89–90,